Contemporary Topics in Immunobiology

VOLUME 15

Immune Complexes
and Human Cancer

Contemporary Topics in Immunobiology

General Editor:
Michael G. Hanna, Jr.
Litton Institute of Applied Biotechnology
Rockville, Maryland

Editorial Board:

Max D. Cooper
University of Alabama
Birmingham, Alabama

John J. Marchalonis
Medical University of South Carolina
Charleston, South Carolina

G. J. V. Nossal
The Walter & Eliza Hall Insitute of Medical Research
Victoria, Australia

Victor Nussenzweig
New York University School of Medicine
New York, New York

George W. Santos
Johns Hopkins University
Baltimore, Maryland

Ralph Snyderman
Duke University Medical Center
Durham, North Carolina

Osias Stutman
Sloan-Kettering Institute for Cancer Research
New York, New York

Noel L. Warner
Becton Dickinson & Co.
Mountain View, California

William O. Weigle
Scripps Clinic and Research Foundation
La Jolla, California

A Continuation Order Plan is available for this series. A continuation order will bring delivery of each new volume immediately upon publication. Volumes are billed only upon actual shipment. For further information please contact the publisher.

Contemporary Topics in Immunobiology

VOLUME 15

Immune Complexes and Human Cancer

Edited by
Fernando A. Salinas
Cancer Control Agency of British Columbia and
University of British Columbia
Vancouver, British Columbia, Canada

and

Michael G. Hanna, Jr.
Litton Institute of Applied Biotechnology
Rockville, Maryland

PLENUM PRESS • NEW YORK AND LONDON

Library of Congress Cataloging in Publication Data

Main entry under title:

Immune complexes and human cancer.

  (Contemporary topics in immunobiology; v. 15)
  Includes bibliographies and index.
  1. Cancer — Immunological aspects. 2. Immune complexes. I. Salinas, Fernando A.
II. Hanna, M. G. (Michael G.), 1936–   . III. Series. [DNLM: 1. Antigen-Antibody
Complex. 2. Neoplasms — immunology. W1CO77 v.15/QZ 200 I324]
QR180.C632 vol. 15   574.2'9 s   85-6315
[RC268.31   [616.99'4079]
ISBN 978-1-4684-4933-4   ISBN 978-1-4684-4931-0 (eBook)
DOI 10.1007/978-1-4684-4931-0

© 1985 Plenum Press, New York
Softcover reprint of the hardcover 1st edition 1985

A Division of Plenum Publishing Corporation
233 Spring Street, New York, N.Y. 10013

Contributors

Joe P. Balint
Immune Response Program
Pacific Northwest Research Foundation
Seattle, Washington 98104
and Imré Corporation
Seattle, Washington 98109

Kim Bennett
Department of Internal Medicine
University of Nevada School of Medicine
Reno, Nevada 89520

Didier Cupissol
Department of Chemo-immunotherapy and
Laboratory of Tumor Immunopharmacology INSERM U-236
ERA-CNRS No. 844, Centre Paul Lamarque
BP 5054, 34 033 Montpellier Cedex, France

Mehmet F. Fer
Section of Hematology/Oncology
University of Kentucky Medical Center
Lexington, Kentucky 40536

Rishab K. Gupta
John Wayne Clinic and Armand Hammer Laboratories
Division of Oncology
Department of Surgery
UCLA Medical School
University of California
Los Angeles, California 90024

Stephen W. Hall
Department of Internal Medicine
University of Nevada School of Medicine
Reno, Nevada 89520

Ingegerd Hellström
Oncogen
Seattle, Washington 98121
and Department of Microbiology and Immunology
University of Washington
Seattle, Washington 98195

Karl Erik Hellström
Oncogen
Seattle, Washington 98121
and Department of Pathology
University of Washington
Seattle, Washington 98195

Thomas V. Holohan *Food and Drug Administration*
United States Public Health Service
Rockville, Maryland 20857
and Immunochemistry Laboratory
George Washington University Medical Center
Washington, D.C. 20037

Frank R. Jones *Imré Corporation*
Seattle, Washington 98109
and Immune Response Program
Pacific Northwest Research Foundation
Seattle, Washington 98104

Stefan Korac *Medical Oncology Division*
Georgetown University Hospital
Washington, D.C. 20007

F. Roy MacKintosh *Department of Internal Medicine*
University of Nevada School of Medicine
Reno, Nevada 89520

Newton S. More *Immunochemistry Laboratory*
George Washington University Medical Center
Washington, D.C. 20037

Donald L. Morton *John Wayne Cancer Clinic and Armand Hammer Laboratories*
Divison of Oncology
Department of Surgery
UCLA Medical School
University of California
Los Angeles, California 90024

Robert K. Oldham *Biological Therapy Institute*
Franklin, Tennessee 37064

Terence M. Phillips *Immunochemistry Laboratory*
George Washington University Medical Center
Washington, D.C. 20037

William D. Queen *Immunochemistry Laboratory*
George Washington University Medical Center
Washington, D.C. 20037

Prasanta K. Ray *Department of Immunobiology*
Industrial Toxicology Research Center
Lucknow 226001, India

Fernando A. Salinas *Advanced Therapeutics Department*
Cancer Control Agency of British Columbia
Vancouver, British Columbia V5Z 4E6, Canada
and Department of Pathology
University of British Columbia
Vancouver, British Columbia V6T 1W5, Canada

Bernard C. Serrou *Department of Chemo-Immunotherapy and*
Laboratory of Tumor Immunopharmacology INSERM U-236
ERA-CNRS No. 844, Centre Paul Lamarque
BP 5054, 34 033 Montpellier Cedex, France

Hulbert K. Silver

Advanced Therapeutics Department
Cancer Control Agency of British Columbia
Vancouver, British Columbia V5Z 4E6, Canada
and Department of Medicine
University of British Columbia
Vancouver, British Columbia V6T 1W5, Canada

Harry W. Snyder, Jr.

Imré Corporation
Seattle, Washington 98109
and Immune Response Program
Pacific Northwest Research Foundation
Seattle, Washington 98104

Christian Thierry

Department of Chemo-Immunotherapy and
Laboratory of Tumor Immunopharmacology INSERM U-236
ERA-CNRS No. 844, Centre Paul Lamarque
BP 5054, 34 033 Montpellier Cedex, France

Kian H. Wee

Advanced Therapeutics Department
Cancer Control Agency of British Columbia
Vancouver, British Columbia V5Z 4E6, Canada

Preface

Immune Complexes and Human Cancer, the fifteenth volume of Contemporary Topics in Immunobiology, is a compilation of information derived from recent studies on the role of circulating immune complexes (CIC) in the pathogenic manifestations of a variety of human cancers. Technical improvements in the detection of CIC in body fluids have resulted in data that indicate that CIC do occur in different types of cancer. In addition, tumor-associated antigens and antibodies have been detected in immune complexes of cancer patients' sera. Until recently the exact role and clinical relevance of immune complexes have been the subject of debate, partially because of the problems encountered in measuring immune complexes. But these problems are being confronted as more accurate measurement protocols are developed. Technical refinements, along with strict protocols, have provided evidence of heterogeneity in CIC, a factor that makes accurate detection of immune complexes in cancer patients difficult. Recent insights indicate that the measurement of immune complexes in cancer patients may be clinically useful not only as a tumor marker, but also in regard to the deranged immune response of tumor-bearing hosts and other disorders such as nephrotic syndrome, immune anemias, and clotting dysfunction.

A panel of international experts have been selected to contribute relevant and up-to-date information to this volume, which is designed not only for immunopathologists and oncologists but also for physicians, health professionals, and immunobiology students. The introductory chapters review basic concepts and provide insight into the methodology used to determine the characteristics and nature of immune complexes in cancer. The isolation of tumor-associated antigens and their concentrations with regard to recurrences, monitoring of tumor burden, and disease prognosis are also described in the first two chapters. Chapters 3–6 detail immune complex interactions with immune system components, to account for their involvement in immunoregulation and their role in the pathogenesis of cancer. These chapters and Chapters 7 and 8 critically review experimental approaches for immune intervention, such as extracorporeal immunoadsorption, a tool for removal of immune complexes and other putative blocking factors. Also included are critical reviews of protein A immunoadsorption as a form of serotherapy, with emphasis on its clinical effects as well as implications for modes of action.

All the chapters have been prepared by experts who are actively engaged in research relevant to the topics covered. Efforts have been made to encourage differences of opinion among authors on any given topic to allow continued developments in areas of controversy.

In summary, we have presented a comprehensive yet nonexhaustive review of immune complexes as initiators of injury, their role in homeostasis, involvement in several immunoregulatory mechanisms, and, finally, the prospects for serotherapy, an as yet provocative and controversial approach to cancer treatment that requires further understanding.

The preparation of this volume involved the work of many individuals, each of whose contributions was of great importance. We wish to thank the authors for their stimulating and informative contributions; Kirk Jensen, Senior Editor for Life Sciences, and Peter Strupp, Assistant Managing Editor, at Plenum Publishing Corporation, who encouraged every author and supervised production; and Linda Wood and Miriam Weismiller, for their secretarial assistance.

Fernando A. Salinas
Michael G. Hanna, Jr.

Contents

Chapter 3

The Pathophysiology of Circulating Immune Complexes: Their Role in Host–Tumor Interactions and Removal by Immunoadsorption Therapy

Terence M. Phillips, Thomas V. Holohan, Stefan Korac,
Newton S. More, and William D. Queen

Contents

Chapter 4

Immune Complexes in Patients Bearing Solid Tumors

Didier Cupissol, Christian Thierry, and Bernard C. Serrou

Chapter 5

Immunosuppressor Control as a Modality of Cancer Treatment: Effect of Plasma Adsorption with *Staphylococcus aureus* Protein A

Prasanta K. Ray

Chapter 6

**Blocking (Suppressor) Factors, Immune Complexes, and Extracorporeal
Immunoadsorption in Tumor Immunity**

> *Karl Erik Hellström, Ingegerd Hellström, Harry W. Snyder, Jr.,
> Joe P. Balint, and Frank R. Jones*

Chapter 7

**Trials of Staphylococcal Protein A-Treated Plasma Infusions in Cancer
Therapy: Clinical Effects and Implications for Mode of Action**

F. Roy MacKintosh, Kim Bennett, and Stephen W. Hall

Chapter 8

Protein A Immunoadsorption/Immunoactivation: A Critical Review

Mehmet F. Fer and Robert K. Oldham

Chapter 1

Clinical Significance and Nature of Circulating Immune Complexes in Melanoma Patients

Rishab K. Gupta and Donald L. Morton

John Wayne Cancer Clinic and Armand Hammer Laboratories
Division of Oncology
Department of Surgery
UCLA Medical School
University of California
Los Angeles, California 90024

I. INTRODUCTION

Most human malignant tissues express tumor antigens. Mechanisms whereby molecules that can act as tumor antigens may appear on the cell surface and make them autoantigenic have been proposed by Cochran (1978). It was proposed that neoantigens on tumor cells may appear by (1) reexpression of repressed molecules, (2) modification of existing molecules, (3) uncovering of masked molecules, and (4) deletion of existing molecules. There are many reports in the literature regarding the existence of certain tumor antigens that are immunogenic in the autologous and allogenic host. Though the biological and chemical natures of many of these antigens are not completely known, they are recognized as tumor-associated antigens (TAA). Humoral immune responses to TAA in melanoma patients have been summarized in recent reviews (Aryan, 1979; Old, 1981; Reisfeld and Ferrone, 1982).

In view of the presence of surface-bound immunoglobulins (Ig) on biopsy specimens of various types of human malignant tissues (Gunven *et al.*, 1980; MacSween and Eastwood, 1980; Seth and Balachandran, 1980), it is conceivable that the serologic reactions observed *in vitro* between sera from cancer patients and cultured tumor cells (Dent and Liao, 1982; R. K. Gupta and Morton, 1982*a*) could also occur *in vivo* as well. Though Ig may bind to the surface of tumor

1

cells in various ways (Tonder *et al.*, 1976), there is enough evidence to suggest that at least some Ig do bind to antigenic determinants on tumor cells *in vivo* by antigen–antibody interaction. In some cases tumor-cell-bound antibodies have been eluted by low-pH and high-salt treatments, and the eluted antibodies were found to react with the same or similar cells (Phillips and Lewis, 1971; R. K. Gupta and Morton, 1975; Witz, 1977). We observed that the antigenic activity of the biopsy melanoma cells to autologous serum increased significantly after elution of Ig, and the eluted antibodies were of IgG and IgM classes. Therefore, tumor-bound Ig detected on biopsy specimens may be considered as evidence of their immunologic interaction *in vivo* with the corresponding antigens. The antigen–antibody complexes formed on the cell surface may be internalized by the cell or they may be released into the surroundings by mechanisms similar to those described for *in vitro* antigen modulation, capping, and shedding after exposing the tumor cells to antibody (Leong *et al.*, 1979). The released immune complexes may be responsible for many of the pathological conditions that have been described by various investigators (Haakenstad and Mannik, 1977; Zubler and Lambert, 1977; Barnett *et al.*, 1979; Benveniste *et al.*, 1979; Theofilopoulos and Dixon, 1979; Kabat, 1980; Lamers, 1981). A number of other possible mechanisms that might result in release of tumor antigens into the circulation— i.e., cell death, surface bleeding, sublethal autolysis, or secretion from cells—have been proposed by Price and Robins (1978). Spontaneous shedding of tumor antigens into culture medium has been documented by a number of investigators (Grimm *et al.*, 1976; Reisfeld *et al.*, 1977; R. K. Gupta *et al.*, 1979*d*; R. K. Gupta and Morton, 1983*b*; Leong *et al.*, 1978; Bystryn, 1980; Heaney-Kieras and Bystryn, 1982). This may be similar to *in vivo* antigen shedding by tumor cells. Part or all of the antigens shed into circulation may combine with humoral antibodies and result in circulating immune complexes (CIC).

Many serum factors that modify cellular and humoral immune responses have been described (Nelson and Gatti, 1976; StC. Sinclair, 1979; Rossen and Morgan, 1981; Salinas and Wee, 1983). However, circulating free antigen and/or immune complexes have received special attention with respect to their interaction with lymphoid cells (Haakenstad and Mannik, 1974; Halpern, 1974). It can now be postulated that some of the serum factors that block *in vitro* cell-mediated immunity against melanoma cells (Hellström *et al.*, 1971; Happner *et al.*, 1973) are antigen–antibody complexes (Sjögren *et al.*, 1971; Baldwin *et al.*, 1973; Theofilopoulos and Dixon, 1978; R. K. Gupta *et al.*, 1979*c*). Recent developments suggest that an assessment of CIC levels in cancer patients may be of significance for diagnosis, prognosis, and monitoring the clinical course of their disease (Baldwin and Robins, 1980; R. K. Gupta and Morton, 1981; Rossen and Barnes, 1978; Dent *et al.*, 1980; Salinas *et al.*, 1983). However, a comparative evaluation of immune complex detection assays for the diagnosis of human cancer revealed them to be of little value (Herberman *et al.*,

1981; Angello, 1978; Barnett *et al.*, 1979; Haakenstad and Mannik, 1977; Kabat, 1980; Williams, 1980). Many of the inconsistencies could be explained by differences in size of the immune complexes detectable by various assays and by the ability of the immune complexes to bind complement. Furthermore, it is obvious that almost all of the CIC detection assays applied in the area of human tumor immunology were antigen-nonspecific and that immune complexes in circulation may arise from causes other than tumor activity (Espinoza, 1983). Therefore, mere detection of CIC by such assays in cancer patients could not be an accurate tumor marker for diagnosis and evaluation of the clinical status of the disease. For these reasons, it becomes necessary to determine the nature of the antigen(s) in the immune complexes of CIC-positive patients. Although progress in this direction has been slow, the antigen portion of the immune complexes isolated from cancer patients has been identified in some cases (Maidment *et al.*, 1981; Stein *et al.*, 1980; Staab *et al.*, 1980; Faldt and Ankerst, 1980).

In this chapter we attempt to review (1) the analysis of CIC; (2) the significance of such analysis in relation to (a) disease stage, (b) tumor burden, and (c) recurrence rate; and (3) the nature of CIC in melanoma patients. Attention is also directed to the methodologies that can be applied for characterization of immune complexes isolated from melanoma patients.

II. CIC DETECTION METHODS IN CANCER

A number of highly sensitive assays have been developed for the detection of CIC in sera of humans suffering from various clinical disorders (Theofilopoulos and Dixon, 1980), and new ones are constantly described in the literature (Espinoza, 1983; R. K. Gupta *et al.*, 1982; Johny *et al.*, 1980; Chautenoud *et al.*, 1979; Kauffmann *et al.*, 1981). The development of these sensitive assays has revealed the usefulness of CIC measurements in clinical manifestations of the immune complexes in diseases that originally were not considered to be conditions with disordered immune functions; nevertheless the relationship between the results of the assays has not been clear since conflicting results have been reported (World Health Organization, 1977). These problems are attributed to the unavailability of and difficulty of preparing standardized reagents, and to the heterogeneous nature of antibody, antigen, and secondary factors (i.e., complement) that form and determine the size of the complexes (Salinas and Wee, 1983).

Despite the availability of more than 50 immune complex detection assays, only a few have been applied in the areas of human tumor immunology and only some of these—e.g., Raji cell, Cq binding, and polyethylene glycol (PEG) precipitation assays—have been used relatively widely. Different laboratories have become experts in one or the other assay. Given many possible choices, a non-expert is usually left to follow either the most recent, as yet unconfirmed, publication or his own anecdotal experience (Nydegger and Davis, 1980).

Most of the techniques used for assaying CIC in cancer patients have been antigen-nonspecific. These techniques have relied on physiochemical characteristics, interaction with complement and conglutinin, interaction with rheumatoid factors, and interaction with cellular receptors (Baldwin and Robins, 1980; Theofilopoulos, 1982). The assays based on physiochemical properties of CIC are precipitation with PEG, ultracentrifugation, and gel filtration chromatography. Of these the PEG-precipitation technique has been used frequently because of its ease of performance and the small amount of sample required. In addition, PEG precipitation has been used in combination with other assays (Grangeot-Keros et al., 1978) or as a pretreatment for serum samples to enrich the CIC for subsequent analysis.

The techniques based on interaction with complement components include complement consumption, C1q precipitation in gel, C1q binding, C1q deviation, C1q solid phase, C1q latex agglutination inhibition, and C3 binding assays. The principles behind and procedures for these assays can be found in recent reviews (Nydegger and Davis, 1980; Espinoza, 1983). Techniques using radiolabeled C1q have been used widely because of their sensitivity and ability to provide quantitative results. Rossen et al. (1978) compared the C1q binding and C1q deviation tests for their ability to detect immune-complex-like materials in sera of cancer patients. Through the results of the two tests in general correlated significantly, more sera from cancer patients were identified as likely to have immune complexes by the C1q binding assay than by the C1q deviation assay. However, the number of sera from cancer patients tested by the two assays was small, and it was concluded that the results did not necessarily suggest that the C1q binding assay was more sensitive than the C1q deviation test. Despite the fact that the C1q deviation assay detected lower concentrations of aggregated human IgG than did the C1q binding assay (Sobel et al., 1975), the former assay identified immune-complex-like material in about 50% of sera from more than 400 patients with various types of malignant diseases (Teshima et al., 1977; Gropp et al., 1980).

Based on the fact that rheumatoid factors (RhF) (IgG or IgM antibodies) have an affinity for immune-complexed IgG, a number of assays using rheumatoid RhF have been developed. These include RhF precipitation in gel, RhF latex agglutination inhibition, and soluble and solid phase RhF binding inhibitions. Monoclonal RhF (MRhF) present in the sera of patients with lymphoproliferative disorders and Waldenström's macroglobulinemia exhibit higher affinity than polyclonal RhF (Espinoza, 1983). The interaction between immune complexes and RhF can be quantitated by inhibition of agglutination of IgG-coated latex particles or inhibition of $[^{125}I]$-MRhF that binds to an insoluble substrate like IgG-Sepharose. Such assays can detect complexes of IgG as small as 8 S, irrespective of their complement-fixing activity. However, the results may be influenced by the presence of high concentrations of monomeric IgG in the test serum (Baldwin and Robins, 1980).

Purified bovine conglutinin has been used to develop a very sensitive immune complex detection assay (Eisenberg *et al.*, 1977). Conglutinin, an unusual protein with a molecular weight of 750,000 that is found only in the sera of some members of the bovine species, binds to C3b present on immune complexes. The assay is performed by incubating the test serum in conglutinin-coated polystyrene tubes to allow C3-carrying immune complexes to bind the conglutinin. The amount of immune complex that reacts with the conglutinin is detected by radiolabeled or enzyme-linked antiglobulins. This assay detects only large immune complexes that are complement-fixing.

As opposed to the fluid phase immune complex receptors, e.g., complement, conglutatin and RhF assays have been developed that involve cellular receptors. A variety of cells—e.g., Raji cells, platelets, macrophages, murine leukemia cells, and bovine spermatozoa—have been used for this purpose (Espinoza, 1983). Of these, the Raji cell assay has gained the most popularity. Raji is a B lymphoblastoid cell line derived from Burkitt's lymphoma. These cells lack membrane-bound Ig but have receptors for Fc and complement components. It has been demonstrated that the majority of complement-fixing immune complexes bind to Raji cells via receptors of C3b and C3d (Theofilopoulos *et al.*, 1976). This assay is simple, reproducible, and sensitive, and it is able to detect complexes of various sizes. However, like other cellular assays, it suffers from the drawback that false positivity may occur owing to the presence of antilymphocyte antibodies in the test serum. However, using anti-HLA antibodies that frequently occur after multiple pregnancies or renal transplantation, Dasgupta *et al.* (1982) observed that sera containing these antibodies did not result in significant false positives under the operational conditions of the Raji cell assay. An enzyme-linked immunosorbent version of the Raji cell assay has been reported by Cunningham-Rundles *et al.* (1980).

In addition to the assays already mentioned, staphylococcal protein A (McDougal *et al.*, 1979) and fetal liver cell radioimmunossay (FLC-RIA) (Salinas *et al.*, 1981a) have been used successfully to measure immune-complex-like materials in sera of cancer patients. Though comparison of the results of the FLC-RIA with those of the Raji cell assay revealed a general agreement, the FLC-RIA appeared to be more sensitive for quantitation of CIC in serum samples where fewer and smaller immune complexes were present (Salinas *et al.*, 1981a).

There has been a lack of development of antigen-specific CIC detection assays for cancer patients. This is mainly due to the unavailability of well defined tumor antigen in the pure form. Attempts are now being made in this direction, and these will be reviewed in the subsequent sections.

III. INCIDENCE OF CIC IN MELANOMA PATIENTS

Increased incidence of elevated CIC in the sera of patients with cancer, including malignant melanoma, has been reported by various investigators (Dorval and Pross, 1983). Several different assays have been used to assess the incidence and level of CIC. As indicated in Table I, the incidence of CIC in melanoma patients varied from 7 to 92%. These incidences differed not only from assay to assay but also from laboratory to laboratory even when the same CIC detection assay was used. In some cases there was variation when the same assay was used in the same laboratory but on a different set of serum samples. For example, Rossen *et al.* (1977) reported an 83% incidence of CIC in sera of melanoma patients by the C1q binding assay, but in a subsequent study using another group of serum samples the incidence was reported to be only 34% (Rossen *et al.*, 1978). Though wide discrepancies in the incidence of CIC positivity reported by various investigators could be due to the use of different assays, it must be realized that random selection of patients and the time of serum sampling are equally likely explanations. The latter factors are perhaps additionally responsible for the discrepancies observed within the same laboratory when the same assay but different samples were used. It is known that the formation, fate, and physiochemical and biological properties of the immune complexes are governed by the nature of the antibody class and antigens involved (Haakenstad and Mannik, 1977; Barnett *et al.*, 1979). Furthermore, the molar ratio of antibody to antigen is equally important in determining these properties of the immune complexes (VanEs *et al.*, 1979).

Table I. Incidence of CIC in Sera of Patients with Melanoma and of Normal Controls as Assessed by Various Methods and Investigators

		Incidence of CIC positivity	
Assay	References[a]	Melanoma	Normal
C1q binding	Hoffken *et al.* (1977)	83%	—[b]
	Rossen *et al.* (1977)	83%	5%
	Schrohenloher *et al.* (1978)	10%	—
	Rossen *et al.* (1978)	34%	5–7%
	Norris *et al.* (1980)	62%	0%
	Carpentier and Miescher (1983)	14%	0%
	Phillips *et al.* (1982)	44%	Not reported
	Ruell *et al.* (1982)	17%	5%
	R. K. Gupta *et al.* (1982)	17%	5%
	Krapf *et al.* (1982)	33–56%	Not reported
C1q deviation	Teshima *et al.* (1977)	45%	0%
	Shepherd (1979)	11%	0%
C1q inhibition	Gabriel and Angello (1977)	25%	5%
	Angello (1978)	25%	0%
	Yoshida and Zawadzki (1980)	32%	0%
C1q-PEG	Shepherd (1979)	45%	0%
Raji cell	Eisenberg *et al.* (1977)	64%	4%
	Theofilopoulos *et al.* (1977)	48%	19%
	Schrohenloher *et al.* (1978)	10%	—

Table I. (*Continued*)

Assay	References[a]	Incidence of CIC positivity	
		Melanoma	Normal
Raji cell	R. C. Gupta *et al.* (1979)	71%	Not reported
	Persson *et al.* (1981)	29%	0%
	Olberding *et al.* (1981)	70%	4–9%
	Phillips *et al.* (1982)	34%	Not reported
Conglutinin	Eisenberg *et al.* (1977)	7%[c]	4%
	Krapf *et al.* (1982)	33–56%	Not reported
	Lodola *et al.* (1981)	39%	10%
Complement	R. K. Gupta *et al.* (1979a)	44%	7%
consumption	R. K. Gupta *et al.* (1979b)	45%	10%
	R. K. Gupta *et al.* (1979c)	41%	14%
	Kristensen *et al.* (1980)	19%	Not reported
	R. K. Gupta and Morton (1981)	43%	13%
	R. K. Gupta *et al.* (1982)	53%	Not reported
PEG precipitation	Gauci *et al.* (1978)	90%	0%
	Phillips *et al.* (1982)	33%	Not reported
	Bentwich *et al.* (1982)	15%	Not reported
	Krapf *et al.* (1982)	33–56%	Not reported
PEG nephelometry	Krapf *et al.* (1982)	38–45%	5%
K562 radiometric	R. K. Gupta *et al.* (1982)	67%	5%
	Bentwich *et al.* (1982)	52%	Not reported
EA-rosette	Sztaba-Kania *et al.* (1981)	68%	20%
inhibition			
Monoclonal RhF	Gabriel and Angello (1977)	75%	0%
	Schrohenloher *et al.* (1978)	26%	–
	Angello (1978)	75%	0%
	Yoshida and Zawadski (1980)	23%	4%
	Ruell *et al.* (1982)	11%	3%
In vivo	Persson *et al.* (1981)	58%	10%
phagocytosis	Persson *et al.* (1981)	33%	Not reported
Cryoprecipitation	Norris *et al.* (1980)	92%	0%
Fetal liver cell	Salinas *et al.* (1981a)	84%	5–7%

[a] Not an exhaustive compilation.
[b] Normal samples used to establish the baseline.
[c] Represents incidence of CIC in various types of malignancies including malignant melanoma.

It has been pointed out by Salinas and Wee (1983) that the clearance of CIC is dependent on several factors that generally interact. Deregulation of any of the factors may result in increased concentration of CIC. A high concentration of CIC has been known to lead to an increase in immune complex size, thus effectively reducing the CIC number (Salinas *et al.*, 1981a,b). Analysis of sera from cancer patients by sedimentation techniques for immune complex size and concentration revealed that elevated levels of CIC were associated with small immune complexes, whereas large immune complexes were associated with low CIC levels (Salinas *et al.*, 1981*b*,*c*). To be cleared from the circulation immune complexes must reach a critical size that allows them to be picked up by the reticuloendothelial system. When there is an excess of antigen or when the affinity of the antibody is low, the size of the immune complex is too small and its elimination is delayed. Therefore, it can be inferred that the persistence of immune complexes in circulation may also depend on the immune status of the host (Masson, 1978).

Not only have different criteria been used for the positivity of test samples, but standardized reagents have not been available for comparison. In some assays (though not in all), the handling and storage of the samples are critical factors that can influence the results (Rossen *et al.*, 1978). The presence and involvement of anti-Ig can also affect the CIC level in a given serum sample by altering their molecular characteristics and modifying their intravascular survival (Phillips *et al.*, 1982; Rossen and Morgan, 1981).

Despite the inconsistencies in results obtained by various assays, it is obvious that CIC do occur in melanoma patients, though they may represent a spectrum of complexes (Rossen and Morgan, 1981). In general, their incidence in cancer is lower than in autoimmune diseases—e.g., rheumatoid arthritis, systemic lupus erythematosus—but consistently greater than in apparently normal controls.

IV. CLINICAL APPLICATION OF CIC ANALYSIS IN MELANOMA

Despite the fact that the presence of elevated CIC could not be correlated from assay to assay and laboratory to laboratory, some reports indicate that elevated levels of CIC represent a poor prognosis in cancer patients (including melanoma), and that fluctuations in CIC levels as detected by C1q deviation and monoclonal RhF radioimmunoassay correlate with response to therapy (Jerry *et al.*, 1976). Patients with active melanoma have been reported to have higher levels of CIC than those with no clinical evidence of disease; furthermore, patients who were considered cured after surgery had lower incidences and levels of CIC than those considered not cured (Theofilopoulos *et al.*, 1977). Thus, evaluation of CIC levels in melanoma patients appears to have some clinical significance.

A. Diagnostic Significance of CIC

Because virtually all of the CIC detection assays used thus far have been antigen-nonspecific, and because CIC may arise from causes other than tumor growth, at present these assays do not appear to have direct diagnostic significance. Baldwin and Robins (1980) have suggested a possible diagnostic value of the C1q binding test in breast carcinoma. In their preliminary studies only 2 of 17 benign breast patients had elevated C1q binding activity as opposed to 18 of 23 breast carcinoma patients. However, it was pointed out that false diagnosis based on CIC detection might occur because of intercurrent infections and a range of inflammatory of autoimmune diseases. In view of these precautions, the C1q binding assay can best be used for differential diagnosis (Rossen *et al.*, 1977; Papsidero *et al.*, 1978). Even though significantly higher levels of CIC have been detected in cancer patients than in controls using more than one assay, their diagnostic significance is limited (Ruell *et al.*, 1982). It has now become apparent that elevated levels of CIC do not necessarily mean that the complexes are comprised of tumor antigen and antibody (Salinas *et al.*, 1982b). If elevated CIC levels that are determined by an antigen-nonspecific assay are to be used as diagnostic markers for malignancy, it is absolutely necessary to determine the presence of tumor antigen in the immune complexes. Studies along these lines have been undertaken by Salinas and co-workers. These investigators observed that immune complexes of certain CIC-positive melanoma and breast carcinoma patients contained TAA and IgG antibody (Salinas *et al.*, 1981b, 1982b). Presence of TAA in immune complexes circulating in melanoma patients has also been documented in our laboratory (R. K. Gupta *et al.*, 1983a,b). Yet these constitute only a few studies performed on a limited number of samples. At present, therefore, the data on CIC levels in melanoma patients or patients with other types of cancer should be evaluated very carefully in the light of other clinical parameters for diagnosis.

B. Prognostic Significance of CIC

Despite inconsistencies in the literature on detection of CIC levels in cancer patients and the antigen-nonspecific nature of the assay systems, a number of reports have suggested correlations between immune complex levels and tumor size, survival rate, and treatment modality. In this section we will attempt to review such studies, dealing specifically with malignant melanoma. However, caution must be exercised in judging the significance of CIC detection until it is proven that CIC contain tumor antigen or until antigen-specific CIC detection assays are developed. In view of the information available thus far, it appears possible that analysis of sera from melanoma patients for CIC could provide an additional immune parameter for prognosis and for the management of their disease.

1. Relationship between CIC and Clinical Stage of Disease

The criteria used in the Division of Surgical Oncology at UCLA and at other institutions for the clinical staging of malignant melanoma are as follows: stage

I, localized disease; stage II, metastases to regional lymph nodes; and stage III, metastases to distant organs or skin.

Dorval and Pross (1983) analyzed 129 melanoma patients belonging to various stages of the disease by a modified Fc_γ-receptor-bearing cell and staphylococcal protein A assay for CIC. Comparison of CIC level [expressed as micrograms of aggregated human IgG (AHG) per milliliter] with stage of the disease revealed a great variation among individual patients' results, but no significant differences in CIC levels were observed among patients with stage I, II, or III disease. Though statistically not significant, the mean CIC level in stage II (12.9 μg AHG/ml, $N = 25$) was slightly higher than those in stage I (10.1 μg AHG/ml, $N = 70$) and stage III (10.7 μg AHG/ml, $N = 34$). The standard deviations were quite large. Comparisions of CIC level with tumor stage have been made in other types of malignancies (Yoshida and Zawadzki, 1980; Ristow et al., 1979). It has also been reported that marked fluctuations in CIC levels were observed within individuals belonging to the same stage (Dorval and Pross, 1983). Obviously, diagnostic or therapeutic manipulations or infections may contribute to such fluctuations in CIC levels assessed by the antigen-nonspecific assays (Jerry et al., 1976; Pesce et al., 1980; Teshima et al., 1977).

Kristensen et al. (1980) analyzed serum samples obtained preoperatively from 32 melanoma patients with stage I (23 patients) and stage II (9 patients) disease for CIC. The presence of CIC was evaluated by two different assays, namely complement consumption and C1q-protein A. These investigators observed that all 9 patients with stage II disease were positive for CIC as detected by complement consumption, whereas only 2 were positive by the C1q-protein A assay. In contrast, only 7 of 23 stage I patients were positive for CIC by the complement consumption assay, and only 2 were positive by the C1q-protein A assay. Thus, the incidence of CIC in stage I patients was significantly lower than that in stage II patients, at least as measured by the complement consumption assay. It must be realized that in this study serum samples were taken before surgical resection of the tumor. These investigators also reported that none of the 14 patients whose serum samples were analyzed postoperatively and thus were free of disease clinically was positive for CIC. Thus, presence of CIC may be related to tumor burden and not to the clinical stage in melanoma. The discrepancy between the results of the two assays was explained on the basis of the antibody class involved in the immune complexes: The C1q-protein A assay detected immune complexes that were composed of IgG antibody and the complement consumption assay detected immune complexes that were composed of both IgG and IgM antibodies.

Norris et al. (1980) studied 13 randomly selected melanoma patients for CIC levels by the C1q binding assay. In 11 patients serum samples were taken after removal of the *primary* tumor. The incidence of CIC positively was 20% (1/5) in stage, 1, 50% (1/2) in stage II and 40% (2/5) in stage III. Though the number of patients in each stage group was too small for statistical comparison, it can be noted that the incidence of CIC positivity increased with increasing stage. Since the serum samples were taken after removal of the primary tumor only, the stage II and stage III patients could still have had clinically undetectable tumor, and could have represented a larger tumor mass compared to the stage I patients.

Low levels of CIC and no positive correlations with clinical stage of melanoma in 34 patients were observed by D'Amelio et al. (1982). Again with the exception of three patients in stage I, all serum samples were obtained after surgical excision of the tumor. Thus, these patients possibly had very little or no tumor.

Ruell et al. (1982) analyzed sera obtained before surgery from 132 melanoma patients in stages I, II, and III for CIC by C1q RIA and by IgM MRhF assay. Though little concordance between the C1q RIA and MRhF assays was observed, the incidence of CIC was the highest (27%) in stage III patients. Stage I patients had only 6% CIC incidence as compared to 18% in stage II. Serum samples containing CIC as measured by either of the two assays were considered positive. The incidence of CIC-positive patients in stage I melanoma did not differ from that of normal controls. The incidence of CIC in stage I and II melanoma patients did not change significantly after surgery. These investigators suggested that the higher incidence of CIC in stage III patients could be due to immune complexes resulting from the presence of rheumatoid factors or anti-idiotype antibodies (Lewis et al., 1976; Morgan et al., 1979).

We analyzed serum samples for CIC from randomly selected 129 melanoma patients before any treatment. The incidence of CIC was determined by the complement consumption assay. The results were correlated with clinical stage of the disease (R. K. Gupta et al., 1979a). Results presented in Table II indicate that 36% stage I, 47% stage II, and 42% stage III melanoma patients were positive for CIC. However, despite the large number of patients in each group, the differences in the incidence of positive CIC were not statistically significant. Because the serum samples were obtained at the time of the first visit to the John Wayne Cancer Clinic, before any treatment (including surgery), and because

Table II. Incidence of CIC in Melanoma Patients at Various Clinical Stages[a]

Clinical stage	No. tested	No. positive	Percent positive	P value
I	50	18	36	0.298
II	36	17	47	
III	43	18	42	0.562

[a]Incidence of CIC was determined by the complement consumption assay as described by R. K. Gupta et al. (1979a).

Table III. Relationship of CIC Positivity to Tumor Burden at Various Clinical Stages in Melanoma Patients[a]

Clinical stage[b]	Tumor burden	No. patients tested	No. patients positive	Percent positive
I	NED[c] or <1 g	46	15	33
	1–100 g	4	3	75
II	NED or <1 g	22	9	41
	1–100 g	12	8	67
	>100 g	2	0	0
III	NED or <1 g	3	0	0
	1–100 g	10	7	70
	>100 g	30	11	37

[a] CIC was analyzed by the complement consumption assay (R. K. Gupta et al., 1979a).
[b] Regional lymph nodes of stage II patients were histopathologically positive for malignant melanoma, and those of stage I patients were negative.
[c] NED, no evidence of disease.

many of the patients in stage I had localized tumor, the results were reevaluated on the basis of tumor burden in each stage of the disease. The tumor burden at the time of serum sampling for each patient was estimated by determining the number and size of tumor nodules that were palpable or that were visible on radiological films, scans, and tomograms. It was arbitrarily assumed that a 1-cc nodule weighed about 1 g. It was observed that the incidence of CIC was consistently higher in patients with a 1- to 100-g tumor burden than in those with no evidence of disease or less than 1.0 g of tumor in stages I and II, and than those with a large (>100-g) tumor burden (Table III). Thus, incidence of CIC appeared to correlate with tumor burden rather than with clinical stage of the disease. Similar observations have been reported in other types of solid tumors (R. K. Gupta et al., 1979a). In view of these observations CIC analysis may not be applicable for clinical staging of malignant melanoma.

2. Relationship between CIC and Tumor Burden

In evaluate the relationship between CIC and tumor burden in human malignant melanoma, Rossen et al. (1983) evaluated 53 patients. The CIC were analyzed by the C1q binding assay. Ninety-four percent of sera from 13 patients that had no evidence of disease and remained so for 41 months did not contain CIC. On the contrary, 32% of samples from 40 patients with varying tumor burdens were positive. Evaluation of the data by the odds-product ratio test revealed a value of 8, suggesting a high association between the presence of CIC and evidence of tumor in the patients. Measurement of CIC in initial serum samples was helpful in identifying those stage IV (equivalent to clinical stage III by our definition) patients who had unfavorable prognosis. Furthermore, patients whose disease had metastasized to the regional lymph nodes or to distant organs (clinical stages II and III) but who underwent surgical removal and thus were tumor-free did not have abnormal levels of CIC. Gauci *et al.* (1981) documented that CIC composed of IgG and IgM antibodies were significantly higher in patients with evident disease. Thus, the studies of Rossen *et al.* (1983) and those of Gauci *et al.* (1981) corroborated our findings as described previously.

Ruell *et al.* (1982) reported a higher incidence of CIC, as assessed by the C1q-RIA and MRhF assays, in sera of melanoma patients taken after surgical resection of tumor than in sera taken before surgery. Clinically, these patients belonged to stages I and II; however, some patients demonstrated recurrence of their disease when followed for about 12 months, but the false positive rate was 73%. In view of the kinetics of immune complex formation, size of immune complexes, and tumor burden (Salinas *et al.*, 1982c), a 12-month period of follow-up may not be sufficient to assess the prognostic significance of CIC analysis. Furthermore, a significantly lower incidence of CIC in melonoma patients with no evidence of disease than in those with localized or metastatic disease was reported by Sztaba-Kania *et al.* (1981). In addition, the high levels of CIC or a tendency for them to increase in most cases was associated with dissemination of the disease. In a comparative study between the PEG precipitation and K562 radiometric assays, it was reported that the K562 radiometric assay was far superior to the PEG precipitation assay in its correlation with the presence or absence of tumor in melanoma patients (Bentwich *et al.*, 1982), and the two assays correlated poorly with each other (correlation coefficient = 0.33). Thus, the type of CIC detection assay used could also account for the discrepant relationships between CIC and tumor burden reported by some investigators. This notion is supported by the report of Yoshida and Zawadzki (1980). They observed that discrepant incidences of CIC in melanoma patients were observed by the C1q inhibition and MRhF inhibition assays (correlation coefficient = 0.295), and that, though the incidence of CIC in melanoma patients with metastatic disease was higher than that in patients with localized disease by both assays, the differences were not statistically significant. On the contrary, Rossen *et al.* (1977) reported that the incidence of CIC detectable by the C1q binding assay was significantly higher in cancer patients with evidence of disease than the incidence in those with no evidence of disease. However, with respect to malignant melanoma 92% (12/13) patients with evidence of disease and 78% (18/23) patients with no evidence of disease were positive for CIC. The data of Kristensen *et al.* (1980) also suggest that the presence of CIC in the preoperative phase of melanoma patients may reflect a high tumor burden.

Theofilopoulos *et al.* (1977) reported significantly lower levels of CIC in

Table IV. Relationship between CIC Positivity and
Tumor Burden in Malignant Melanoma Patients[a]

Tumor burden	No. patients	No. CIC patients	CIC incidence (%)
NED or <1 g	71	24	34
1–10 g	14	9	64
10–100 g	12	8	67
100–1000 g	20	9	45
>1000 g	12	3	25

[a]CIC was determined by the complement consumption assay
(R. K. Gupta et al., 1979a).

cancer patients with no evidence of disease than in those with metastatic disease. However, in patients with malignant melanoma CIC were detectable irrespective of the tumor mass, and patients with large tumors had significantly higher levels of CIC compared with those with smaller tumors. The CIC were analyzed by the Raji cell radioimmunoassay. In subsequent investigations, we (R. K. Gupta et al., 1979a) observed that the incidence of CIC positivity was dependent on tumor burden (Table IV). The patients were carefully grouped on the basis of clinically detectable tumor burden irrespective of their clinical stage. As shown in the table, the incidence of CIC was the highest in patients with 1- to 100-g tumor burdens. It was significantly lower in patients with <1-g or >100-g tumor burdens. Our findings have been confirmed by Gauci et al. (1981), who reported that within certain limits the CIC in cancer patients would increase proportionately with tumor growth, but that a continued increase in tumor burden resulted in a fall in CIC level.

The lower incidences of CIC in patients with very low or very high tumor burdens than in those with moderate tumor burdens can possibly be explained by the assumption that patients with very low tumor burdens had immune complexes in antibody excess and that patients with very large tumor burdens had immune complexes in antigen excess. The quantity and/or composition of immune complexes in these extreme groups could have been such that they were not detected by the complement consumption assay. Validation for such an assumption comes from the elegant series of investigations performed by Salinas and associates. These investigators observed in malignant melanoma cases that patients with no evidence of disease and patients with advanced disease had significantly lower CIC levels than patients who had intermediate tumor burdens (Salinas et al., 1980). Though FLC-RIA was used to assess the CIC levels, their results are in close agreement with those reported by us (R. K. Gupta et al., 1979a), despite the fact that we used a different assay.

Because the relationship between CIC level and tumor burden was not linear,

Salinas *et al.* (1981*c*) analyzed serum samples of selected melanoma patients by density gradient ultracentrifugation and polyacrylamide gel electrophoresis (PAGE) to determine the size of CIC. Serum samples from patients with no evidence of disease were found to have medium-size (10–15 S) immune complexes; sera of patients with intermediate tumor burden had small (7–9 S), medium, and large (>16 S) immune complexes; and sera of patients with advanced disease had small and large immune complexes. In subsequent studies, these investigators were able to generate immune complexes *in vitro* by admixing selected sera containing either xenogeneic oncofetal antigen (XOFA) or melanoma-associated antigen (MAAg) (Salinas *et al.*, 1982*a*). Analyses of the immune complexes formed *in vitro* between XOFA and antibodies from sera of melanoma patients showed that the absolute and relative levels of the reactants regulated the concentration, size, and composition of associated immune complexes (Salinas *et al.*, 1981*c*). Similar studies were performed using MAAg that was isolated from each melanoma serum by the Raji cell bound immune complex method (Theofilopoulos *et al.*, 1978). When MAAg was mixed at optimal concentration with autologous melanoma serum, a growth in immune complex size was followed by their breakdown to *de novo* limiting-size moieties (Salinas *et al.*, 1983). Addition of allogeneic MAAg resulted in an increase in immune complex size in sera from patients with no evidence of disease and in sera from patients with intermediate tumor burden; however, a decrease in immune complex size was observed in sera from patients with advanced disease. Thus it was suggested that sera of patients with no evidence of disease had CIC with moderate excess of antibody and that sera of patients with advanced disease had CIC with antigen excess, whereas CIC in sera of patients with intermediate tumor burden exhibited antigen-antibody equivalence. We have shown that admixing early (antibody-rich) with late (antigen-rich) serum during the clinical course of a single patient results in the formation of immune complexes (R. K. Gupta *et al.*, 1979*b*). Thus, as suggested by Salinas *et al.* (1983), the fluctuating CIC observed in melanoma patients during the clinical course of their disease could be due to changes in tumor burden or to changes in the dynamic equilibrium of the immune reactants.

3. Relationship between CIC and Disease Recurrence

As discussed previously, the level of CIC in the sera of melanoma patients correlated well with tumor burden in many studies. Patients with intermediate but not exceedingly large tumor burden had the highest incidence of CIC. Thus, it may be deduced that the presence of high levels of CIC in a patient may signal a poor prognosis. A number of studies attest to the validity of such deductions. Some of these reports are reviewed in this section.

Despite a higher incidence and level of CIC in melanoma patients with clinically detectable disease, CIC at low incidence and levels have been observed in patients with no evidence of disease. The presence of CIC in these patients could be due to a subclinical amount of tumor. This assumption is supported by the report that melanoma patients receiving bacillus Calmette–Guérin (BCG) plus melanoma tumor cell vaccine had significantly higher levels of CIC than those receiving BCG alone or no treatment. Furthermore, in some patients who received BCG alone, CIC levels were stable but increased shortly after initiation of the tumor cell vaccine (Theofilopoulos *et al.*, 1977).

We observed that 26% (6/23) of melanoma patients who were positive for CIC and had no evidence of disease had recurrence of their disease within 3 months of the serum analysis. On the contrary, 92% (34/37) of patients who were negative for CIC and showed no evidence of disease remained free of disease up to 6 months after the serum analysis (R. K. Gupta and Morton, 1983*a*). Sztaba-Kania *et al.* (1981) observed that high levels of CIC or their increase in the face of no therapy accompanied the progression or recurrence of malignant melanoma. The stabilization of CIC at a low level was found to be a prognostically favorable sign. However, in 5 patients the levels of CIC decreased drastically as their disease progressed. The unexpected drop in the CIC level in these patients probably was caused by the deposition of the immune complexes in tissues, by systemic anergy (Nydegger, 1979; Theofilopoulos and Dixon, 1979; Jerry *et al.*, 1976), or by antigen excess (Salinas *et al.*, 1983). Kristensen *et al.* (1980) reported that 4/7 (57%) stage I melanoma patients who were CIC-positive had a recurrence within the period of observation. No recurrence was observed in 16 stage I patients who were negative for CIC during the preoperative period. Only one of the 14 patients who were negative for CIC postoperatively, when clinically disease-free, had a recurrence. Gauci *et al.* (1978) also observed that increased levels of CIC are associated with tumor recurrence in malignant melanoma; however, concomitant infection may give rise to increased levels of CIC. Despite this limitation they felt that the results of their investigation were sufficiently encouraging to continue their studies. Though a difference in recurrence rate between CIC-positive (75%) and CIC-negative (40%) patients was observed by Norris *et al.* (1980), the frequency of recurrence was not significantly different between the two groups because of the small number of melanoma patients in each group. Ruell *et al.* (1982) reported that of 160 melanoma patients who were clinically free of disease, CIC were detected at some time in 62 patients during their sequential follow-up. Twenty-one percent (13/62) of the CIC-positive patients developed a recurrence within 12 months. On the contrary, in those patients who were CIC-negative, the disease recurred in 19 patients within 3 months of the last negative assay.

Dorval and Pross (1983), in a prospective study of stage I melanoma patients, observed that the CIC levels of those patients whose disease did not progress tended to be lower than the CIC levels of the patients who eventually progressed. A similar pattern was observed with stage II patients. These investigators

Table V. Correlation between CIC and Recurrence of Disease in Clinically and Histologically Proven Stage I Malignant Melanoma Patients[a]

	No. patients		
Disease course	CIC-positive	CIC-negative	Total
Recurrence[b]	10	4	14
No recurrence[c]	4	11	15
Total	14	15	29

[a] Serum samples for CIC were analyzed by the complement consumption assay (R. K. Gupta et al., 1979a).
[b] Mean recurrence time from wide excision and lymphadenectomy was 27 months.
[c] All patients remained disease-free for at least 4 years.

also reported that, when the CIC levels of the patients with progressive disease were analyzed with respect to the results obtained prior to clinical evidence of disease progression, significantly elevated levels of CIC were observed 4–8 months prior to stage III diagnosis. Patients with rapidly progressing disease had lower levels of CIC compared to those with slowly progressing disease. Similar observations have been reported by Yoshida and Zawadzki (1980). We analyzed CIC levels in sequential serum samples from ten melanoma patients with stage II disease who progressed to stage III during the observation period of 20 months (R. K. Gupta et al., 1979b). In three patients, the CIC level decreased and became undectable as their disease progressed. None of the sequential serum samples from three other patients were positive for CIC despite the presence of low to medium tumor burdens. The other four patients, who had varying tumor burdens during the course of the study, were consistently positive for CIC. The nature of specificity of the antigenic component of the CIC in these patients was not determined.

Ahn et al. (1982) undertook investigations to determine whether the presence of CIC could predict tumor recurrence in patients with deeply invasive stage I malignant melanoma after definitive surgical resection of their disease. Twenty-nine patients, 14 of whom developed recurrence and 15 who remained disease-free for at least 4 years, were selected. All patients had a deeply invasive primary lesion at Clark level III, IV, or V with a >0.65-mm depth of invasion. Each patient was treated with wide excision of the primary and tumor regional lymphadenectomy. Stage I disease was clinically and histologically confirmed at the time of operation. Serum samples obtained 6–8 weeks postoperatively were analyzed by the complement consumption assay (R. K. Gupta et al., 1979a) for CIC levels. The results shown in Table V indicate that 71% of patients in the disease recurrence group were positive for CIC. Conversely, only 27% of the patients in the nonrecurrent group were positive. Statistically, the correlation of CIC with disease recurrence was significant ($P < 0.025$). It was concluded that analysis of serum samples from melanoma patients for CIC could be of prognostic value. However, because of some false-positive results, it is necessary to establish that the CIC do contain putative tumor antigen as one of their constituents.

Rossen et al. (1983) evaluated the prognostic significance of CIC in malignant melanoma patients. CIC levels were determined by the C1q binding assay in serum samples collected sequentially. Patients who were positive for CIC had significantly ($P < 0.004$) shorter mean survival time (4.7 months) than those who were CIC-negative (14.1 months). Thirty-five of 53 patients had distant metastases at the start of the study. Ten of these patients were CIC-positive and their mean survival time was shorter (4.7 months) than that of the other 25 patients, who were CIC-negative (mean survival time = 8.05 months). The mean survival times of patients with localized disease and with metastases to regional lymph nodes were 36 months and 14.9 months, respectively. All these patients were CIC-negative at the time of entry into the study. Reevaluation of the patients on the basis of changes in CIC level in subsequent serum samples revealed that patients who remained CIC-negative had a mean survival time of 15.8 months, patients who became CIC-positive had a mean survival time of 10.3 months, and patients who were persistently CIC-positive had a mean survival time of 4.7 months. Thus, the taking of several CIC measurements appeared to have increased the sensitivity for prognosis.

4. Effect of Treatment Modality on CIC Level

With the exception of a few reports, no systematic investigations have been undertaken to evaluate the effect of various treatment modalities on CIC levels in cancer patients. One may assume that any therapy that potentiates the immune response, especially humoral, should result in elevated CIC when tumor is present. Similarly, any therapy that causes immunosuppression may result in a decrease or abolishment of CIC. For these reasons it is necessary to take into consideration the effect of treatment during analysis of sequential serum samples from cancer patients.

In view of the reports that increases in CIC levels were observed in melanoma patients who received tumor cell vaccine as immunotherapy (Theofilopoulos et al., 1977) and that the presence of CIC may be a sign of poor prognosis, interpretation of CIC results may give rise to false information. In this section we have attempted to gather available information on this subject.

Gauci et al. (1978) reported that an often transient rise in CIC level can occur in patients receiving BCG. The increase in CIC level rarely reaches values similar to those seen in evolutive disease. Fluctuations in levels of CIC in melanoma patients receiving BCG have been reported by Jerry et al. (1976). Though significantly higher incidences and levels of CIC were observed in melanoma patients receiving BCG than in those who received no treatment, they were much higher in patients receiving BCG and tumor cell vaccine (Theofilopoulos *et al.*, 1977). In the report of Sztaba-Kania *et al.* (1981), the CIC levels in a BCG-treated group were not substantially different from those in patients who did not receive BCG. However, the mean rosette inhibition was slightly higher during the first 6 months of immunotherapy with BCG. A significant decrease in CIC levels in some melanoma patients after immunostimulation has been reported by Teshima *et al.* (1977).

While Lodola *et al.* (1981) reported that no significant variations were observed in CIC levels in melanoma patients following surgery, Ruell *et al.* (1982) found that cancer patients, whether melanoma or not, had higher levels of CIC after surgery than before surgery. Furthermore, patients receiving BCG had a greater incidence of CIC before and after surgery than those who did not receive BCG.

Skeem and Olkowski (1981) found that CIC levels remained within normal limits in some melanoma patients during immunotherapy with levamisole. In other patients, however, CIC tended to be higher during the levamisole administration period than during the post-drug observation period. We observed that, in a melanoma patient who had metastases to his liver, the CIC levels were negative. This patient was treated with hepatic artery perfusion and hyperthermia. Following each treatment, his CIC levels increased significantly (Fig. 1); however, the increases were transient (Huth *et al.*, 1982), suggesting tumor destruction with each treatment, which was associated with release of antigenic components into the circulation. These antigenic components then complexed with

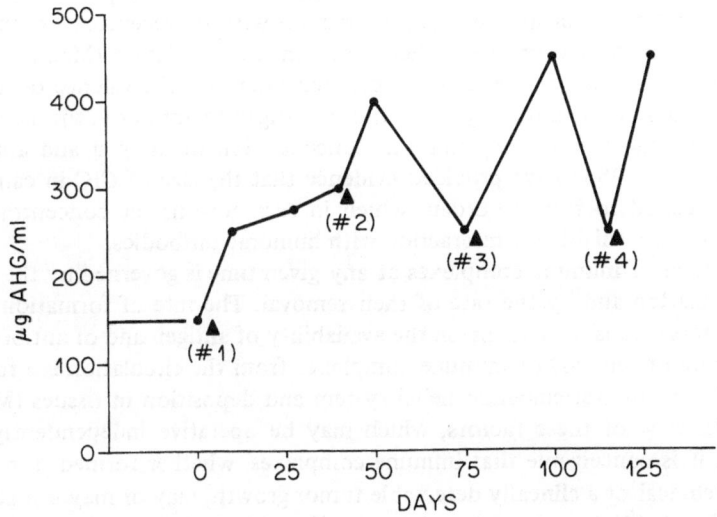

Figure 1. CIC levels during the thermochemotherapy of a patients with malignant melanoma. Points 1, 2, 3, and 4 represent the time of hyperthermia treatment.

humoral antibody and resulted in increased CIC. It was also noted that during this period of time the patient had a dramatic decrease in the extent of his metastatic liver disease and that his liver function tests had returned to normal.

C. Possible Reasons for Poor Correlations

The problems encountered and the inconsistent results obtained thus far in human malignant melanoma can not be due merely to the inadequacy of the technologies applied in the area of CIC detection. Rather, they probably stem from the complexity of the immune response of the host to the tumor and the heterogeneity of the disease. In view of reports on the detection and definition of a number of tumor antigens that are immunogenic in the host, it is logical to assume that their immune reaction products, i.e., immune complexes, must be present in the circulation at one time or another during growth of the tumor. Indeed, CIC have been detected and quantitated in melanoma patients by various investigators. A number of reasons can be envisioned for not finding satisfactory correlations between CIC and the clinical course of disease, and among the results of various investigators. To begin with, the immune complexes that circulate in patients are heterogeneous mixtures of antigen- and antibody-related types (Gauci et al., 1981). Tumors generally vary in their malignant nature and thus in their metastatic potential and growth. As a result CIC levels should vary in relation to the amount of tumor antigens expressed and their shedding.

Apart from the above factors, the nature and properties of immune complexes depend on the nature of the antigen and antibodies of which they are comprised. The size of immune complexes influences their deposition in tissues and their biological properties—i.e., interaction with Fc receptors, complement activation—which in turn affect their levels in the circulation (Mannik, 1980). The size of immune complexes is in turn dependent on the valence of the antigens, the class of the antibody, the ratio of antigen to antibody, the association constant of these reactants, and the concentration of antigen and antibody. Salinas et al. (1983) have provided evidence that the size of CIC in cancer patients is related to tumor burden, which in turn governs the concentration of antigen that is available for interaction with humoral antibodies.

The level of immune complexes at any given time is governed by the rate of their formation and by the rate of their removal. The rate of formation of immune complexes is dependent on the availability of antigen and of antibodies to it. The rate of removal of immune complexes from the circulation is a function of uptake by the reticuloendothelial system and deposition in tissues (Mannik, 1980). In view of these factors, which may be operative independently or in concert, it is conceivable that immune complexes, whether formed in response to a subclinical or a clincally detectable tumor growth, may or may not accumulate in the circulation at concentrations sufficiently high to be detected by the available assays. Furthermore, causes other than tumor growth may result in CIC, and formation of anti-Ig may complicate the situation further. From studies performed to elucidate the prognostic significance of CIC in cancer patients, the necessity of analyzing sequential serum samples has become quite obvious (Rossen et al., 1983).

Despite the reports reviewed here, which are by no means exhaustive, inadequate data are available to delineate conclusively the relationship between CIC level and tumor progression. However, there is sufficient evidence to suggest that estimation of CIC levels or their fluctuations during the course of the malignant disease may predict the outcome of the disease in some if not in all cases.

One of the major drawbacks has been the use of antigen-nonspecific assays for the estimation of CIC. This is not by choice, but is rather due to the unavailability of well defined and characterized specific tumor antigens. Until such reagents are developed, investigators in this area will have to rely on the existing assays.

V. NATURE OF CIC IN MELANOMA PATIENTS

One of the major problems in the area of CIC determination concerns the nature of the immune complexes detected by various antigen-nonspecific assays. Because the final characterization of an immune complex requires the identification of the specific antigen and/or antibody, it has not been possible to prove that the material (CIC) measured by various assays in melanoma patients does indeed represent immune complexes. It is quite possible that some of the material assumed to be CIC may be aggregated IgG, polyamines, or bacterial lipopolysaccharides. The presence of such components in human sera and their ability to bind with C1q has been documented (Angello et al., 1970; Sobel et al., 1975). However, some reports have suggested that the contribution of polyamines and aggregated Ig to the materials that represent immune complexes is not major (Cairns et al., 1980; R. C. Gupta et al., 1979; Heier et al., 1977). Price and Baldwin (1977) have provided evidence that tumor-antigen-containing immune complexes are present in the serum of tumor-bearing animals.

The nature and molecular weight of CIC detected by the C1q binding assay in human malignancy have been determined by Carpentier and Miescher (1983) using the physical and immunochemical properties of the immune complexes. In general, immune complexes detected in sera of cancer patients have been characterized with respect to their size and the presence of angi-Ig, antitumor antibodies, and tumor or other antigens. Some of these studies are reviewed in this section; however, this review is not exhaustive. Of course, the most direct approach to quantitate CIC is to apply antigen-specific assays. In the absence of such assays the use of antigen-nonspecific assays is justified. For this reason it becomes necessary to characterize the CIC. However, before any method of characterization can be applied for the characterization of CIC, these entities must be concentrated and isolated from the serum.

A. Methods for Concentration of CIC

Because of the relatively large size of immune complexes compared to either antigen or antibody alone or most serum proteins, they can be concentrated as an initial step in the separation of CIC from serum samples by such methods as gel filtration chromatography, sucrose density gradient ultracentrifugation, PEG precipitation, or their combinations.

1. Gel Filtration Chromatography

This method has been applied to separate large molecules or complexes from sera of patients with various diseases. Sephacryl S-300, Sephadex G-200, and Sepharose 6B gels have been used for this purpose (R. K. Gupta et al., 1979b; Poulton et al., 1983). The immune complexes are concentrated in the heaviest fraction.

2. Sucrose Density Gradient Ultracentrifugation

Sucrose gradients of, for example, 10–40%, 10–37%, and 5–35% have been used to concentrate heavy IgG from CIC-positive sera of cancer patients. The heavy IgG fractions were then used to demonstrate the immune-complex-like material in the assays initially used to determine the presence of CIC (Rossen et al., 1977; Theofilopoulos et al., 1977; Salinas et al., 1981a), Though gel filtration and gradient centrifugation methods are time-consuming, with the availability of Aifuge the sample processing time can be reduced significantly (Phillips et al., 1981).

3. Precipitation with PEG

PEG has been widely used to concentrate CIC from serum samples because a large number of samples can be processed with ease. A final concentration of 2.5–8% has been applied to precipitate soluble immune complexes. PEG-precipitated material may contain large amounts of other serum proteins; however, because of the solubility of the PEG-precipitated immune complexes, subsequent purification and analysis of their components is easy.

4. Combination of PEG and Sucrose Density Gradient Centrifugation

Male and Roitt (1979) have developed a single-step method by combining PEG and sucrose in a density gradient before ultracentrifugation.

B. Methods for Isolation of CIC

In general, methods for the isolation of immune complexes have been derived from those applied for their detection, with the exception of those assays that are based on phagocytosis, nephelometry, or EA-rosette inhibition. Though all of the CIC isolation methods available have not been applied to human malignant melanoma, they have been used successfully in other types of malignancies and, therefore, have the potential for application in this type of cancer. Some of these methods are now listed.

1. Binding to Complement Components

Though immune complexes containing IgG and IgM can be precipitated by C1q from serum samples or concentrated CIC, the amount of purified C1q required limits the use of this technique in isolating immune complexes (Chenais, 1977). For this reason C1q has been coupled to Sepharose (Svehag et al., 1979) and polymethylmethacrylate beads (Casali and Lambert, 1979) and used in affinity chromatography to isolate immune complexes. After precipitation with PEG and solubilization enough immune complexes can be absorbed and eluted from the C1q column to identify the antigens and antibodies. However, not all immune complexes bind C1q; therefore, this method is limited to the isolation of those immune complexes that can activate the classical pathway of the complement system. It has been reported that immune complexes containing at least three IgG antibody molecules can bind to C1q (Porter, 1980), and thus complexes above a certain minimum size can be isolated. However, Chenais et al. (1977) reported that some immune complexes that activate the classical pathway can be missed because of their saturation with endogenous C1q. To circumvent this problem, ethylenediaminetetraacetic acid (EDTA) can be added to the samples before isolation of the immune complexes by the immobilized C1q method. The binding of immune complexes to C1q is much greater at ionic strengths (e.g., $u = 0.075$) lower than physiological ($u = 0.15$) (Jones and Orlans, 1981).

2. Binding to Conglutinin

Conglutinin, a normal serum protein of many bovine species that binds to human inactivated C3b in the presence of Ca^{2+}, has been immobilized on a solid matrix and used to isolate immune complexes from human sera (Casali and Lambert, 1979). By this method immune complexes that activate complement by both classical and alternate pathways can be isolated; however, they must have C3b bound to them either endogenously or exogenously. Because inactivated C3b in immune complexes is liable to degradation by proteolytic enzymes, addition of inhibitors (e.g., phenyl methyl sulfonyl fluoride at a final concentration of 0.5 mM) to the samples has been recommended (Lachmann and Hobart, 1978). By the conglutinin method the recovery of immune complexes is low, because only undegraded C3b-bound complexes are isolated. Pereira *et al.* (1980) reported that this method isolated some of the low-molecular-weight materials that do not represent immune complexes. They found by sucrose density gradient ultracentrifugation that 7–8 S material bound to solid-phase conglutinin. This material represented IgG antibody that was no longer bound to antigen but retained inactivated C3b.

R. C. Gupta and Tan (1981) have described a three-step procedure to isolate complement-fixing immune complexes from human sera using soluble bovine conglutinin. The serum containing immune complexes was reacted with conglutinin in the presence of 10 mM Ca^{2+}. The conglutinin-bound immune complexes were precipitated using anticonglutinin rabbit serum. After washing the precipitate, the complexes were recovered by treatment with EDTA, which chelates Ca^{2+} and releases C3b-associated immune complexes from conglutinin. Because of the presence of anticonglutinin, the conglutinin remained in the precipitate and the immune complexes (C3b-bound) remained in the supernatant, from which they could be recovered and analyzed further.

3. Binding to Receptors on Cell Surfaces

Raji cells have been used to isolate preformed (either *in vitro* or *in vivo*) immune complexes as model systems (Theofilopoulos *et al.*, 1977, 1978; Tucker *et al.*, 1978). The immune complexes are adsorbed to the surface of Raji cells via C3b and other complement receptors in sufficient amounts to be radiolabeled and eluted for subsequent analysis for antigen and antibody constituents. Tucker *et al.* (1978) pointed out that culturing of sufficient Raji cells was cumbersome and that small immune complexes incapable of fixing complement could be missed. Furthermore, other proteins from the surface of Raji cells were eluted that interfered with antigen identification. Horsfall *et al.* (1981) noted that antibodies to Raji cell-surface antigens could be present in patients' sera and might bind to the Raji cell surface. For these reasons, this method did not see widespread use for the isolation of immune complexes. However, cells with receptors on their surface have been sucessfully used to identify antigen while immune complexes were still bound to their surface using specific fluorescence labeled antibodies (Theofilopoulos *et al.*, 1977; Amoroso *et al.*, 1980). It can thus be postulated that, where the antigenic component of the immune complexes is known or suspected, the use of cells applied for CIC detection (e.g., L1210 or K562) could be feasible for identifying the presence of the specific antigen in the complexes.

4. Binding to Antiimmunoglobulins

Immunoprecipitation or binding to immobilized anti-Ig antibodies can be used to isolate immune complexes from serum samples. However, though practical, this method will also isolate free Ig. Despite this limitation, Jones et al. (1980) have isolated IgM containing immune complexes. This provided a useful preliminary purification step for isotypes other than IgG. Harkiss and Brown (1980) have used low-affinity rabbit IgM anti-Fc to bind IgG complexes after concentration by 2–5% PEG; however, attempts by Chenais et al. (1977) to use immobilized IgM anti-Fc to isolate IgG complexes were not successful because the binding capacity of the columns was lost rapidly. Gilead and Sulitzeanu (1979) reported isolation of immune complexes formed in vitro. These investigators used plastic tubes coated with human polyclonal RhF to isolate tetanus toxoid-human antitoxoid complexes. The complexes, after elution, were contaminated with IgM and nonantibody IgG but contained enough antigen to be detected by autoradiography.

5. Binding to Anticomplement Components

Phillips et al. (1982) have described affinity chromatography procedures to isolate immune complexes by complement binding. Immobilized antibodies directed against human C3, C4, and C5b could be used to capture the complexes via the specific complement components, and they could then be eluted with an appropriate dissociating agent for subsequent characterization of their antigen and antibody components. Scharfstein et al. (1979) have used anti-C3 and -C4 in free solution to isolate immune complexes formed in vitro by subsequent binding of the anti-C3 or -C4 to immobilized protein A. Pereira et al. (1980) used immobilized $F(ab')_2$ of anti-C3 to characterize the antigen in immune complexes. These investigators also reported that the anti-C3 primarily bound a 7–8 S IgG fraction that lacked antigen which could be a misleading factor in subsequent procedures designed to identify the antigen.

Our studies using anti-C1q immunobeads revealed that the removal of immune complexes formed in vitro was a function of the amount of complement added (R. K. Gupta and J. Hillman, unpublished data). The immune complexes were generated by mixing [^{125}I]-melanoma-TAA and allogeneic serum from a melanoma patient. The melanoma-TAA was purified from a melanoma cell line (R. K. Gupta and Morton, 1984a). The goat anti-C1q immunobeads were obtained from Antibodies, Inc., Davis, California. As shown in Fig. 2, in the absence of complement no appreciable binding of [^{125}I]-melanoma-TAA-containing immune complexes to the anti-C1q beads occurred. This binding increases with the addition of complement to the antigen–antibody mixture. The allogeneic serum was decomplemented especially with respect to C1q by heating it at 56°C and passing it through an anti-C1q column. Addition of excess complement, thus C1q, resulted in saturation of the anti-C1q beads and in competition between immune-complex-bound C1q and free C1q. These results suggested that anti-C1q beads may potentially be used to isolate immune complexes from pathologic sera. To determine the feasibility of such an approach, we analyzed a number of serum samples from melanoma patients. As much as 95% of the com-

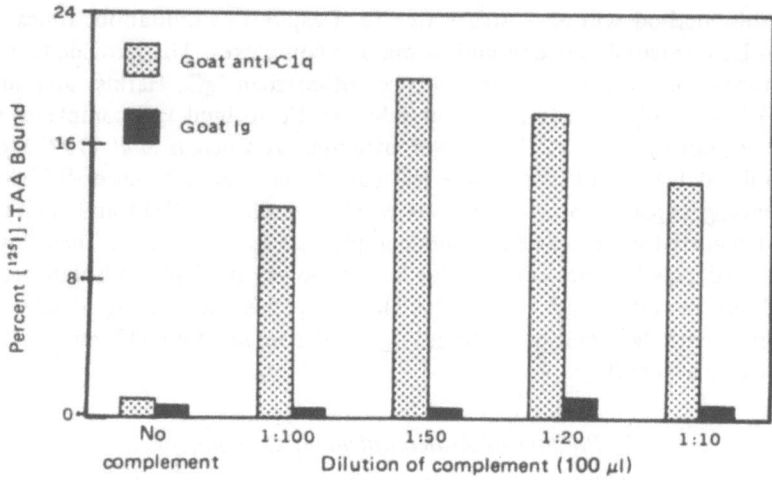

Figure 2. Binding of [^{125}I]-melanoma-TAA to immobilized goat anti-C1q and goat Ig (control) after reacting with allogeneic antimelanoma antibody in the absence and in the presence of various amounts of complement.

plement-fixing immune complexes were removed by the colums. The absorbed immune complexes were recovered by elution with glycine-HCl. Representative results are shown in Table VI; these denote that the recovery of the isolated immune complexes ranged from 12 to ≥100%. The level of CIC was assessed by the complement consumption assay (R. K. Gupta *et al.*, 1979*b*). The greater-than-100% recovery could be due to nonspecific aggregation of antibodies or to breakdown of large immune complexes into smaller ones.

In a comparative study using anti-C1q and anti-C3 immunobead columns and performed immune complexes between melanoma-TAA and allogeneic anti-TAA, we observed that anti-C3 immunobeads bound about twice as much [^{125}I]-melanoma-TAA-containing immune complexes as anti-C1q immunobeads (Fig. 3). Similar results have been reported by Kilgallon *et al.* (1982). These investigators observed that only 15–30% of the total complexes formed between bovine serum albumin (BSA) and anti-BSA in the presence of complement bound to the anti-C1q column. The unbound complexes had a similar molecular weight profile to those that bound to the anti-C1q column. The failure of unbound complexes to bind to the anti-C1q column was not due to saturation of the column; rather it was due to masking of the C1q by other complement components, e.g., C3b. The complexes that could not bind to anti-C1q were able to bind to the anti-C3 column. Comparative study revealed that the anti-C3 column bound three times more immune complexes than the anti-C1q column.

6. Binding to Staphylococcal Protein A

Tucker *et al.* (1978) developed procedures to isolate CIC from samples in a rat tumor model. These procedures involved binding of immune complexes to

Table VI. Isolation and Recovery of CIC from Sera of Melanoma Patients from Anti-C1q Immunobead Columns[a,b]

Sample No.	CIC (μg AHG equiv./ml)		Percent of serum
	Serum	Eluate from column[c]	
1	30	29	97
2	100	22	22
3	56	19	34
4	140	17	12
5	62	15	24
6	84	70	83
7	21	22	104
8	40	42	105
9	40	30	75
10	28	10	36

[a]CIC were determined by the complement consumption assay (R. K. Gupta et al., 1979b).
[b]Goat anti-Clq immunobeads were obtained from Antibodies, Inc., Davis, California; 0.5 ml of beads were packed in 1-ml hypodermic syringes using 24-gauge needles.
[c]The columns were charged with 200 μl of the serum sample and washed with ten volumes of buffer. The absorbed immune complexes were eluted with 0.6 ml of 0.1 M glycine-HCl (pH 2.6). The eluent was collected into 0.2 ml of 0.2 M phosphate buffer. The eluates were checked and adjusted to pH 7.2 before analysis for CIC. The dilution factors were taken into consideration before expressing the CIC results as μg AHG equiv./ml.

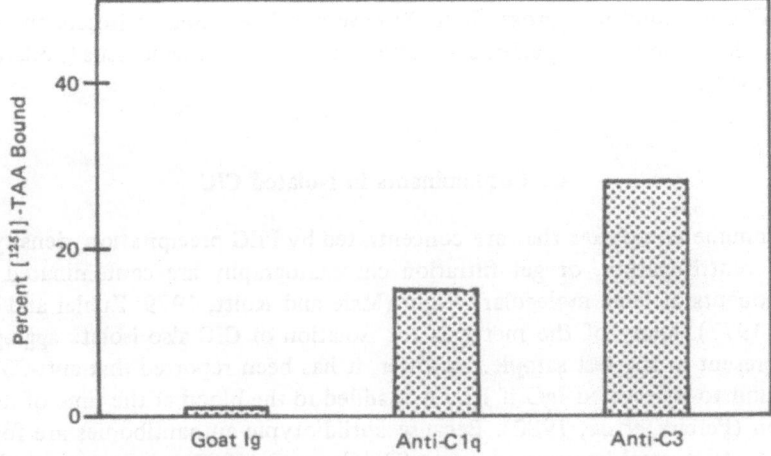

Figure 3. Binding of immune complexes formed in vitro between [125I]-melanoma-TAA and allogeneic anti-TAA in the presence of complement to immobilized goat anti-C1q and -C3. Immobilized goat Ig was included as a control.

protein A–Sepharose and subsequent elution at low pH (2.4). The use of protein A could be restricted by its inability to bind IgG3, IgA, IgM, or IgE. These investigators reported that the use of purified and immobilized protein A could be better than the use of fixed *Staphylococcus aureus* cells because of the large binding capacity of protein A–Sepharose. However, Goding (1978) reported that nonspecific adsorption to protein A immobilized on Sepharose is greater than that to the bacteria. There is some evidence that complement components may interfere with binding of immune complexes to protein A owing to steric hindrance (Nussenzweig, 1980). Despite these limitations, immune complexes have been isolated from the circulation of animals and humans using protein A (Snyder *et al.*, 1982; Maidment *et al.*, 1981). Combinations of protein A, gel filtration, PEG precipitation, and gradient ultracentrifugation have been used to increase the purity of the final product. For example, as much as 50% of the material isolated using the protein A method may not be immune complexes (R. K. Gupta *et al.*, 1983*b*). Furthermore, free IgG molecules are isolated along with immune complexes. This can be minimized by including Sephacryl S-200 or Sephadex G-150 chromatography of the sample as a prestep.

7. Dye–Ligand Chromatography

Recently Quay *et al.* (1983) have isolated CIC in high yield from serum samples of patients with malignant melanoma utilizing a bifunctional [diethylaminoethyl cellulose (DEAE) and Cibracon blue F3GA dye] chromatographic matrix. This matrix binds all normal serum proteins except IgG-containing immune complexes, IgG, and transferrin. The unbound material was subsequently analyzed by PAGE and was found to contain one common and several unique non-Ig proteins. These proteins had molecular weights similar to those of several proteins previously identified as human melanoma antigens. DEAE-Sephacel and Cibracon blue F3GA bound to agarose (Blue A) have also been used to isolate anti-DNA antibodies from sera of patients with systemic lupus erythematosus (Pollard and Webb, 1982).

C. Contaminants in Isolated CIC

Immune complexes that are concentrated by PEG precipitation, density gradient centrifugation, or gel filtration chromatography are contaminated with components of large molecular weight (Male and Roitt, 1979; Zubler and Lambert, 1977). Many of the methods for isolation of CIC also isolate aggregated IgG present in the test sample. However, it has been reported that anti-C3 does not bind to aggregated IgG if EDTA is added to the blood at the time of its collection (Pereira *et al.*, 1980). Because antiidiotypic autoantibodies are formed during any normal immune response (Goidle *et al.*, 1980), the presence of idiotype–antiidiotype complexes in the circulation is to be expected, and their presence has been documented in normal (Morgan *et al.*, 1979) and cancer (Lewis *et al.*, 1976) sera. Complement components in immune complexes isolated by a majority of methods may account for as much as 50% of the total protein (Jones and Orlans, 1981). Table VII, as modified from the report of Jones and Orlans (1981), lists some of the contaminants that have been found in isolated immune complexes.

D. Dissociation of Isolated CIC

A number of methods are available to elute antibodies of antigens from affinity ligands on solid matrix [see Jones and Orlans (1981) for review]. However, regardless of the method selected, the least avid antibodies are dissociated and selectively eluted first, all or part of the antigen or antibody may be modi-

Table VII. Contaminants Generally Found in Immune Complexes Isolated by Various Methods

Isolation method	Contaminants	Representative reference
PEG precipitation	7 S IgG, aggregated IgG, >7 S serum proteins	Zubler and Lambert (1977)
Gel filtration and density gradient centrifugation	Complement components, >7 S serum proteins	Benveniste and Bruneau (1979)
Raji cell	C-reactive protein, antibodies to Raji cell membrane antigens, antibodies to nuclear antigens	Horsfall *et al.* (1981)
C1q	Polyanions, endotoxins, DNA, serum components not specifically bound to the antibody isotypes	Cooper *et al.* (1976)
Conglutinin	IgG antibody associated with C3 fragments, immunoconglutinins	Pereira *et al.* (1980)
Antiimmunoglobulins	Free immunoglobulins of the relevant isotype	Pereira *et al.* (1980)
Anti-C1q, -C3, -C4	Complement components, aggregated IgG (?), IgG antibody associated with C3 fragments	Pereira *et al.* (1980)
Protein A	Antiidiotype antibodies unrelated to immune complexes, 7 S IgG and immunoglobulins of other classes, other serum proteins that can bind to the solid support	Goding (1978)

fied or denatured by the agent, and removal of the agent will result in reassociation of antigen and antibody if they are not physically separated beforehand. The reassociated immune complexes may have altered molar ratios of antigen and antibody. Jones and Orlans (1981) suggested the following factors to consider in choosing a particular method:

1. Affinity of the ligands used to isolate CIC. More powerful agents are needed to elute immune complexes from high-affinity ligands. For example, acid or alkaline buffers are used for protein A and anti-Ig columns. On the contrary, milder agents are employed for lower-affinity ligands, as with the use of 0.02 M EDTA at pH 7.4 for immobilized conglutinin.
2. Requirement to recover intact immune complexes.
3. Optimum recovery of antibody or antigen.
4. Recovery of immunologically active antibody or antigen.

Phillips *et al.* (1982) have reported that acid and chaotropic ion dissociation of immune complexes resulted in immunologically active antibody and antigen; however, the chaotropic agents, e.g., polyvinyl pyrrolidone–iodine, gave better results.

We have observed that both antigen and antibody could be eluted from protein A-bound immune complexes of melanoma patients by treatment with 2.5 M $MgCl_2$ at pH 6.8 and that at least some of the antigen and antibody reassociated after removal of the dissociating agent (R. K. Gupta *et al.*, 1983*b*). We also observed that treatment of immobilized protein A-bound immune complexes with 0.1 M glycine-HCl buffer at pH 3.5 resulted in dissociation of the immune complexes and recovery of the antigen (melanoma-TAA) in the supernatant. The antibody remained bound to the protein A and was later recovered by treatment with 2.5 M $MgCl_2$ (R. K. Gupta *et al.*, 1983*a*).

Hendrick *et al.* (1981) dissociated isolated and purified immune complexes by low-pH treatment and subsequent gel filtration chromatography on Ultrogel AcA34. Citrate–phosphate buffer at pH 3.0 was used as the eluent. Low-pH treatment of the isolated immune complexes from melanoma patients has also been used by Rossen and Morgan (1981). However, they used sucrose density gradient ultracentrifugation at pH 2.9 to separate the antibody from dissociated immune complexes. Carpentier and Miescher (1983) used 0.5 M acetate buffer at pH 3.5 to dissociate the purified immune complexes from a leukemia patient and separated the antigen and antibody by sucrose density gradient ultracentrifugation at pH 3.5. In addition, Phillips *et al.* (1981) reported that agarose block electrophoresis or thin-layer chromatography can be used to separate and recover individual immune complex components.

Though these studies testify to the applicability of various methods of dissociation to immune complexes isolated from cancer patients, other methods—such as 1.0 M ammonia, 3 M NaSCN, 0.1 M lithium diiodosalicylate, 0.2 M 1,4-

diaminobutane, and 0.005 M 2,5-diaminotoluosulfate (Jones and Orlans, 1981)—can also be used, and their practicality has been proven.

E. Detection of Immune Reactants

Ideally, identification in the CIC of the antigen that is associated with the disease process is the best approach to document a relationship between immune complexes in the circulation and the presence of active disease. Even though the presence of antigen and/or antibody in preformed immune complexes has been documented in model systems, identification of suspected constituents in clinical materials poses considerable problems despite the use of the same methods. These problems could be the result of loss of antigenic or antibody activity in the dissociated products of the immune complexes. Furthermore, inadequate separation of the antigen and antibody from dissociated immune complexes could lead to their recombination at neutral pH and isotonicity, thus hindering the recognition of the antigenic sites of the antigen and the detection of the antibody (Jones and Orlans, 1981). Successful attempts have been made to detect the antigens in question in intact immune complexes from melanoma patients bound to Raji cells (Theofilopoulos *et al.*, 1977). Some of the methods used to characterize immune complexes with respect to their antigen and/or antibody constituents are now summarized.

1. Polyacrylamide Gel Electrophoresis

Analysis of isolated immune complexes by sodium dodecyl sulfate (SDS)-PAGE has revealed the presence of components (putative antigens) that are not related to IgG or other serum proteins. For this purpose both one- and two-dimensional PAGE has been used (Tucker *et al.*, 1978; Male and Roitt, 1979; Casali and Lambert, 1979). Recently, Quay *et al.* (1983) revealed by SDS-PAGE the presence of common and unique proteins in the immune complexes isolated from sera of three melanoma patients. Some of the common proteins represented β_2-macroglobulin and the heavy and light chains of IgG, whereas the unique proteins were of varying molecular weights. The reactivity of these unique proteins with antibody of known specificity was not evaluated. It is known that some antigens, especially glycoprotein, are not destroyed by SDS treatment (R. K. Gupta and Morton, 1983b; Anderton and Thorpe, 1980); thus, the antigens in immune complexes separated by PAGE can be transferred from the gel to cellulose nitrate paper for identification by radiolabeled or enzyme-linked antibody (Heimer *et al.*, 1981).

We analyzed, by immunoprecipitation and subsequent SDS-gradient PAGE, the composition of the putative antigen fraction separated from isolated immune complexes of melanoma patients (R. K. Gupta *et al.*, 1983b) and compared it

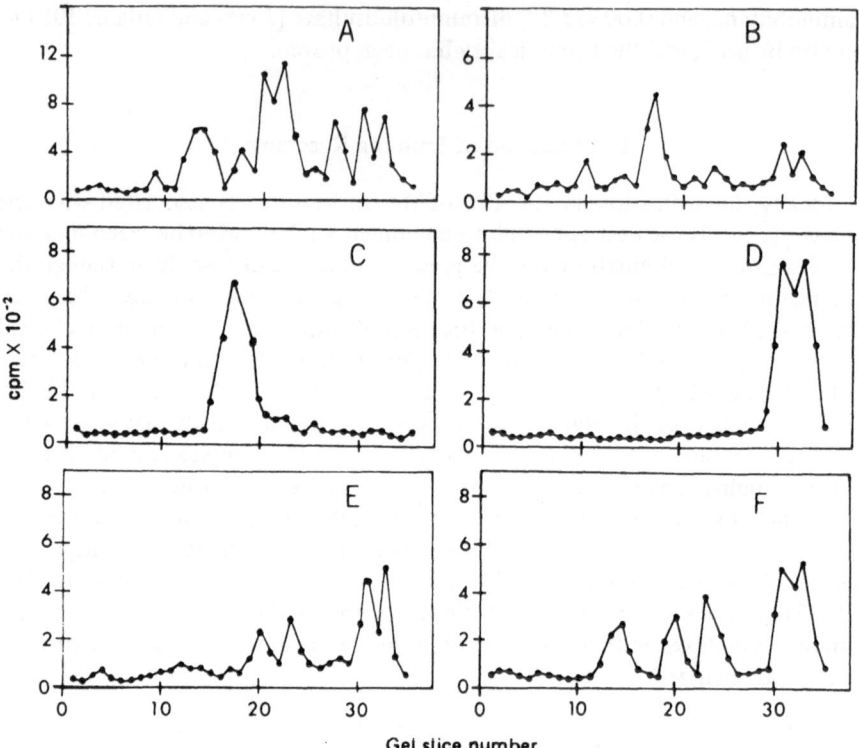

Figure 4. Radioactivity profile after SDS-PAGE of the putative antigen fraction isolated from purified [^{125}I]-immune complexes of a melanoma patient and its immunoprecipitates. (A) Putative antigen fraction. (B) Immunoprecipitate of putative antigen fraction using rabbit antimelanoma serum raised against partially purified spent culture medium of a melanoma cell line (R. K. Gupta *et al.*, 1979*b*). (C) Fetal antigen (R. K. Gupta and Morton, 1983*b*). (D) [^{125}I]-melanoma-TAA (R. K. Gupta and Morton, 1984*a*). (E) Immunoprecipitate of the putative antigen fraction using allogeneic antibody from a melanoma patient. (F) Immunoprecipitate of the putative antigen fraction using autologous antibody.

with the compositions of fetal antigen (FA) (R. K. Gupta and Morton, 1983*b*) and melanoma-TAA (R. K. Gupta and Morton, 1984*a*). The results are shown in Fig. 4. After immunoprecipitation of the putative antigen fraction with rabbit antimelanoma serum that was rendered functionally specific for tumor tissues by absorption with normal tissues (R. K. Gupta *et al.*, 1979*e*), one major and three minor peaks were observed. The major peak corresponded to the FA (R. K. Gupta *et al.*, 1983*b*). Two fast-migrating bands corresponded to the melanoma-TAA. The immunoprecipitates using allogeneic and autologous antibodies revealed four and five bands, respectively. Three bands of these two immunoprecipitates were in the regions of FA and melanoma-TAA, whereas one band of each was in the 50,000- to 70,000-molecular-weight region. The fifth band in the autologous antibody immunoprecipitate was in the molecular weight region of >120,000. These results suggested that the immune complexes isolated from melanoma patients contained at least five components that were recognized by autologous antibody. Some of these components represented at least two of the antigens (FA and melanoma-TAA) that have been isolated and purified from spent culture medium of a human melanoma cell line.

2. Preparative Isoelectric Focusing

Maidment *et al.* (1981) have documented the presence of TAA in the immune complexes of cancer patients. These investigators subjected the isolated immune complexes of breast cancer patients to preparative isoelectric focusing. The dissociated Ig and putative antigens were recovered from the appropriate pH regions. The IgG recovered from the immune complexes reacted with the recovered antigens and with three breast cancer cell lines. The recovered antigens had isoelectric points of between pH 3 and 5 and molecular weights of 20,000 and 42,000. Using the same procedures, these investigators have analyzed the immune complex components of lymphoma, leukemia, colon, and kidney cancer patients.

3. Double Countercurrent Immunoelectrophoresis

This technique was developed by Phillips *et al.* (1982) to document the presence of antibody and antigen of known specificities in immune complexes of melanoma patients. These investigators dissociated the isolated immune complexes with 4 *M* polyvinylpyrrolidone–iodine and subjected them to electrophoresis in an agar gel at pH 8.6. The components thus separated were identified as antigen that migrated toward the anode and antibody that migrated toward the cathode. The immunoreactivity of the antigen component was determined within the gel by the use of antibodies from isolated immune complexes that had previously been typed by immunofluorescence and that of the antibody, by the use of antigens isolated from tumor extracts. With this approach, antitumor antibodies associated with immune complexes have been demonstrated in 16% (54/340) patients and tumor antigens associated with immune complexes in 13% (43/340) of melanoma patients.

4. Indirect Immunofluorescence

Theofilopoulos *et al.* (1977) documented the presence of TAA in the immune complexes of three melanoma patients by binding the immune complexes to Raji cells and by subsequent indirect immunofluorescence. Rabbit antimelanoma serum and fluorescein isothiocyanate (FITC)-conjugated anti-rabbit IgG were used as the detecting reagents. Raji cells reacted with immune-complex-negative melanoma sera, and normal human sera, melanoma cell extracts, and immune-complex-positive nonmelanoma sera, as controls were negative for the presence of melanoma-associated antigen. Phillips *et al.* (1982) showed by indirect immunofluorescence that antibodies separated from immune complexes of melanoma patients reacted with melanoma cells.

5. Radioimmunoassay

In addition to indirect immunofluorescence, Theofilopoulos *et al.* (1977) used ^{125}I-labeled rabbit antimelanoma antibody to document the presence of melanoma-associated antigen in the immune complexes of melanoma patients. They bound immune complexes from sera of 69 melanoma patients to Raji cells. The cells were then reacted with radiolabeled rabbit antimelanoma antibody. The uptake of the radioactivity was 5- to 13-fold greater in 15 instances than in controls. Thus, at least 22% of the melanoma sera contained immune complexes that were composed of melanoma-associated antigen.

Using immobilized protein A, we isolated and dissociated immune complexes from four melanoma patients (R. K. Gupta *et al.*, 1983a,b). The antibodies recovered from the immune complexes showed ractivity with a TAA in a radioimmunoassay (Fig. 5). The binding of radiolabeled melanoma-TAA decreased with decreasing amounts of the antibody isolated from the immune complexes

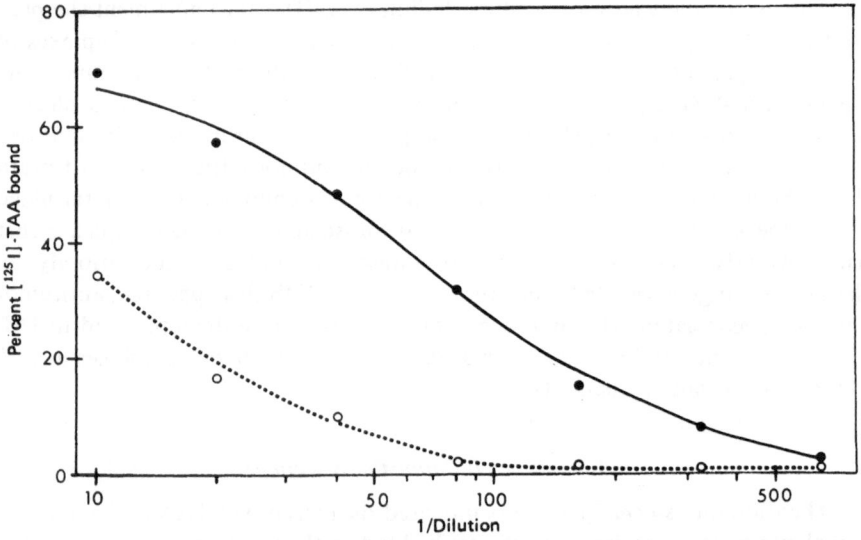

Figure 5. Binding of [125I]-melanoma-TAA (R. K. Gupta and Morton, 1984a) by various dilutions of putative antibody fractions obtained from immune complexes of a melanoma patient. •, Antibody recovered from the immune complexes; o, antibody recovered from the antigen fraction (R. K. Gupta *et al.*, 1983a).

of melanoma patients. Quantitative analysis revealed that of the total protein in the antibody fraction, only 0.15–6% represented anti-TAA activity. In another approach (R. K. Gupta et al., 1983b) the antibodies dissociated by KSCN in the presence of allogeneic antibody from the radiolabeled immune complexes were purified by density gradient ultracentrifugation. The purified radiolabeled antibodies showed immunologic reactivity with cultured cells. This reactivity was inhibited by preincubation of the antibody with purified melanoma TAA and an FA (Table VIII).

We have documented the pesence of an antigen immunologically similar to melanoma-TAA (R. K. Gupta and Morton, 1984a) in the putative antigen fractions of immune complexes isolated from melanoma patients by competitive inhibition in radioimmunoassay (R. K. Gupta et al., 1983a). As illustrated in Fig. 6, the inhibition of binding between [^{125}I]-melanoma-TAA and antimelanoma-TAA decreased in direct proportion to the increased amount of protein of the

Table VIII. Binding of ^{125}I-Labeled Antibodies Isolated from ^{125}I-Labeled Immune Complexes of a Melanoma Patient to Various Cultured Cells and Inhibition of Binding by Preincubation of the Antibodies with Soluble Fetal Antigen and Melanoma-Tumor-Associated Antigen

Target cells	cpm bound without inhibitor[a] (mean ± SD, N = 3)	Percent inhibition of binding after preincubation of labeled antibody with[b]:	
		Fetal antigen	Melanoma-TAA
Melanoma			
UCLA-SO-M7	4890 ± 292	43.4	40.3
UCLA-SO-M14	5500 ± 350	31.4	52.1
UCLA-SO-M16	4839 ± 198	34.4	58.4
UCLA-SO-M21	5473 ± 186	18.8	43.8
Sarcoma			
UCLA-SO-S1	2174 ± 146	81.0	3.3
UCLA-SO-S2	2535 ± 202	82.3	2.5
UCLA-SO-S3	2648 ± 293	82.0	6.5
Normal			
Fibroblast	2040 ± 377	78.4	−3.0

[a]One hundred μl cell suspension (1 × 10^6 cells/ml) were reacted with 200 μl (about 1 × 10^4 cpm) of purified [^{125}I]-antibodies obtained from the dissociation of melanoma immune complexes. The mixtures were incubated at 4°C for 1 hr. Cells were washed three times with RPMI-FCS and analyzed for radioactivity.
[b]The antibody was incubated with 17 μg protein of fetal antigen and 15 μg protein of melanoma-TAA (100-μl volume of each) at 4°C for 1 hr before being subjected to the binding assay. The percent inhibition was calculated by the following formula:

$$\text{Percent inhibition} = \left(1 - \frac{\text{Mean cpm bound after incubation with the inhibitor}}{\text{Mean cpm found without inhibitor}}\right) \times 100$$

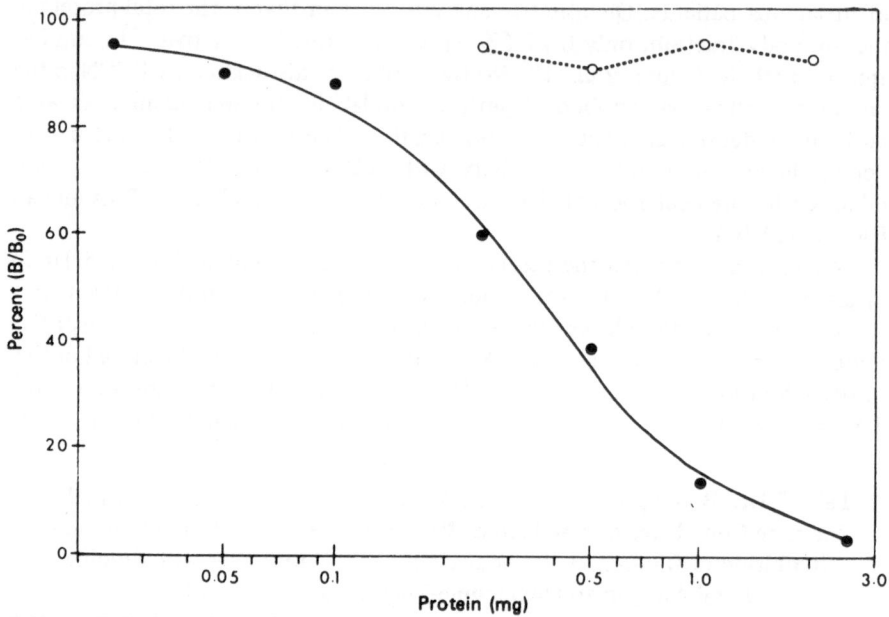

Figure 6. Dose-dependent competitive inhibition of binding between [^{125}I]-melanoma-TAA and allogeneic antibody from a melanoma patient (R. K. Gupta and Morton, 1984*a*) by the putative antigen fractions obtained from immune complexes of a melanoma patient (•) and blood bank plasma (o).

putative antigen fraction. On the contrary, the putative antigen fraction obtained from blood blank plasma did not compete in the radioimmunoassay and no dose dependence was observed. These results indicated that the putative antigen fraction obtained from immune complexes of melanoma patients contained melanoma-TAA as one of the antigens. Quantitative analysis revealed that relative concentration of melanoma-TAA in various putative antigen fractions of melanoma patients ranged from 0.04 to 0.81% of the total proteins (R. K. Gupta *et al.*, 1983a).

6. Antigenic Competition Assay

Because of the availability of a well characterized and radiolabeled melanoma-TAA (R. K. Gupta and Morton, 1984*b,c*), we designed experiments to determine if this antigen would compete with some of the antigen components of the immune complexes isolated from sera of melanoma patients. For this purpose, isolated immune complexes were dissociated with 3.5 *M* KSCN. The ^{125}I-labeled melanoma-TAA was added to the dissociated immune complexes, and the mixtures were dialyzed to remove the dissociating agent and to allow reassociation of the antigen(s) and antibody components. It was anticipated

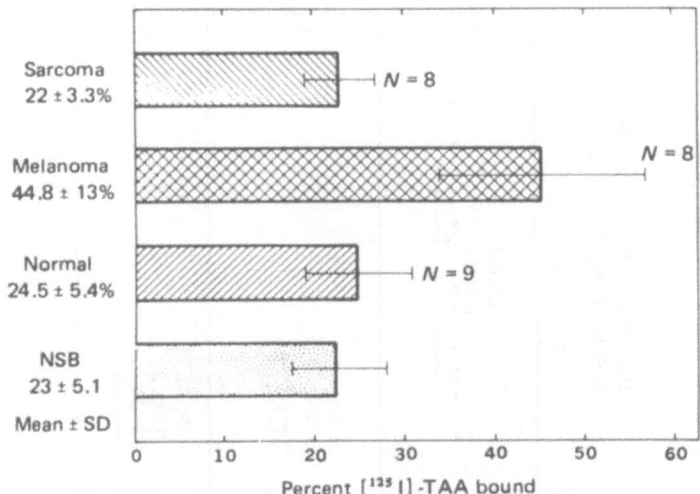

Figure 7. Incorporation of [^{125}I]-melanoma-TAA into isolated immune complexes by the antigenic competition method. Normal group includes patients with connective tissue disease.

that during reassociation the radiolabeled melanoma-TAA would compete with the dissociated antigen for antibody only if the immune complexes contained immunologically similar or cross-reacting antigens. The dialyzed materials were then treated with immobilized protein A. The sediments, after washing with Triton X-100 (0.5%) containing buffer, were analyzed for the incorporation of radioactivity into the reassociated immune complexes. Controls containing immune complexes from patients with connective tissue disease and from patients with malignancy other than melanoma were included to establish the baseline for nonspecific sedimentation of radioactivity. Results shown in Fig. 7 revealed that incorporation of [^{125}I]-melanoma-TAA into immune complexes of melanoma patients was significantly higher than incorporation into immune complexes of sarcoma or connective tissue disease patients (R. K. Gupta et al., 1981). To determine if the incorporation of radiolabeled melanoma-TAA into the isolated immune complexes was due specifically to reaction with a particular antibody or to nonspecific aggregation with other serum components, the reaction mixture after antigenic competition was separated by 5–30% sucrose density gradient ultracentrifugation. A 0.5-ml fraction of gradient was treated with immobilized protein A and the radioactivity in the sediments was determined. The ratio between counts migrated to a density of 1.0218–1.0259 (high) and a density of 1.087–1.137 (low) was calculated for each sample. As shown in Fig. 8, this ratio was 1.1 ± 0.2 for immune complexes of sarcoma patients and 1.04 ± 0.22 for immune complexes of connective tissue disease patients. None of these samples had a ratio of >1.5. Using this value as the baseline, the immune com-

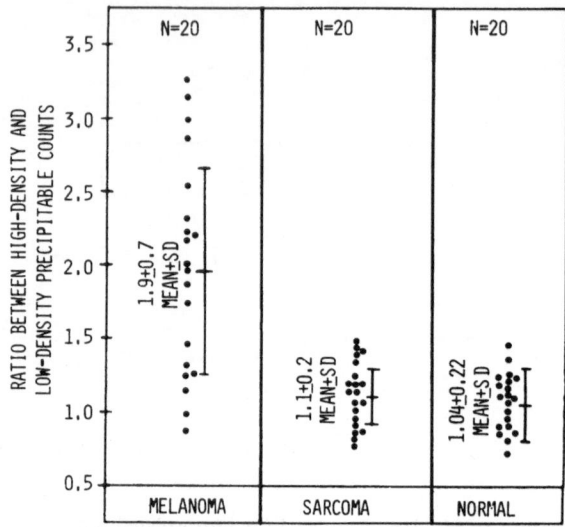

Figure 8. Distribution of radioactivity ratio of [^{125}I]-melanoma-TAA between high-density and low-density regions of sucrose density gradient ultracentrifugation after subjecting it to antigenic competition using immune complexes isolated from CIC-positive sera of melanoma, sarcoma, and connective tissue disease (normal) patients.

plexes of 65% (13/20) of the melanoma patients contained antigen that was immunologically similar to melanoma-TAA. The mean ±SD ratio for this group was 1.9 ± 0.7 (R. K. Gupta and Morton, 1982b).

7. Use of Monoclonal Antibody Directed to Tumor Antigen

Morgan and Reisfeld (1982) observed reactivity between a monoclonal antibody that was developed against a melanoma-associated oncofetal glycoprotein of 94,000 molecular weight and normal human sera. Gel filtration analysis revealed a heterogeneous distribution of the reactive components in the sera, which ranged from 200,000 to 2,000,000 daltons. The reactive components could be precipitated with PEG, suggesting the presence of the 94,000-dalton MAAg in the form of immune complexes in these sera. With the use of reverse sandwich enzyme-linked immunosorbent assay (ELISA), these investigators conclusively demonstrated that the antigen was associated with both IgG and IgM classes of antibodies. Thus, it was concluded that the melanoma-associated oncofetal antigen was present and that it elicits a humoral immune response in humans. From these results it could also be inferred that the determinant(s) recognized by the hosts' antibodies were different from those recognized by the mouse monoclonal antibody. Thus, monoclonal antibodies developed against human tumor antigens can be used as potential reagents to characterize the CIC in cancer patients, thus improving the diagnostic and prognostic usefulness of CIC analysis.

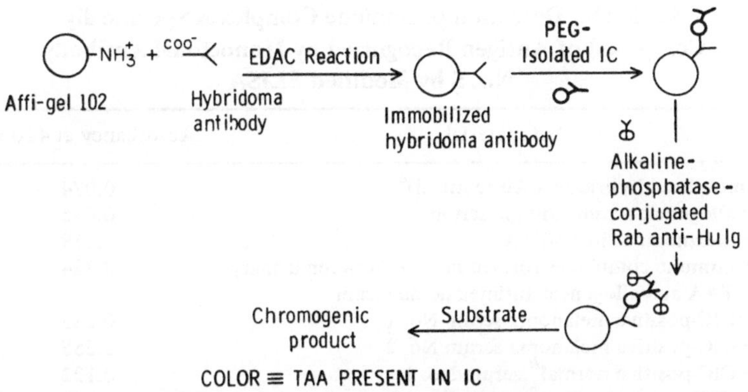

Figure 9. Outline of the procedure to characterize immune complexes by the use of immobilized hybridoma antibody and modified ELISA.

Along these lines, we developed a mouse monoclonal antibody (No. 5) to a urinary-TAA isolated from a melanoma patient (M. Kasai, R. K. Gupta, and D. L. Morton, unpublished data) and used in a modified ELISA. As illustrated in Fig. 9, the monoclonal antibody No. 5 immobilized to Affi-gel 102 beads was reacted with immune complexes isolated from sera of patients with melanoma and connective tissue disease, and with immune complexes formed *in vitro*. After washing, the beads were reacted with alkaline-phosphatase-conjugated rabbit anti-human Ig. The binding of the enzyme conjugate to the beads, which in turn was due to the presence of human Ig in immune complexes bound to the beads initially, was determined using *p*-nitrophenyl phosphate as the substrate. Results listed in Table IX show that the immune complexes, either generated *in vitro* or isolated from melanoma patients, had higher ELISA readings than the immune complexes isolated from sera of connective tissue disease patients or immune reagents by themselves used to generate the *in vitro* immune complexes.

Other variations of this type of approach using immobilized anti-human IgG and protein A have been successful in our laboratory in detecting the presence of TAA by monoclonal antibody (R. K. Gupta, unpublished data). The isolated immune complexes were bound to rabbit anti-human IgG immunobeads and the presence of specific TAA in the immune complexes was determined by the monoclonal antibody No. 5 using ELISA. However, with the procedure just described, detection of classes of immunoglobulins associated with the specific immune complexes is feasible by the use of the enzyme-conjugated second antibodies that are specific for the human Ig class.

F. Summary of TAA Detected in CIC of Melanoma Patients

Despite significant advances in the characterization of CIC with respect to their antigen and antibody constituents in patients with solid neoplasms, rela-

Table IX. Detection of Immune Complexes Specifically
Composed of Antigen Recognized by Monoclonal Antibody
No. 5 by Modified ELISA

Test material	Absorbancy at 410 nm
Immobilized hybridoma Ab (control)[a]	0.074
+ allogeneic antimelanoma serum	0.095
+ melanoma urinary-TAA	0.059
+ immune complexes formed in vitro between urinary- TAA and allogeneic antimelanoma serum	0.324
+ CIC-positive melanoma serum No. 1	0.285
+ CIC-positive melanoma serum No. 2	0.255
+ CIC-positive normal[b] serum No. 1	0.122
+ CIC-positive normal[b] serum No. 2	0.113

[a]Hybridoma antibody No. 5 was immobilized on Affi-gel 102.
[b]Represents serum from patient with connective tissue disease.

tively little has been reported for malignant melanoma. This is mainly due to the lack of availability of melanoma antigens in purified form that are immunogenic in the host. Some investigators have purified immune complexes from sera of melanoma patients and documented the presence of unique and common components after analyzing them by SDS-PAGE. Documentation of the immunoreactivity of these components with defined antibodies is lacking in such studies. On the other hand, some reports provide evidence for immunoreactivity of the putative antigen fractions isolated from purified immune complexes. Though not exhaustive, Table X summarizes the nature of the antigens and antibodies detected in the immune complexes of melanoma patients. It is obvious that unique and common components that are associated with human malignant melanoma have been detected as immune complex constituents in some cases. Only a few reports available in the literature have documented that the antigen component of isolated immune complexes could react with antibody of defined specificity and that at least a fraction of the antibodies recovered from the immune complexes reacted with cultured tumor cells or purified soluble antigen. Certainly, the putative antibody fraction of the immune complexes has been shown to contain anti-Ig (antiidiotypes).

The CIC in melanoma patients may be composed of either IgG or IgM antibodies or both; however, antibodies of the IgG type are more prevalent. The antigen portion of immune complexes has been shown to contain TAA and FA. Such observations do provide affirmative answers to some of the questions posed by Rossen and Morgan (1981): Do CIC in melanoma patients contain antibodies that can react with autologous or allogeneic tumor cells? Are the putative antigens in CIC the products of tumor cells? Application of monoclonal antibody to detect the presence of defined antigens in CIC of melanoma patients should provide information on the origin of the CIC.

Table X. Characteristics of Antigen and Antibody Constituents of Immune Complexes Isolated and Purified from Sera of Melanoma Patients

Antigen		Antibody		
Characteristics	Origin	Type	Biological activity	References[a]
>350,000-dalton protein	Not reported	IgG	Not reported	Hendrick et al. (1981)
15,000-dalton glycoprotein, melanoma-associated	Membrane	IgG	Anti-MAAg	Hersey and Isbister (1981)
Tumor-associated	Membrane	IgG, membrane-directed	Anti-MAAg	Phillips et al. (1982)
	Cytoplasm	IgG, cytoplasm-directed	Anti-TAA	
Associated with medium complex	Cytoplasm	Antibody 1	Directed to common cytoplasmic antigen	MacDonald et al. (1981)
	Membrane	Antibody 2	Individually specific to melanoma surface antigen	
—	—	Antiimmuno-globulins	Rheumatoid factor (anti-Fc) Anti-F(ab')$_2$ Anti-antigen receptor (autoantiidiotype)	Phillips et al. (1982)
Melanoma-associated antigen	Serum	IgG	Anti-MAAg	Salinas et al. (1983)

(Continued)

Table X. (Continued)

Antigen		Antibody		
Characteristics	Origin	Type	Biological activity	References[a]
80,000-dalton protein (common antigen)	Not present on autologous fibroblasts	IgG	Not reported	Quay et al. (1983)
41,000-dalton melanosomal protein	Unique to melanoma?	IgG	Not reported	Quay et al. (1983)
330,000-dalton melanosomal protein	Unique to melanoma?	IgG	Not reported	Quay et al. (1983)
94,000-dalton glycoprotein	Membrane-associated, oncofetal	IgG, IgM	Not reported	Morgan and Reisfeld (1982)
60,000- to 70,000-dalton glycoprotein	Fetal antigen, membrane, cytoplasm?	IgG, IgM	Anti-FA	R. K. Gupta et al. (1983b)
180,000-dalton lipoprotein	Membrane, cytoplasm?	IgG	Anti-melanoma-TAA	R. K. Gupta et al. (1983a)
—	—	IgG-anti-globulin (anti-idiotypes)	Block cytotoxic antibody to tumor and fetal cells	Morgan et al. (1982)
		IgG	Cytotoxic to fetal and tumor cells	

[a]Not an exhaustive compilation.

VI. CONCLUDING REMARKS

Although the pesence of CIC in melanoma patients at incidences and levels higher than in normal controls has been reported by various investigators using different assays, the correlations with the clinical course have not been unequivocal. As explained previously, a number of factors could account for the lack of observed correlations, including (1) the selection of patients and the time of serum sampling, (2) the type of antibody and the nature of the antigen involved in the formation of immune complexes, (3) the amount and types of antigens expressed by the tumor cells, (4) the rate of antigen shedding or modulation after interaction with antibody, (5) the immune status of the patients, which can be influenced by the treatment modality, (6) the tumor burden, and (7) intercurrent subclinical infections or autoimmune phenomena.

The CIC detected in a patient at a given time by an antigen-nonspecific assay may represent a spectrum of complexes that could arise from causes other than tumor growth. In addition, some of the CIC may be the result of the formation of anti-Ig. Therefore, CIC determination cannot be envisioned to have any direct primary diagnostic significance. Even if an antigen-specific CIC detection assay were available for melanoma, it could only be applied for differential diagnosis.

Despite the inconsistencies and the drawback that the antigen component of the immune complexes has not been identified in each and every case, it has been observed by various investigators that increased levels of CIC represent a poor prognosis for malignant melanoma patients. The presence of CIC during remission or disease-free periods in melanoma patients has been observed. Follow-up of these patients revealed that they had shorter disease-free intervals compared to those who were CIC-negative during their disease-free periods (Morton et al., 1985). Therefore, it is conceivable that the presence of CIC during tumor-free periods may have represented the residual subclinically active disease. It has been reported that, in some melanoma patients who recurred after a long tumor-free period, CIC were present at some point prior to the recurrence of the disease (Rossen et al., 1983). Such observations could be interpreted to mean that the appearance or increase in the level of CIC could indicate proliferation of otherwise inactive tumor cells in the host. In this regard, Carpentier and Miescher (1983) have suggested a temporal relationship between CIC and malignant cell proliferation.

It has been observed repeatedly that CIC levels fall in human malignant melanoma as the disease progresses. This could be due to saturation of all available antibodies in circulation with the tumor antigen shed by the progressing tumor (high tumor burden). A similar situation can also be observed during treatment of the patients with chemotherapeutic agents that are immunosuppressive. On the contrary, treatment modalities that result in potentiation of immune response, e.g., immunotherapy with tumor cell vaccine, have resulted in significantly increased levels of CIC. The results obtained with BCG immunotherapy have been equivocal. That is, higher incidences of CIC were observed by Ruell *et al.* (1982) in patients receiving BCG than in those who did not receive BCG, whereas Gauci *et al.* (1978) observed only a transient rise and fluctuations in CIC levels in patients receiving this immunotherapeutic agent. One possible explanation for such discrepancies could be that BCG, in general, acts as a potentiator of cellular immune response and that humoral antibodies elicited to BCG cells do not result in the formation of soluble immune complexes.

There is sufficient evidence in the literature to indicate that measurement of CIC levels or their fluctuation during the clinical course of the disease of melanoma patients may be used to prognosticate the outcome of their disease. When applied in conjunction with measurement of other immune parameters—e.g., presence of antibody or antigen, concurrent infection, therapeutic modality—the analysis of CIC should be of value to the physician for the management of malignant melanoma.

Although characterization of the Ig component of the immune complexes has been achieved in many reports, it has not been possible to identify the antigen(s) present in CIC of melanoma patients. To establish the specificity of the antibody and to identify the antigens present in CIC are extremely difficult tasks. The methods employed to isolate immune complexes and in subsequent analysis of the complexed antigen(s) and antibodies may pose several limitations. The antibody component may be denatured during dissociation of CIC and thus lose its immunoreactivity with the corresponding antigens. The procedure may yield antibodies from clinical samples in such small amounts that they may not be enough for its specificity analysis. The antibody component isolated from CIC may be of selectively low affinity. The antigen component may not be stable under conditions of isolation and dissociation of the immune complexes. Despite these limitations, progress has been made in these directions. The antigen and antibody constituents of immune complexes isolated from melanoma patients have been characterized by some investigators. In selected cases it has been documented that melanoma patients with low tumor burdens contain CIC in antibody excess, whereas patients with high tumor burdens contain CIC in antigen excess. This was documented by isolating the MAAg from immune complexes and establishing its reactivity with allogeneic and autologous antibody (Salinas *et al.*, 1983). The presence of multiple antigens (e.g., FA, melanoma-TAA and autoantigens) in immune complexes that reacted with allogeneic, autologous, and heterologous antibody has been documented in our laboratories. The antibodies isolated from immune complexes of melanoma patients have been found to react with tumor cells and soluble tumor antigens. In light of these advancements, it is conceivable that procedures could be developed to apply to clinical samples on a small scale, and that antigen-specific assays could be developed to detect and quantitate specific CIC in melanoma patients using monoclonal antibodies.

ACKNOWLEDGMENTS

These investigations were supported by USPHS Grants R01 CA30019, CA12582, and CA29605 awarded by the National Cancer Institute (DHEW) and by the Jonsson Comprehensive Cancer Center, the Committee to Cure Cancer through Immunization, and the Cancer Research Coordinating Committee of the University of California. We gratefully acknowledge the technical assistance of Mr. Zacarias Leopoldo and Mr. William J. Lappen.

VII. REFERENCES

Ahn, S. S., Gupta, R. K., and Morton, D. L., 1982, Predictive value of circulating immune complexes for tumor recurrence in stage I malignant melanoma, *Surg. Forum* 33:415.

Amoroso, P., Vergani, D., Wojcicka, B. M., McFarlane, I. G. Eddlestone, A. L. W. F., Tee, D. E. H., and Williams, R., 1980, Identification of biliary antigen in circulating immune complexes in primary biliary cirrhosis, *Clin. Exp. Immunol.* 42:95.

Anderton, B. H., and Thorpe, R. C., 1980, New methods of analysing for antigens and glycoproteins in complex mixtures, *Immunol. Today* 1:122.

Angello, V., 1978, Pitfalls in the use of biologic reagents for detection of immune complexes, in: *Protides of the Biological Fluids* (H. Peeters, ed.), Vol. 26, p. 15, Pergamon Press, Elmsford, New York.

Angello, V., Winchester, R. J., and Kunkel, H. G., 1970, Precipitin reactions of the C1q component with aggregated γ-globulin and immune complexes in gel diffusion, *Immunology* 19:909.

Aryan, S., 1979, Immunological aspects of malignant tumors, *Clin. Plast. Surg.* 6:125.

Baldwin, R. W., and Robins, R. A., 1980, Circulating immune complexes in cancer, in: *Cancer Markers* (S. Sell, ed.), p. 507, Humana Press, Clifton, New Jersey.

Baldwin, R. W., Bower, J. A., and Price, M. R., 1973, Detection of circulating hepatoma D23 antigen and immune complexes in tumor bearer serum, *Br. J. Cancer* 28:111.

Barnett, E. V., Knutson, D. W., Abrass, C. K., Chia, D. S., Young, L. S., and Leibling, M. R., 1979, Circulating immune complexes: Their immunohistochemistry, detection, and importance, *Ann. Intern. Med.* 91:430.

Bentwich, Z., Fahey, J., Gupta, R. K., Golub, S., Chia, D., and Barrett, E., 1982, Comparison of assays for circulating immune complexes in human diseases, in: *Progress in Rheumatology* (I. Machtey, ed.), p. 23, John Wright, PSA Inc., Boston.

Benveniste, J., and Bruneau, C., 1979, Detection and characterization of circulating immune complexes by ultracentifugation: Technical aspects, *J. Immunol. Methods* 26:99.

Benveniste, J., Mencia-Huesta, J. M., and Camussi, G., 1979, Immune mechansim of immune complex deposition, *Adv. Inflam. Res.* 1:353.

Bystryn, J.-C., 1980, Shedding and degradation of cell-surface macromolecules and melanoma-associated antigens, *Fed. Proc.* 39:351.

Cairns, S. A., London, A., and Mallick, P., 1980, The value of three immune complex assays in the management of systemic lupus erythematosus: An assessment of immunochemical properties in relation to disease activity and manifestations, *Clin. Exp. Immunol.* 40:273.

Carpentier, N. A., and Miescher, P. A., 1983, The clinical relevance of circulating immune complexes in cancer, kidney transplantation and pregnancy, in: *Immunology of Trans-*

plantation, Cancer and Pregnancy (P. K. Ray, ed.), p. 375, Pergamon Press, Elmsford, New York.

Casali, P., and Lambert, P. H., 1979, Purification of soluble immune complexes from serum using polymethylmetacrylate beads coated with conglutinin or C1q, *Clin. Exp. Immunol.* 37:295.

Chautenoud, L. M., DePavoda, F., and Bainchi, G., 1979, Critical review of the methods employed for circulating immune complex detection, *Haematologica* 64:494.

Chenais, F., Virella, G., Patrick, C. C., and Feudenberg, H. H., 1977, Isolation of soluble immune complexes by affinity chromatography using staphylococcal protein A as substrate, *J. Immunol. Methods* 18:183.

Cochran, A. J., 1978, *Man, Cancer and Immunity*, p. 66, Academic Press, New York.

Cooper, N. R., Jensen, F. C., Welsh, R. M., and Oldstone, 1976, Lysis of RNA tumor viruses by human serum: Direct antibody-dependent triggering of the classical complement pathway, *J. Exp. Med.* 144:970.

Cunningham-Rundles, C., Brandies, W. E., Zacharczuk, T., Good, R. A., and Day, N. K., 1980, Quantitation of circulating immune complexes in serum by Raji cell using an enzyme-linked immunosorbent assay, *Clin. Exp. Immunol.* 40:411.

D'Amelio, R., Cooke, B., and Hobbs, J. R., 1982, Circulating immune complexes in human malignant melanoma, *Tumori* 68:469.

Dasgupta, M. K., Kovithavongs, T., Schaut, J., Longenecker, B. M., and Dossetor, J. B., 1982, Antibody-mediated cellular cytotoxicity against Raji cell ADCC(Raji): Evaluation of false positives in the detection of circulating immune complexes by Raji cell assay, *J. Clin. Immunol.* 2:197.

Dent, P. B., and Liao, S. K., 1982, Heterogeneity of melanoma-associated antigens revealed by alloantisera and xenoantisera, in: *Melanoma Antigens and Antibodies* (R. A. Reisfeld and S. Ferrone, eds.), p. 101, Plenum Press, New York.

Dent, P. B., Louis, J. A., McCullock, P. B., Dunnett, C. W., and Cerottini, J. C., 1980, Correlation of elevated C1q binding activity and carcinoembryonic antigen levels with clinical features and prognosis in bronchiogenic carcinoma, *Cancer* 45:130.

Dorval, G., and Pross, H., 1983, Immune complexes in cancer, in: *Circulating Immune Complexes: Their Clinical Significance* (L. R. Espinoza and C. K. Osterland, eds.), p. 161, Futura, New York.

Eisenberg, R. A., Theofilopoulus, A. N., and Dixon, F. J., 1977, Use of bovine conglutinin for the assay of immune complexes, *J. Immunol.* 118:1428.

Espinoza, L. R., 1983, Assays for circulating immune complexes, in: *Circulating Immune Complexes: Their Clinical Significance* (L. R. Espinoza and C. K. Osterland, eds.), p. 21, Futura, New York.

Faldt, R., and Ankerst, J., 1980, Possibly specific immune complexes in sera of patients with untreated acute myelogenous leukemia, *Int. J. Cancer* 26:309.

Gabriel, A., and Angello, V., 1977, Detection of immune complexes: The use of radioimmunoassays with C1q and monoclonal rheumatoid factors, *J. Clin. Invest.* 59:990.

Gauci, L., Ursule, E., Pujol, H., and Serrou, B., 1978, Clinical implications of elevated levels of circulating immune complexes in patients with malignant melanoma, in: *Protides of the Biological Fluids* (H. Peters, ed.), Vol. 26, p. 349, Pergamon Press, Elmsford, New York.

Gauci, L., Caraux, J., and Serrou, B., 1981, Immune complexes in the context of the immune response in cancer patients, in: *Immune Complexes and Plasma Exchanges in Cancer Patients* (B. Serrou and C. Rosenfeld, eds.), p. 37, Elsevier/North-Holland, New York.

Gilead, Z., and Sulitzeanu, D., 1979, A technique for the purification of immune complexes using rheumatoid factor, *J. Immunol. Methods* 30:11.

Goding, J. W., 1978, Use of staphylococcal protein A as an immunological reagent, *J. Immunol. Methods* **20**:241.

Goidle, E. A., Schrater, A. F., Thorbecke, G. J., and Siskind, G. W., 1980, Production of auto-anti-idiotype antibody during the normal immune response. IV. Studies of the primary and secondary responses to thymus-dependent and -independent antigens, *Eur. J. Immunol.* **10**:810.

Grangeot-Keros, L., Segond, P., Capel, F., Iscaki, S., and Pillot, J., 1978, Detection of immune complexes: A simple assay based on characterization of the *in vivo* bound C1q (PEG-C1q immunodiffusion test), *J. Immunol. Methods* **23**:349.

Grimm, E. A., Silver, H. K. B., and Roth, J. A., Chee, D. O., Gupta, R. K., and Morton, D. L., 1976, Detection of tumor-associated antigen in human melanoma cell line supernatants, *Int. J. Cancer* **17**:559.

Gropp, C., Havemann, K., Scherfe, T., and Ax, W., 1980, Incidence of circulating immune complexes in patients with lung cancer and their effect on antibody-dependent cytotoxicity, *Oncology* **37**:71.

Gunven, P., Klein, G., Klein, E., Norin, T., and Singh, S., 1980, Surface immunoglobulins on Burkitt's lymphoma biopsy cells from 91 patients, *Int. J. Cancer* **25**:711.

Gupta, R. C., and Tan, E. M., 1981, Isolation of circulating immune complexes by conglutinin and separation of antigen from dissociated complexes by immobilized protein A, *J. Immunol. Methods* **46**:9.

Gupta, R. C., McDuffie, F. C., Huston, K. A., Tappeiner, G. Meurer, M., Jordan, R. E., Luthra, H. S., Hunder, G. G., and Ilstrup, D., 1979, Comparison of three immunoassays for immune complexes in rheumatoid arthritis, *Arthritis Rheum.* **22**:433.

Gupta, R. K., and Morton, D. L., 1975, Suggestive evidence for *in vivo* binding of specific anti-tumor antibodies of human melanomas, *Cancer Res.* **35**:58.

Gupta, R. K., and Morton, D. L., 1981, Possible clinical significance of circulating immune complexes in melanoma patients, in: *Fundamental Mechanisms in Human Cancer Immunology* (J. P. Sanders, J. Daniels, B. Serrou, D. Rosenfeld, and C. Denney, eds.), p. 305, Elsevier/North-Holland, Amsterdam.

Gupta, R. K., and Morton, D. L., 1982*a*, Clinical significance of tumor-associated antigens and anti-tumor antibodies in human malignant melanoma, in: *Melanoma Antigens and Antibodies* (R. A. Reisfeld and S. Ferrone, eds.), p. 139, Plenum Press, New York.

Gupta, R. K., and Morton, D. L., 1982*b*, Nature of circulating immune complexes in melanoma patients, *Fed. Proc.* **41**:323.

Gupta, R. K., and Morton, D. L., 1983*a*, Tumor antigens, in: *Immunobiology of Transplantation, Cancer and Pregnancy* (P. K. Ray, ed.), p. 113, Pergamon Press, Elmsford, New York.

Gupta, R. K., and Morton, D. L., 1983*b*, Immunochemical characterization of fetal antigen isolated from spent culture medium of a human melanoma cell line, *J. Natl. Cancer Inst.* **70**:993.

Gupta, R. K., and Morton, D. L., 1984*a*, Studies of a melanoma tumor-associated antigen detected in spent culture medium of a human melanoma cell line by allogeneic antibody. I. Purification and development of a radioimmunoassay, *J. Natl. Cancer Inst.* **72**:67.

Gupta, R. K., and Morton, D. L., 1984*b*, Studies of a melanoma tumor-associated antigen detected in spent culture medium of a human melanoma cell line by allogeneic antibody. II. Immunobiological characterization, *J. Natl. Cancer Inst.* **72**:75.

Gupta, R. K., and Morton, D. L., 1984*c*, Studies of a melanoma tumor-associated antigen detected in spent culture medium of a human melanoma cell line by allogeneic antibody. III. Physicochemical properties, *J. Natl. Cancer Inst.* **72**:83.

Gupta, R. K., Golub, S. H., and Morton, D. L., 1979*a*, Correlation between tumor burden and anticomplementary activity in sera from cancer patients, *Cancer Immunol. Immunother.* **6**:63.

Gupta, R. K., Theofilopoulos, A. N., Dixon, F. J., and Morton, D. L., 1979*b*, Circulating immune complexes as possible cause for anticomplementary activity in humans with malignant melanoma, *Cancer Immunol. Immunother.* **6**:211.

Gupta, R. K., Golub, S. H., Rangel, D. M., and Morton, D. L., 1979*c*, Inhibition of mitogen-induced lymphocyte proliferation correlated to anticomplementary activity in sera from melanoma patients, *Cancer Immunol. Immunother.* **5**:221.

Gupta, R. K., Irie, R. F., Chee, D. O., Kern, D. H., and Morton, D. L., 1979*d*, Demonstration of two distinct antigens in spent culture medium of a human malignant melanoma cell line, *J. Natl. Cancer Inst.* **63**:347.

Gupta, R. K., Silver, H. K. B., and Morton, D. L., 1979*e*, Production and characterization of xenogeneic antisera to tumor-associated antigens, *J. Surg. Oncol.* **13**:75.

Gupta, R. K., Huth, J. F., and Morton, D. L., 1981, Characterization of antigen component of immune complexes isolated from sera of melanoma patients, *Proc. Am. Assoc. Cancer Res.* **22**:293.

Gupta, R. K., Huth, J. F., and Golub, S. H., 1982, Application of cultured human myeloid cells (K562) for detection of immune complexes in human sera, *Immunol. Commun.* **11**:401.

Gupta, R. K., Leitch, A. M., and Morton, D. L., 1983*a*, Detection of tumor-associated antigen in eluates from protein A columns used for *ex vivo* immunoabsorption of plasma from melanoma patients by radioimmunoassay, *Clin. Exp. Immunol.* **53**:589.

Gupta, R. K., Leitch, A. M., and Morton, D. L., 1983*b*, Nature of antigens and antibodies in immune complexes isolated by staphylococcal protein A from plasma of melanoma patients, *Cancer Immunol. Immunother.* **16**:40.

Haakenstad, A. O., and Mannik, M., 1974, Saturation of the reticuloendothelial system with soluble immune complexes, *J. Immunol.* **112**:1939.

Haakenstad, A. O., and Mannik, M., 1977, The biology of immune complexes, in: *Autoimmunity* (N. Talal, ed.), p. 277, Academic Press, New York.

Halpern, B., 1974, Role of reticuloendothelial system in the clearance of macromolecules, in: *Enzyme Therapy in Lysosomal Storage Disease* (J. M. Tager, G. J. M. Hooghwinkel, and W. Th. Daems, eds.), p. 111, Elsevier/North-Holland, Amsterdam.

Happner, G. A., Stolbach, I., Byrne, M., Cummings, J. J., Donough, E., and Calabresi, P., 1973, Cell mediated and serum blocking reactivity to tumor antigens in patients with malignant melanoma, *Int. J. Cancer* **11**:245.

Harkiss, G. D., and Brown, D. L., 1980, The Use of C1q, conglutinin and low affinity rabbit IgM antibody to human FC in a ligand cocktail radioassay for detecting and characterizing immune complexes in pathological sera, *Clin. Exp. Immunol.* **39**:576.

Heaney-Kieras, J., and Bystryn, J.-C., 1982, Identification and purification of a M_r 75,000 cell surface human melanoma-associated antigen, *Cancer Res.* **42**:2310.

Heier, H. E., Carpentier, N., Lange, G., Lambert, P. H., and Godal, T., 1977, Circulating immune complexes in patients with malignant lymphomas and solid tumors, *Int. J. Cancer* **20**:887.

Heimer, R., Abruzzo, J. L., and Ulick, D., 1981. The detection of antigens in immune complexes, *Scand. J. Immunol.* **13**:441.

Hellstrom, I., Sjogrnen, H. O., Warner, G. A., and Hellstrom, K. E., 1971, Blocking of cell mediated immunity by sera from patients with growing neoplasmas, *Int. J. Cancer* **7**:226.

Hendrick, J. C., Zangerle, P. F., Franchimont, P., Samak, R., and Israel, L., 1981, Isolation of immune complexes from cancerous patients and antigen characterization, in: *Immune Complexes and Plasma Exchanges in Cancer Patients* (B. Serrou and C. Rosenfeld, eds.), p. 29, Elsevier/North-Holland, New York.

Herberman, R. B., Bordes, M., Lambert, P. H., Luthra, H. S., Robins, R. A., Sizaret, P., and Theofilopoulos, A. N., 1981, A report on international comparative evaluation of possible value of assays for immune complexes for diagnosis of human breast cancer, *Int. J. Cancer* 27:569.

Hersey, P., and Isbister, J. P., 1981, Developments in immune complex therapy and its application to cancer, in: *Immune Complexes and Plasma Exchanges in Cancer Patients* (B. Serrou and C. Rosenfeld, eds.), p. 135, Elsevier/North-Holland, New York.

Hoffken, K., Meridith, I. D., Robins, R. A., Baldwin, R. W., Davies, C. J., and Blamey, R. W., 1977, Circulating immune complexes in patients with breast cancer, *Br. Med. J.* 2:218.

Horsfall, A. C., Venables, P. J. W., Mumford, P., and Maine, R. N., 1981, Interpretation of the Raji cell assay in sera containing antinuclear antibodies and immune complexes, *Clin. Exp. Immunol.* 44:405.

Huth, J. F., Gupta, R. K., and Morton, D. L., 1982, Relationship between circulating immune complexes and urinary antigen in human malignancy, *Cancer* 49:1150.

Jerry, L. M., Rowden, G., Cano, P. O., Phillips, T. M., Deutsch, G. F., Copeck, A., Hartman, D., and Lewis, M. G., 1976, Immune complexes in human melanoma: A consequence of deranged immune regulation, *Scand. J. Immunol.* 5:845.

Johny, K. V., Dasgupta, M. K., Singh, B., and Dossetor, J. B., 1980, Radioconglutinin binding assay for circulating immune complexes: A new method, *Clin. Exp. Immunol.* 40:459.

Jones, V., and Orlans, E., 1981, Isolation of immune complexes and characterization of their constituent antigens and antibodies in some human diseases: A review, *J. Immunol. Methods* 44:249.

Jones, V. E., Cowley, P. J., Allen, C., and Elson, C. J., 1980, The isolation of immune complexes containing IgM rheumatoid factor and recovery of IgG rheumatoid factor from the complexes, *J. Immunol. Methods* 37:1.

Kabat, E. A., 1980, Basic principles of antigen–antibody reactions, *Methods Enzymol.* 70A:3.

Kauffman, R. H., VanEs, L. A., and Daba, M. R., 1981, The specific detection of IgA immune complexes, *J. Immunol. Methods* 40:117.

Kilgallon, W., Amlot, P. L., and Williams, B. D., 1982, Anti-C1q column: Ligand specific purification of immune complexes from human serum or plasma: Analysis of the interaction between C1q and immune complexes, *Clin. Exp. Immunol.* 48:705.

Krapf, F., Renger, D., Schedel, I., Leiendecker, K., Leyssens, H., and Deicher, H., 1982, A PEG-precipitation laser nephelometer technique for detection and characterization of circulation immune complexes in human sera, *J. Immunol. Methods* 54:107.

Kristensen, E., Brandslund, I., Nielsen, H., and Svehag, S. E., 1980, Prognostic value of assays for circulating immune complexes and natural cytotoxicity in malignant skin melanoma (stages I and II), *Cancer Immunol. Immunother.* 9:31.

Lachmann, P. J., and Hobart, M., J., 1978, Complement technology, in: *Handbook of Experimental Immunology* (D. M. Weir, ed.), p. 5A.1, Blackwell, Oxford.

Lamers, C. M., 1981, Factors influencing the development of immune complex diseases, *Allergy* 36:527.

Leong, S. P. L., Copperband, S. R., Sutherland, C. M., Krementz, E. T., and Deckers, P. J., 1978, Detection of human melanoma antigens in cell-free supernatants, *J. Surg. Res.* 24:245

Leong, S. P. L., Cooperband, S. R., Deckers, P. J., Sutherland, C. M., Cesane, J. F., and Krementz, E. T., 1979, Antibody-induced movement of common melanoma membrane antigens on the surface of unfixed human melanoma cells, *Cancer Res.* 39:2125.

Lewis, M. G., Hartmann, D., and Jerry, L. M., 1976, Antibodies and anti-antibodies in human malignancy: An expression of deranged immune regulation, *Ann. N.Y. Acad. Sci.* 276:316.

Lodola, M. A., Villa, M. L., Masserini, C., and Clerici, E., 1981, Immunocomplexes in nor-
    mal blood donors and in melanoma patients, *Immunol. Lett.* **2**:327.
MacDonald, J. S., Phillips, T. M., Smith, F. P., Lewis, M., and Israel, L., 1981, Effect of
    aggressive plasma exchange on immune complex levels in plasma of patients with
    metastatic cancer, in: *Immune Complexes and Plasma Exchanges in Cancer Patients*
    (B. Serrou and C. Rosenfeld, eds.), p. 243, Elsevier/North-Holland, New York.
McDougal, J. S., Redecha, P. B., Inman, R. D., and Christian, C. L., 1979, Binding of
    immunoglobulin G aggregates and immune complexes in human sera to Staphylococci
    containing protein A, *J. Clin. Invest.* **63**:627.
MacSween, J. M., and Eastwood, S. L., 1980, Immunoglobulins associated with human tu-
    mors *in vivo:* IgG concentration in eluates of colonic carcinomas, *Br. J. Cancer* **42**:503.
Maidment, B. W., Pepsidero, L. D., Nemoto, T., and Chu, T. M., 1981, Recovery of im-
    munologically reactive antibodies and antigens from breast cancer immune complexes
    by preparative isoelectric focusing, *Cancer Res.* **41**:795.
Male, D., and Roitt, I. M., 1979, Analysis of the components of immune complexes, *Mol.
    Immunol.* **16**:197.
Mannik, M., 1980, Physicochemical and functional relationships of immune complexes, *J.
    Invest. Dermatol.* **74**:333.
Masson, P., 1978, Are circulating immune complexes the key to immunopathology? in:
    Protides of the Biological Fluids (H. Peeters, ed.), Vol. 26, p. 3, Pergamon Press, Elms-
    ford, New York.
Morgan, A. C., and Reisfeld, R. A., 1982, Detection and characterization of a monoclonal
    antibody-defined melanoma associated antigen within circulating immune complexes
    in normal donor sera, *Fed. Proc.* **41**:410.
Morgan, A. C., Rossen, R. D., and Twomey, J. J., 1979, Naturally occurring circulating im-
    mune complexes: Normal human serum contains idiotype-antiidiotype complexes dis-
    sociable by certain Ig antiglobulins, *J. Immunol.* **122**:1672.
Morgan, A. C., Rossen, R. D., McCormick, K. J., Stehlin, J. S., and Giovenella, B. C., 1982,
    "Hidden" cytotoxic antibodies that react with allogeneic cultured fetal and tumor cells
    contained in soluble immune complexes from normal human sera, *Cancer Res.* **42**:881.
Morton, D. L., Gupta, R. K., and Huth, J. F., 1985, New horizons in surgical oncology:
    Malignant melanoma, in: *Basic Mechanisms and Clinical Treatment of Tumor Metastasis*
    (M. Torisu and T. Yashid, eds.), pp. 561–572, Academic Press, Orlando, Florida.
Nelson, D. S., and Gatti, R., 1976, Humoral factors influencing lymphocyte transformation,
    Prog. Allergy **21**:261.
Norris, D. A., Huff, J. C., Swinehart, J. M., Carr, R. I., Thorne, E. G., Weston, W. L., and
    McIntosh, R. M., 1980, Cryoglobulinemia and decreased monocyte chemotaxis in malig-
    nant melanoma, *J. Invest. Dermatol.* **75**:219.
Nussenzweig, V., 1980, Interaction between complement and immune complexes: Role of
    complement in containing immune complex damage, in: *Immunology 80* (M. Fougereau
    and J. Dausset, eds.), p. 1044, Academic Press, New York.
Nydegger, V. E., 1979, Biological properties and detection of immune complexes in animal
    and human pathology, *Rev. Physiol. Biochem. Pharmacol.* **85**:63.
Nydegger, V. E., and Davis, J. S., IV, 1980, Soluble immune complexes in human disease,
    CRC Crit. Rev. Clin. Lab. Sci. **12**:123.
Olberding, P., Koldovsky, P., Goenz, G., and Mark, H., 1981, Immune complexes in sera
    from melanoma patients, in: *Third European Workshop on Melanin Pigmentation*, Sept.
    28–Oct. 1, 1981, p. 128, Czechoslovak Medical Society, Prague, Czechoslovakia.
Old, L. J., 1981, Cancer immunology: The search for specificity (G. H. A. Clowes Memorial
    Lecture), *Cancer Res.* **41**:361.
Papsidero, L. D., Nemoto, T., Snyderman, M. C., and Chu, T. M., 1978, Immune complexes
    in breast cancer patients as detected by C1q binding, *Cancer* **44**:1636.

Pereira, A. B., Theofilopoulus, A. N., and Dixon, F. J., 1980, Detection and partial characterization of circulating immune complexes with solid-phase anti-C3, *J. Immunol.* 125:763.

Persson, B., Eldh, J., Lindholm, L., and Rudenstam, C. M., 1981, Immunocomplexes in patients with malignant melanoma, WHO Seminar on Malignant Melanoma, June 24, 1981, Gothenburg, Sweden, p. 35.

Pesce, A. J., Phillips, T. M., Ooi, B. S., Evans, A., Shank, R. A., III, and Lewis, M. G., 1980, Immune complexes in transitional cell carcinoma, *J. Urol.* 123:486.

Phillips, T. M., and Lewis, M. G., 1971, A method for elution of immunoglobulin from the surface of living cells, *Rev. Eur. Stud. Clin. Biol.* 16:1052.

Phillips, T. M., MacDonald, J. S., and Lewis, M. G., 1981, Towards tumor antibody isolation and characterization in immune complexes, in: *Immune Complexes and Plasma Exchanges in Cancer Patients* (B. Serrou and C. Rosenfeld, eds.), p. 3, Elsevier/North-Holland, New York.

Phillips, T. M., Queen, W. D., and Lewis, M. G., 1982, The significance of circulating immune complexes in patients with malignant melanoma, in: *Melanoma Antigens and Antibodies* (R. A. Reisfeld and S. Ferrone, eds.), p. 289, Plenum Press, New York.

Pollard, K. M., and Webb, J., 1982, Partial purification of anti-DNA antibodies from systemic lupus erythematosus serum by dye–ligand chromatography, *J. Immunol. Methods* 54:81.

Porter, R. R., 1980, The complex proteases of the complement system, *Proc. R. Soc. Lond.* B210:477.

Poulton, T. A., Mooney, N. A., Nineham, L. J., and Hay, F. C., 1983, Characterization of immune complexes detectable by two independent assays in gynecological malignancies, *Clin. Exp. Immunol.* 53:573.

Price, M. R., and Baldwin, R. W., 1977, Shedding of tumor cell surface antigens, in: *Dynamic Aspects of Cell Surface Organization* (G. Poste and G. L. Nicolson eds.), p. 423, Elsevier/North-Holland, New York.

Price, M. R., and Robins, R. A., 1978, Circulating factors modifying cell-mediated immunity in experimental neoplasia, in: *Immunological Aspects of Cancer* (J. E. Castro, ed.), p. 155, University Park Press, Baltimore.

Quay, S. C., Murphy, G. F., and Mihm, M. C., Jr., 1983, Biochemical studies of immune complexes. II. Purification of immune complexes from sera of patients with malignant melanoma, *Clin. Immunol. Immunopathol.* 26:318.

Reisfeld, R. A., and Ferrone, S. (eds.), 1982, *Melanoma Antigens and Antibodies*, Plenum Press, New York.

Reisfeld, R. A., David, G. S., Pellegrino, M. A., and Holmes, E. C., 1977, Approaches for the isolation of biologically functional tumor-associated antigen, *Cancer Res.* 37:2860.

Ristow, S. S., Rossen, R. D., Fryd, D. S., and McKhann, C. F., 1979, Circulating immune complexes in colon cancer patient sera, *Cancer* 43:1320.

Rossen, R. D., and Barnes, B. C., 1978, Measuring serum immune complexes in cancer (editorial), *Ann. Int. Med.* 88:570.

Rossen, R. D., and Morgan, A. C., 1981, Blockage of the humoral immune response: Immune complexes in cancer, in: *Humoral Immunity in Relation to Cancer* (H. Waters, ed.), p. 209, *Handbook of Cancer Immunology*, Vol. 9, Garland STPM Press, New York.

Rossen, R. D., Reisberg, M. A., Hersh, E. M., and Gutterman, J. V., 1977, The C1q binding test for soluble immune complexes: Clinical correlations obtained in patients with cancer, *J. Natl. Cancer Inst.* 58:1205.

Rossen, R. D., Zubler, R. H., Day, N. K., Reisberg, M. A., Morgan, A. C., Gutterman, J. U., and Hersh, E. M., 1978, Detection of immune complex-like material in cancer patients' sera: A comparative study of results obtained with the C1q deviation and C1q binding tests, *J. Lab. Clin. Med.* 91:191.

Rossen, R. D., Crane, M. M., Morgan, A. C., Giannini, E. H., Giovanella, B. C., Stehlin, J. S., Twomey, J. J., and Hersh, E. M., 1983, Circulating immune complexes and tumor cell cytotoxins as prognostic indicators in malignant melanoma: A prospective study of 53 patients, *Cancer Res.* 43:422.

Ruell, P., Murray, E., McCarthy, W. H., and Hersey, P., 1982, Evaluation of assays to detect immune complexes as an immunodiagnostic aid in patients with melanoma, *Oncodev. Biol. Med.* 3:1.

Salinas, F. A., and Wee, K. H., 1983, Immune complexes and human neoplasia, *Biomed. Pharmac. Ther.* 37:119.

Salinas, F. A., Wee, K. H., and Silver, H. K. B., 1980, Xenogeneic oncofetal antigen (XOFA) and its relationship with tumor burden in malignant melanoma (MM) patients' sera, *Am. Assoc. Cancer Res. Proc.* 21:225.

Salinas, F. A., Wee, K. H., and Silver, H. K., 1981a, Immune complexes and human neoplasia: Detection and quantitation of circulating immune complexes by the fetal liver cell assay, *Cancer Immunol. Immunother.* 12:11.

Salinas, F. A., Wee, K. H., and Silver, H. K. B., 1981b, Modulation of lymphocyte activation by plasmapheresis in advanced malignant melanoma, in: *Proceedings of Mechanism of Lymphocyte Activation* (K. Resch, ed.), p. 4790, Elsevier/North-Holland, Amsterdam.

Salinas, F. A., Wee, K. H., and Silver, H. K. B., 1981c, Malignant melanoma tumor burden and its relationship to antigen concentration, size, and composition of immune complexes, *Proc. Am. Assoc. Cancer Res.* 20:181.

Salinas, F. A., Wee, K. H., and Silver, H. K. B., 1982a, Xenogeneic oncofetal antigen (XOFA) immunoregulation in malignant melanoma, *Proc. Int. Cancer Congress* 13:309.

Salinas, F. A., Wee, K. H., Silver, H. K. B., and Ragaz, J., 1982b, Circulating immune complexes and associated antigen in breast carcinoma, *Proc. Am. Assoc. Cancer Res.* 23:250.

Salinas, F. A., Wee, K. H., and Silver, H. K. B., 1982c, Immune reactants' changes and their relationship to tumor burden in malignant melanoma, *Proc. Am. Soc. Clin. Oncol.* 1:35.

Salinas, F. A., Wee, K. H., and Silver, H. K. B., 1983, Immune complexes and human neoplasia, *Biomed. Pharmacother.* 37:211.

Scharfstein, J., Correa, E. B., Gallo, G. R., and Nussenzweig, V., 1979, Human C4-binding protein: Association with immune complexes *in vitro* and *in vivo*, *J. Clin. Invest.* 63:437.

Schrohenloher, R. E., Balch, C. M., and Volanakis, J. E., 1978, Detection of circulating immune complexes by radioimmunoassay with monoclonal rheumatoid factor: Comparison with C1q binding and Raji cell radioassay in cancer, in: *Protides of the Biological Fluids* (H. Peeters, ed.), Vol. 26, p. 43, Pergamon Press, Elmsford, New York.

Seth, P., and Balachandran, N., 1980, Elution of herpes simplex virus-specific cytotoxic antibodies from squamous cell carcinoma of uterine cervix, *Nature* 286:613.

Shepherd, P. S., 1979, A comparison of two ^{125}I-C1q binding tests to detect soluble immune complexes in serum of patients with malignant disease, *Clin. Exp. Immunol.* 36:250.

Sinclair, N. R., StC., 1979, Modulation of immunity by antibody, antigen–antibody complexes and antigen, *Pharmacol. Ther.* 4:355.

Sjögren, H. O., Hellstrom, I., Bansal, S. C., and Hellstrom, K. E., 1971, Suggestive evidence that the "blocking antibodies" to tumor bearing animals may be antigen–antibody complexes, *Proc. Natl. Acad. Sci. USA* 68:1372.

Skeem, M. J., and Olkowski, Z. L., 1981, Circulating immune complexes in melanoma patients treated with levamisole following surgery, *Rev. Latinoam. Oncol. Clin.* 13:5.

Snyder, H. W., Jr., Jones, F. R., Day, N. K., and Handy, W. D., 1982, Isolation and characterization of circulating feline leukemia virus-immune complexes from plasma of persistently infected pet cats removed by *ex vivo* immunoabsorption, *J. Immunol.* 128:2726.

Sobel, A. T., Botisch, V. A., and Muller-Eberhardt, H. J., 1975, C1q deviation test for the detection of immune complexes, aggregates of IgG and bacterial products in human serum, *J. Exp. Med.* 142:130.

Staab, J. K., Andever, F. A., Stumpf, E., and Fischer, R., 1980, Are circulating CEA immune complexes a prognostic marker in patients with carcinoma at the gastrointestinal tract? *Br. J. Cancer* 42:26.

Stein, P. C., Christensen, M., and Char, D. H., 1980, Characterization of retinoblastoma immune complexes, *Invest. Opthalmol. Vis. Sci.* 189:302.

Svehag, S.-E., Husby, S., Glikmann, G., and Nielson, H., 1979, Methodological approaches for identification of disease-related and new antigens in soluble immune complexes, *Scand. J. Immunol.* 10:381.

Sztaba-Kania, M., Jassem, J., Piskorzynska, M., and Kondrat, W., 1981, Circulating immune complexes in patients with melanoma, *Neoplasma* 28:491.

Teshima, H., Wanebo, H., Pinsky, C., and Day, N. K., 1977, Circulating immune complexes detected by ^{125}I-Clq deviation test in sera of cancer patients, *J. Clin. Invest.* 59:1134.

Theofilopoulos, A. N., 1982, Immune complexes in cancer (editorial), *N. Engl. J. Med.* 307: 1208.

Theofilopoulos, A. N., and Dixon, F. J., 1978, Immune complexes associated with neoplasia, in: *Immunodiagnosis of Cancer* (R. B. Herberman, ed.), p. 896, Marcel Dekker, New York.

Theofilopoulos, A. N., and Dixon, F. J., 1979, The biology and detection of immune complexes, *Adv. Immunol.* 28:89.

Theofilopoulos, A. N., and Dixon, F. J., 1980, Detection of immune complexes: Techniques and implications, *Hosp. Pract.* 15:107.

Theofilopoulos, A. N., Wilson, C. B., and Dixon, F. J., 1976, The Raji cell radioimmuno assay for detecting immune complexes in human sera, *J. Clin. Invest.* 57:169.

Theofilopoulos, A. N., Andrews, B. S., Urist, M. M., Morton, D. L., and Dixon, F. J., 1977, The nature of immune complexes in human cancer sera, *J. Immunol.* 119:657.

Theofilopoulos, A. N., Eisenberg, R. A., and Dixon, F. J., 1978, Isolation of circulating immune complexes using Raji cells: Separation of antigens from immune complexes and production of antiserum, *J. Clin. Invest* 61:1570.

Tonder, O., Krishnan, E. C., Jewell, W. R., More, P. A., and Humphrey, L. J., 1976, Tumor Fc receptors and tumor-associated immunoglobulins, *Acta Pathol. Microbiol. Scand.* 84:105.

Tucker, D. F., Begent, R. H., and Hogg, N. M., 1978, Characterization of immune complexes in serum by absorption on staphylococcal protein A: Model studies and application to sera of rats bearing a gross virus-induced lymphoma, *J. Immunol.* 121:1644.

VanEs, L. A., Knutson, D. W., Kayser, B. S., and Glassock, R. J., 1979, Soluble oligovalent antigen–antibody complexes. I. The effect of antigen valence and combining ratio on the composition of fluorescein-carrier antifluorescein complexes, *Immunology* 37:485.

Williams, R. C., Jr., 1980, *Immune Complexes in Clinical and Experimental Medicine*, Harvard University Press, Cambridge, Massachusetts.

Witz, I. P., 1977, Tumor-bound immunoglobulins: In situ expressions of humoral immunity, *Adv. Cancer Res.* 25:95.

World Health Organization, 1977, The role of immune complexes in disease, Technical Report, Series 606, World Health Organization, Geneva.

Yoshida, R., and Zawadzki, Z. A., 1980, Circulating immune complexes in patients with neoplastic disorders, *Oncology* 37:152.

Zubler, R. H., and Lambert, P. H., 1977, Immune complexes in clinical investigation, in: *Recent Advances in Clinical Immunology* (R. A. Thomson, ed.), p. 125, Churchill Livingstone, New York.

Chapter 2

Clinical Relevance of Immune Complexes, Associated Antigen, and Antibody in Cancer

Fernando A. Salinas, Kian H. Wee, and Hulbert K. Silver

Advanced Therapeutics Department
Cancer Control Agency of British Columbia
Vancouver, British Columbia V5Z 4E6, Canada
and Departments of Pathology and Medicine
University of British Columbia
Vancouver, British Columbia V6T 1W5, Canada

I. INTRODUCTION

During the past 15 years there has been an increased interest in tumor-associated antigens (TAA) and the potential clinical role their immunologically oriented markers may play in the management of human cancer. One such immunological test for human tumor-associated markers, the identification of circulating immune complexes (CIC), is the subject of this volume.

Historically, the prominent role of CIC as initiators of mechanisms of tissue injury is well established. Antigen–antibody complexes result from noncovalent binding of an antigen with a specific antibody. An individual elicits specific antibodies when exposed to most antigens. The formation of CIC represents one component of the physiological response of the organism designed to eliminate foreign antigens. CIC are normally removed by the mononuclear phagocytic cells. However, CIC formation or their defective clearance under certain circumstances becomes detrimental to the host, resulting in pathological deposition, altering host immunological response and leading to inflammation and tissue injury.

Since the pathogenic significance of CIC was first suggested by Von Pirquet (1911), further confirmation and elaboration of the pathogenic mechanisms involved in overt clinical manifestations during disease has been provided by Dixon

55

et al. (1958, 1961) and Germuth *et al.* (1957, 1973). Recent *in vitro* and *in vivo* results have provided further insight into the mechanisms and factors involved in CIC formation, localization, deposition, and phagocytosis, and in the CIC-induced inflammatory reaction (Salinas and Wee, 1983; Salinas *et al.*, 1983*b*). In addition, it has become evident that CIC play an important role in the modulation of cellular and humoral immune effector mechanisms through their interaction with subpopulations of B, T, and natural killer cells, as well as macrophages. Besides the intrinsic interaction of CIC with antigen and antibodies, this modulation appears to be mediated mainly via Fc and complement receptors, to account for either suppressive or enhancing humoral-to-cell and cell-to-cell immune effects (Salinas *et al.*, 1983*b*).

Interest in the relationship of CIC to cancer was generated in part by reports of a number of often "unrelated" observations. Among such studies, those dealing with the ability of serum factors to modulate the host response to autologous tumor growth (Currie, 1973; Rossen and Morgan, 1981; Zubler and Lambert, 1977), along with data suggesting that these factors may be antigen-antibody complexes, stimulated both basic and clinical investigations (reviewed in Penn, 1981; Rossen and Morgan, 1981). Other information that directly influenced this field included early work on the role of CIC in the host response, as derived from studies on immunological enhancement in response to tumor and tissue allografts (Salinas *et al.*, 1983*b*).

Since the early association of CIC with the onset and course of serum sickness owing to toxic factors generated by the host circulating antibody and antigen (Von Pirquet, 1911), extensive experimental confirmation and elaboration of this pathogenetic role of CIC have been provided (Barnett *et al.*, 1979; Cochrane and Koffler, 1973; Dixon *et al.*, 1958; Halpern, 1974). The association of CIC with many pathological conditions has been described (Zubler and Lambert, 1977). Since few efforts have until now been reported, there is as yet no fully accepted criterion for the pathogenetic involvement of antigen–antibody complexes in a given disease condition. Initially, establishment of the presence of these complexes was listed as a substantiation step, since their association with certain neoplastic and systemic or multisystemic inflammatory diseases offered unique diagnostic and therapeutic considerations (Salinas *et al.*, 1983*b*; Salinas and Wee, 1983). Thereafter, an attempt to establish a classification was made (Steward and Devey, 1981), and the basic requirements for the pathogenetic role of CIC were as follows: (1) Supporting evidence that CIC detected by different tests are of high molecular weight and dissociable. (2) Demonstration of antigen, antibody, and activated complement in the reactive CIC. (3) Demonstration of CIC or their components deposited at the lesions of the disease to prove conclusively the pathogenetic involvement of CIC.

The variety of diseases in which CIC have been implicated include autoimmune disease; neoplastic disease; infectious disease caused by bacteria, viruses, and parasites; and other unclassified disorders. Since extensive listings have been compiled (Theofilopoulos and Dixon, 1979; Steward and Devey, 1981; Nydegger *et al.*, 1983), we have excluded a complete list of specific conditions, in keeping with our complementary rather than exhaustive intent. It will suffice to indicate that the most common clinical manifestations observed in cases in which a pathogenic role of CIC is suspected include vasculitis, nephritis, and joint involvement. Other prevalent disorders in which increased levels of CIC have been observed include systemic lupus erythematosus, rheumatoid arthritis, polyarthritis nodosa, viral hepatitis, acute glomerulonephritis, and human malignancies (Barnett *et al.*, 1979; Cochrane and Koffler, 1973; Grandeis *et al.*, 1980; R. C. Williams, 1980; World Health Organization, 1977). Furthermore, it has become evident that tumor-associated antigen–antibody complexes may play a significant pathogenetic role in several human neoplastic diseases. CIC deposits were demonstrated in renal glomerular membranes of tumor-bearing patients and in analogous animal models (reviewed by Salinas and Wee, 1983; Salinas *et al.*, 1983*a,b*; Dorval and Pross, 1983). Thereafter, CIC, including those containing oncofetal antigens, were implicated in blocked host immune responses. With the advent of technical improvements in the highly sensitive detection of low-level CIC in body fluids, it became possible to determine how measurement of CIC in cancer patients might be clinically useful for monitoring the course of disease activity, for detection of residual tumor, and for evaluating prognosis.

Interestingly, the still expanding literature on methodology for CIC detection could be a sign of preliminary progress in this field. The emergence of techniques to isolate and characterize CIC-associated antigens, and the eventual use of isolated antigens for monoclonal antibody production, led us to the development of new approaches to CIC concentration by protein A or Raji cells, and to the isolation of CIC-derived antigens by isoelectrofocusing or monoclonal antibodies. These studies have fulfilled a long-standing need to demonstrate TAA as an integral component of CIC in several human tumor types. These procedures have yielded sufficient TAA to allow their physicochemical and functional characterization (Salinas *et al.*, 1984; Gupta *et al.*, 1984*a*; Chu *et al.*, 1983). In addition, the clinical significance of CIC in cancer patients—with regard to localization, tissue injury, and modulation of host immune response, as well as interaction with the clotting, kinin, fibrinolytic, and C' systems—has been noted (Phillips *et al.*, 1982; Salinas *et al.*, 1983*b*). Despite difficulties encountered in the transfer of technology from the bench site to the bedside, the preliminary steps into potential serotherapeutic application, such as monoclonal antibodies or the still controvertible immunoadsorption therapy, appear to be a direct spinoff that may eventually find a definitive place in clinical oncology. An overview of the progress achieved in the area of CIC in cancer patients appears to fulfill many of the recommended general criteria for tumor marker usefulness, with the exception of the specificity requirement and its clinical diagnostic application (Herberman, 1982). Although these tumor markers may be helpful in diagnosis, they deserve greater or at least equal merit as monitors of tumor burden in following disease recurrence or response to treatment. When used solely as monitors of tumor burden, markers need not be tumor-specific. Indeed, tumor markers with relatively broad specificity should be identified and evaluated for use in human cancer (Silver *et al.*, 1979). CIC represent one such marker.

In view of current research emphasis, and the impact that new technical developments may have on the clinical management of cancer patients, the following aspects of CIC will be emphasized in this chapter: (1) Their role in diagnosis, clinical prognosis, and assessment of patients at high risk of recurrence. (2) Their role as monitors of tumor burden in following disease response to treatment. (3) Their role as *in vivo* regulatory factors involved in the mechanisms that facilitate tumor growth. (4) Their nature and composition as factors that influence progression or regression of underlying disease.

The current methodology available for the detection of CIC has been extensively reviewed (Barnett *et al.*, 1979; Haakenstad and Mannik, 1977; V. E. Jones and Orlans, 1981; Kabat, 1980; Peeters, 1979; Theofilopoulos and Dixon, 1979; Rossen and Morgan, 1981). In the interest of brevity we will discuss assay methodology only as it relates to underlying pathophysiology, prognosis, and monitoring of therapy.

II. INCIDENCE OF IMMUNE COMPLEXES IN CANCER

The occurrence of increased CIC or CIC-like macromolecules in the sera of patients with various forms of cancer is now well established (Salinas *et al.*, 1983*b*; Salinas and Wee, 1983; Carpentier and Miescher, 1983). Most if not all CIC results reported until now have been obtained by antigen-nonspecific methods, and such assays are only capable of discriminating macromolecular aggregates from monomeric immunoglobulin. Nonetheless, technical improvements in CIC detection in body fluids have made possible two important steps, namely the isolation and characterization of CIC-derived TAA and the assessment of how measurement of CIC in the sera of cancer patients may be useful for clinical monitoring.

Despite the variety of methodologies reported, none of the described assays has been entirely satisfactory for clinical use (World Health Organization, 1977; Gupta *et al.*, 1979; Rossen and Morgan, 1981; Salinas and Wee, 1983). The problem is compounded by the difficulty of obtaining suitable standards for CIC and by assay idiosyncracies (Zubler *et al.*, 1976; Heimer and Per, 1982). Furthermore, it is known that not all CIC are damaging, since low levels have been reported in people with no apparent disease (Salinas *et al.*, 1981*b*; Salinas and

Wee, 1983) and during pregnancy (Gleicher and Siegel, 1981; Theofilopoulos and Dixon, 1979). Food protein absorption, with its concurrent increased IgA-CIC formation, has been reported in infants and normal adults as well as atopic subjects (Delire et al., 1978; Paganelli et al., 1979). In addition, serial measurement of CIC by multiple assays in healthy subjects and in normal rats has demonstrated heterogeneity of the CIC detected, indicating that both their level and their composition change continuously (Puskas et al., 1982). We have detected comparable heterogeneity and suggested that it may account for a degree of inconsistency in relating CIC concentration to the clinical status of cancer patients (Salinas et al., 1981b,c, 1983b, 1984). Hence, we have suggested that, for effective management of cancer patients, CIC analysis requires knowledge of not only the number of CIC but also their composition and size. This information may permit the assignment of a more uniformly predictable pathological role for detected CIC in cancer patients (Kristensen et al., 1980; Rossen and Morgan, 1981; Salinas et al., 1980b, 1981b-d; Theofilopoulos et al., 1978; World Health Organization, 1977).

The idiosyncracies of various assays, the initial insufficient identification of the antigens involved in CIC, and the fact that different assays do not consistently correlate with each other often resulted in a controversial decade of studies which indicated that CIC prevalence varies in patients with cancer of different types (Salinas et al., 1983b; Rossen and Morgan, 1981; Carpentier and Miescher, 1983). While increased efforts have been dedicated to identify an optimal assay or simultaneous assay combination, insufficient attention has been given to the demonstrated differences among assays (Rossen and Barnes, 1978; Salinas et al., 1981b; Salinas and Wee, 1983). Such "inconsistencies" may in fact be explained by the heterogeneity in molecular size and composition of CIC, as recently reviewed by Salinas and Wee (1983). [Detailed descriptions of the over 50 assays described in the literature can be found in Chapters 1, 3, and 6 of this volume, and in other extensive reviews (Agnello, 1981; Gupta and Morton, 1981; Rossen and Morgan, 1981; Salinas et al., 1983b; Theofilopoulos and Dixon, 1979; Dorval and Pross, 1983; Zubler and Lambert, 1977).] Our experience with a large number of single and serial determinations of CIC in patients with malignant melanoma and breast and ovarian carcinoma (Salinas et al., 1980a, 1981c, 1982b) is in overall agreement with CIC incidence reported by others (Table I). In addition we noted a consistent and significant correlation in four different simultaneous assays comprising solid-space Clq (SP-Clq) (Hay et al., 1976), fetal liver cell radioimmunoassay (FLC-RIA) (Salinas et al., 1981b), Raji cell assay (Theofilopoulos et al., 1977), and polyethylene glycol precipitation assay (PEG/IgG, C3) (Chia et al., 1979). There appears to be no doubt concerning the occurrence of CIC in cancer patients, and reported incidence rates have ranged from 20 to 80% of cases studied. It is noteworthy that there have been circumstances, such as in certain leukemias, where CIC appear to be orphans in seach of

Table I. CIC Occurrence in Cancer Patients

Tumor type	No. of cases	No. elevated/ total (%)	Mean value	Range
Malignant melanoma	262	128 (49)	38	1–163
Breast carcinoma	195	47 (24)	24	1–101
Ovarian carcinoma	142	68 (48)	37	1–139
Colon carcinoma	12	9 (75)	84	15–224
Lung carcinoma	17	5 (29)	18	10–80
Testicular carcinoma	4	3 (75)	92	14–210
Sarcoma	43	21 (49)	42	1–131
Total	675	281 (42)	35	1–180
Control normal serum	139	7 (5)	7	1–20

an association with demonstrable injury or pathogenic significance (Winchester, 1983). Such an association has been recently reported (Schupbach *et al.*, 1984).

As suggested by WHO (Lambert *et al.*, 1978), detection of CIC by the use of simultaneous multiple tests could improve discrimination rates in the assessment of the relative incidence of true- to false-positive and -negative results. By selecting two or more tests with different detection mechanisms (e.g., conglutinin, Clq, or FLC-RIA), additive or synergistic effects for improving their detection and discriminatory efficiency may be achieved. Indeed, this was proven to be the case in some studies. By simultaneous use of three different assays (Clq, conglutinin, and PEG precipitation followed by quantitative determination of immunoglobulins) to determine CIC, diagnostic sensitivity increased from 33–56% by any single test to 85% in malignant melanoma and breast carcinoma sera, and to 77% by simultaneous use of three different tests. There was a doubling of the predictive value of CIC calculated for 100 breast cancer patients' sera. Despite the twofold increase in predictive value observed, the authors suggested that for practical reasons this approach appears not to be suitable for tumor screening. Predictive value depends mainly on prevalence, and it is known that increased incidence of CIC occurs in other chronic diseases, e.g., rheumatoid arthritis (Krapf *et al.*, 1983). Although they suggested that further work on the composition of CIC will enhance the usefulness of CIC determination in malignant disease, the authors failed to contemplate alternative nondiagnostic clinical applications in which such reported CIC observations may have greater merit as monitors of tumor burden in the follow-up of disease recurrence or response to treatment (Salinas *et al.*, 1983*b*).

Recent advances in the fields of CIC, tumor progression, drug resistance, tumor cell heterogeneity, and metastasis have resulted in a renewed interest in the development of nonspecific immunotherapeutic modalities (Frost and Kerbel, 1983; Spremulli and Dexter, 1983). We are confronted not by a single

Table II. Components of Cancer Patients' CIC

Component	References
1. Tumor-associated antigens	Cronin et al. (1982) Gupta et al. (1983a,b) Salinas et al. (1984) Maidment et al. (1981) Kilgallon et al. (1983)

2. Oncofetal antigens	Salinas et al. (1980b, 1984),
	   F. A. Salinas and K. H. Wee
	   (unpublished results)
	 Gupta et al. (1983a,b)
	 Staab et al. (1980)

3. Virus-related malignancies	Lachmann et al. (1981) Schupbach et al. (1984)
4. Idiotype/antiidiotype	Koprowski et al. (1984) Jaffers et al. (1983)
5. Altered self components	Day et al. (1976) Ozawa et al. (1971) Lewis and Pelgrum (1978) Higgens et al. (1974) Ceriani et al. (1982) Dorval and Pross (1983)
6. Other materials	Lewis and Pelgrum (1978) Day et al. (1976)

type of immune complex, but rather by the expression of different CIC resulting from the host's immune reactivity to different antigenic components (Winchester, 1983). Our experience (Salinas et al., 1984) and that of others (Chee et al., 1983; Koprowski et al., 1984; Krapf et al., 1983) indicate that the antigenic makeup of CIC in cancer patients reflects the host's immune response to a variety of often overlapping antigenic stimuli. Thus the composition of CIC varies for different diseases and individuals. An outline of those antigens included in the antigenic makeup of cancer patients' CIC is given in Table II. If these results are further substantiated (as some limited evidence already indicates), the demonstration that no single CIC test has proven entirely satisfactory for clinical use will come as no surprise. The overall consensus is that only a small percentage of the detected CIC in vivo represent TAA complexed with antibodies. The bulk of CIC most likely represent autoantibodies or the reaction to denatured self proteins, microorganisms, normal lymphocyte antigens, renal tubular epithelial antigen, and nuclear antigen (Day et al., 1976; Ozawa et al., 1971; Lewis and Pelgrum, 1978; Higgens et al., 1974).

III. ETIOLOGY OF IMMUNE COMPLEXES

The etiology of CIC- or antigen–antibody-complex-associated disease is the result of a physiological disarray caused by interaction of a number of factors that normally regulate CIC concentration. The specific cause(s) for such a disarray expressed by increased CIC in a given individual is not yet fully known. However, there is increasing experimental and clinical evidence to substantiate specific features that result in CIC deposition leading to inflammation and tissue/cell damage. Such an outcome is the most common and prominent pathogenetic indicator of host CIC-mediated detrimental effect. Factors that influence the biological properties of CIC include antigenic makeup, mode and rate of formation, composition, fate, and deposition. In addition, the interaction of CIC with immune and nonimmune cellular and humoral factors will determine their involvement in many of the known pathogenetic effects associated with host CIC-mediated pathological manifestations.

A. Source of Immune Reactants

The formation of antigen–antibody complexes is the result of noncovalent binding of an antigen with a specific antibody, and represents the host's physiological and immunological defense response in eliciting specific antibodies upon exposure to most antigenic substances, whether neoantigens or autoantigens. The nature of participating antigen–antibody reactions has attracted considerable attention and has been reviewed extensively (Peeters, 1979; Theofilopoulos and Dixon, 1979; Haakenstad and Mannik, 1977). The kinetics and thermodynamics of the antigen–antibody reaction have been highlighted by Berzofsky and Berkower (1984) and Rossen and Morgan (1981). Our attention will be focused on those characteristics of both the antigen and the antibody components of immune complexes that have been reported to influence directly or indirectly their ultimate biological and pathogenetic properties.

1. Importance of Antigen Type and Nature

The nature of the interaction occurring between antigen and antibody and resulting in immune complex formation depends on whether binding of the reactants takes place at the cell surface, intracellularly, in the interstitial fluid, or within the circulation. Some observations concerning each of these *in vivo* sites are listed below in an attempt to bring their differences into focus.

a. Cell-Bound Antigens. These antigens may result from infectious agents expressed on the cell surface or from the expression of new antigens on the surface of infected or transformed cells. They may occur at the cell surface or intracellularly, and upon interaction with antibody may be subsequently released to the extracellular compartment. An example of a structural antigen that interacts with antibody is the basement membrane; their interaction induces antibasement-membrane disease, as often observed in glomerulonephritis (Germuth and Rodriguez, 1973), Goodpasture syndrome (B. D. Williams et al., 1979), and tubulointerstitial nephritis (Wilson and Dixon, 1981). Other examples of structural/cellular antigen sites of interaction have been reported in tumor-bearing patients and analogous animal models (Salinas et al., 1983b; Houghton et al., 1983). In addition, it has been suggested that immune complexes in parasitic diseases are formed at the site of parasitic localization (Nydegger et al., 1983).

b. *Cell-Free Antigens.* These antigens are represented by bacterial, viral, and parasitic interaction *in vivo* with antibody either in the interstitial fluids or at intravascular sites. At the former site antibody interacts with secreted or injected antigen, resulting in the classical Arthus reaction and those reactions observed in thyroiditis and following vasectomy (Salinas and Wee, 1983). Conversely, at the latter site antibody interacts with soluble antigens to form CIC that are usually removed by phagocytes, such as Kupffer cells (Benacerraf et al., 1959; Haakenstad and Mannik, 1974).

The physicochemical properties of CIC-associated antigen (i.e., composition, valence, number and location of antigenic sites) may directly affect the composition and size of the resulting immune complexes, which in turn determine their pathogenetic potential (Salinas and Wee, 1983; Steward and Devey, 1981). Several important biological substances contain either carbohydrates or protein-polypeptide antigenic determinants. Of the former group, those most frequently observed are glycolipids, e.g., bacterial cell walls and major blood group antigens, and glycoproteins, e.g., Rh blood groups. The members of the protein–polypeptide antigenic determinant group are generally amino acid residues in a particular three-dimensional array. Besides the primary sequence, the three-dimensional configuration represents the other contributing factor that defines a protein antigenic determinant, and these configurations have been classified as either sequential or conformational according to their role in binding (Sela, 1969; Berzofsky and Berkower, 1984).

As a result of the progressive expansion of knowledge in the field of immune complexes, another leap forward has been achieved in the isolation and characterization of antigen, the least well known component of CIC. In human malignancy successful isolation of TAA has been accomplished by the concentration of CIC-associated antigen from body fluids, followed by the application of dissociation procedures to recover both antigen and antibody. A representative group of such procedures has been selected and reviewed below.

1. Preparative isoelectric focusing is a method that has been used for the re-

covery and characterization of immunologically reactive antibodies and antigens from breast cancer immune complexes. The method involved a 2.5% PEG fractionation and affinity chromatography on protein A:Sepharose CL-4B. Isolated immune complexes were then subjected to isoelectric focusing, and the TAA thus detected were reported to have isoelectric points (pI) of 3.0–5.0 and molecular weights (M_r) of 20 to 42 kd (Maidment *et al.*, 1981).

2. Successful isolation of immunologically reactive immune-complex-associated antigens and antibodies from malignant melanoma patients and of cell antigens from human melanoma cell lines (Gupta *et al.*, 1983*a,b*; Gupta and Morton, 1984*a–c*) has been recently reported. In a rather impressive and comprehensive manner Gupta *et al.* have provided evidence on the nature and clinical significance of both malignant-melanoma-associated antigens (MAA) and antibodies. One of the approaches developed by this group consisted briefly of the following sequence: (1) Immobilized nonviable *Staphylococcus aureus* protein A was used in *ex vivo* immunoadsorption of plasma from malignant melanoma patients to concentrate immune complexes. (2) Both MAA and anti-MAA antibodies were eluted from the protein A using 0.1 M glycine-HCl buffer (pH 3.5) and 2.5 M MgCl$_2$. (3) Eluted MAA were characterized by sodium dodecyl sulfate-polyacrylamide gel electrophoresis (SDS-PAGE), while the anti-MAA antibody was determined by its binding activity to a radiolabeled MAA extracted from the spent culture medium of a human melanoma cell line. (4) The activity and specificity of the eluted MAA were determined by a competitive inhibition radioimmunoassay using [^{125}I]-MAA and allogeneic serum from a melanoma patient. An estimation of anti-MAA ranging from 0.15% to 7.8% of total protein in the respective eluates and a linear dose-dependent inhibition of MAA in the radioimmunoassay were reported. Quantitative analysis of MAA from various fractions revealed a concentration of less than 1% of total protein in the eluates.

3. Another approach consisted of an analysis of the antigenic heterogeneity observed in immune-complex-associated antigens isolated from human solid tumors, including malignant melanoma and breast and ovarian carcinoma. The procedures for malignant melanoma sera selected for examination, include qualitative and quantitative analysis of CIC in selected patients' sera before and after interaction with isolated MAA or human oncofetal antigen (HOFA) (Salinas *et al.*, 1984; F. A. Salinas and K. H. Wee, unpublished results).

c. Malignant-Melanoma-Associated Antigens. MAA have been isolated from sera of patients with clinically objective evaluable tumor burden and histopathological confirmation of diagnosis. Patients were selected from an ongoing study to maintain continuity with earlier data and were grouped by tumor burden as previously described (Salinas *et al.*, 1980*c*, 1984). Briefly, Group I included patients with no evidence of disease at the time of serum sampling. Group II patients had relatively small tumor burdens consisting of primary melanoma, local recurrence, or intransit metastases estimated at less than 5 g. Group III patients all had relatively advanced regional or distant metastatic disease, with tumor burdens clearly greater than 5 g. The procedure for isolation of MAA has been described (Salinas *et al.*, 1984) and briefly consisted of the following sequence: (1) CIC from patients' sera were concentrated by use of Raji cell receptors. (2) Cellbound CIC were eluted with isotonic citrate buffer (pH 3.2) or by solubilization with Triton X-100 in Tris-HCl ethylenediaminetetraacetic acid (EDTA)-buffered saline. (3) Subsequent separation of antigen from antibody moieties was achieved by sucrose density gradient fractionation (SGF) or by SDS-PAGE.

The recovered MAA was a glycoprotein containing 3-4% carbohydrate with no evidence of sialic acid residue. MAA showed a common predominant M_r of 54 kd as determined by SDS-PAGE and SGF with a pI of 4.3. The yield of protein averaged 0.43, 0.55, and 0.36 mg/ml of serum for Group I, II, and III patients with increasing tumor burden. The isolated MAA demonstrated similar physiochemical and functional characteristics in all patients tested, suggesting common MAA. A preliminary estimate of the percentage of MAA isolated from CIC of melanoma patients was derived from the recovery yield. Free MAA in patients' sera was excluded from this calculation. As shown in Table III, the MAA concentration was estimated at less than 1% of the total protein recovered. Information on the heterogeneity and concentration of antigen(s) was derived from *in vitro* interaction of MAA and HOFA with patients' sera.

An analysis of CIC detected in selected melanoma patients' sera, grouped

Table III. Recovery of Melanoma-Associated Antigens

Patient serum[a]	CIC (Raji-RIA) (μg/ml)	Extracted protein[b] (mg/ml)	MAA (% of total CIC protein)
Group 1			
A	118.4	0.39	0.04
B	118.4	0.58	0.03
C	160.0	0.31	0.08
Group 2			
D	105.6	0.41	0.04
E	160.0	0.69	0.03
F	96.0	0.20	0.07
Group 3			
G	128.0	0.29	0.07
H	96.0	0.45	0.03
I	105.6	0.33	0.05

[a] Patient sera grouped according to tumor burden.
[b] As per Raji cell technique.

Table IV. Estimated Melanoma-Associated Antigen Occurrence in CIC upon Interaction with MAA

Source of antigen used[a]	CIC levels (Raji cell assay) ($\mu g/ml$)			Estimated MAA (% of total CIC protein)
	Pre	Post	Change	
Group I				
A	118.4	110	−8.4	0.1
B	105.6	123	17.4	2.4
C	128.0	203	7.5	5.5
Group II				
D	118.4	59.2	−59.2	7.4
E	105.6	224.0	118.4	7.8
F	128.0	160.0	32.0	3.0
Group III				
G	118.4	80.0	−38.4	4.8
H	105.6	272.0	116.4	9.0
I	128.0	208	80.0	5.7

[a]Extracted from melanoma patients' sera, grouped according to tumor burden.

according to tumor burden, upon interaction with isolated MAA was undertaken. By use of an *in vitro* model to generate and dissociate CIC, the levels of CIC were evaluated and their molecular compositions were estimated. *In vitro* titration experiments indicated that 3 μg MAA rendered optimal immune complex formation. The reaction mixture was analyzed for lattice size by 5–35% isopycnic SGF, and fractions containing aggregates of estimated molecular size were CIC-determined. This *in vitro* model allowed us to examine the influence of added antigen on total CIC. The occurrence of MAA was estimated to range from 0.1% to 9.0% (Table IV), and that of HOFA to range from 1.7% to 3.6% (Table V) of the total CIC protein (Salinas *et al.*, 1984; F. A. Salinas and K. H. Wee, unpublished results). Analysis of nine selected unreacted patient sera for

Table V. Estimated Human Oncofetal Antigen Occurrence in CIC upon Interaction with HOFA

Patient serum group[a]	CIC levels (Raji cell assay) ($\mu g/ml$)			HOFA (% of total CIC protein)
	Pre	Post	Change	
1	118.4	96.0	−22.4	1.7
2	105.6	176.0	70.4	3.6
3	128.0	176.0	48.0	2.5

[a]Malignant melanoma patients' sera, grouped according to tumor burden.

Table VI. Concentration and Size of Immune Complexes Formed
in Vitro with MAA (II)

IC size (SGF) (S)	Estimated molecular ratio		Concentration of CIC (Raji cell assay) (μg/ml)[a]			Control normal sera
			Group 1	Group 2	Group 3	
7-9	Ag_2	Ab_1	17	49	39	3
10-12	Ag_4	Ab_2	80	50	87	5
13-15	Ag_6	Ab_3	51	78	49	3
16-18	Ag_{10}	Ab_5	24	41	27	1
19-25	Ag_{12}	Ab_6	128	84	96	4

[a]Each point represents the mean of triplicate determinations.

lattice size demonstrated heterogeneous CIC occurrence. Peak CIC were of medium size (10-15 S) for Group 1; small (7-9 S), medium, and large (>16 S) for Group 2; and small and large for Group 3 patients' sera. All autologous combinations with MAA resulted in significant ($P \leqslant 0.001$ by Mann–Whitney test) formation of common-size (7.7 S) *de novo* CIC as compared to unreacted serum samples. Conversely, in allogenic combination MAA Groups I and II resulted in increased CIC size, and MAA from Group III resulted in unchanged or reduced CIC size. The only exceptions noted were those with less apparent breakdown of large to small CIC for MAA Group III reacting with Group 1 serum (not depicted), and breakdown of large to small CIC for MAA Group III reacting with Group 2 serum (Table VI).

An overview of results from criss-cross combinations of Group I, II, and III MAA and patients sera demonstrated that the prevalent CIC size is MAA-dependent (Fig. 1). This schematic represents an attempt to summarize the kinetics of malignant melanoma CIC size changes resulting from multiple MAA autologous and allogenic combinations. The CIC size changes are represented by three cyclical outlines based on the origin of the MAA. The unidirectional changes of observed CIC size are depicted by arrows, the tail ends of which represent initial and the head ends final sizes. It was noted that the resulting changes in CIC lattice size showed significant correlation to patients' tumor burden, and indirectly to the origin of the serum autoantigen involved (Salinas *et al.*, 1984). Representative illustrations of CIC size and concentration changes observed upon interaction with Group I, II, and III MAA (3 μg) reacted in both autologous and allogenic combinations with patients' sera are given in Figures 1 and 2 and Table VI. No significant change was noted when similar combinations were performed with normal control sera. An attempt to estimate the molecular ratio of antigen to antibody was undertaken based on anti-MAA antibody and MAA molecular weights (Table VI). These *in vitro* simulations of tumor burden changes with observed changes in CIC size and concentration are in keeping with

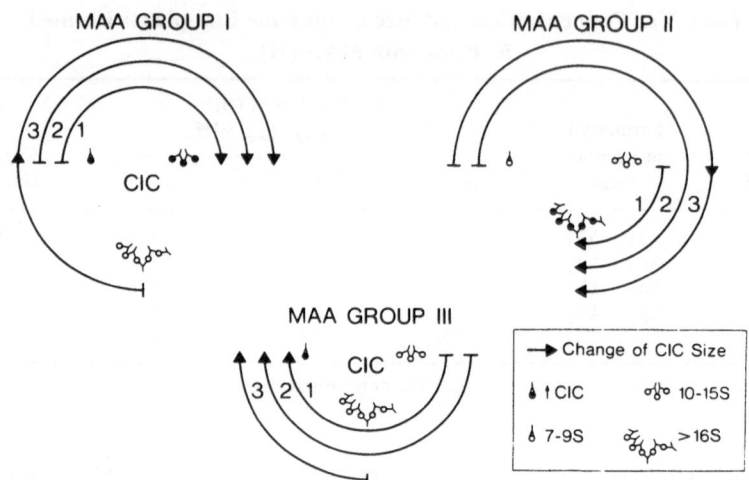

Figure 1. Schematic results upon reacting Group I, II, and III MAA (3 μg) with patients' sera (50 μl 1:8 diluted) from Groups 1, 2, and 3. The observed CIC size changes are depicted by arrows, with tail ends representing initial and head ends final CIC sizes.

other reported observations that indirectly correlated CIC levels with tumor burden (Gupta and Morton, 1981), and with our earlier reports on malignant melanoma single- and serial-sample CIC determinations (Salinas *et al.*, 1980*c*, 1981*a,c*).

In summary (1) An *in vitro* model was used for evaluating how malignant melanoma tumor burden relates to MAA and the size and composition of CIC (precluding treatment interference). (2) The observed CIC size changes correlated with tumor burden. (3) The unidirectional CIC size changes noted were primarily dependent on the origin of MAA. (4) The results on CIC levels, sizes, and composition provide an improved perspective on their correlation with clinical disease.

   d. Human Oncofetal Antigen.   Procedures used for the isolation and purification of HOFA have been previously reported (Salinas *et al.*, 1980*b*, 1982*a*). Briefly, HOFA was found to be composed primarily of 15-kd molecules, as analyzed by SDS-PAGE and SGF. It contained 3% carbohydrate and showed no evidence of sialic acid residues (Salinas *et al.*, 1985). The interaction of isolated HOFA with cancer patients' sera was essentially similar to the reported procedures described for MAA (Salinas *et al.*, 1984). An analysis of CIC size changes resulting from the addition of an optimal amount of $[^{125}I]$-HOFA (3 μg) to selected malignant melanoma sera was undertaken. SGF and SDS-PAGE analysis demonstrated major uptake at 8 S CIC size for Group 1 sera, 16 S for Group 2, and 14 S for Group 3, while a 1.5 S peak was observed for $[^{125}I]$-HOFA with or

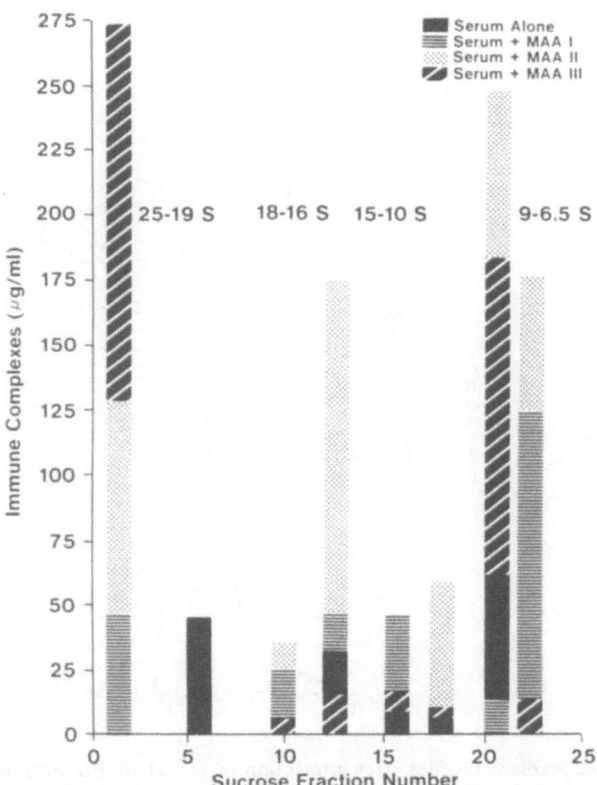

Figure 2. CIC size and concentration changes before and after interaction of Group I, II, and III MAA with patients' sera in autologous and allogenic combinations. CIC concentrations were determined by the Raji cell assay, and CIC sizes (S) were determined by linear sucrose gradient fractionation (5–35% w/v). Each point represents the mean of triplicate determinations.

without added normal control sera (Fig. 3). Immune complexes size changes showed a significant relationship to patients' tumor burden ($P \leqslant 0.001$ by Spearman's test). Parallel sucrose gradient fractions using unlabeled HOFA were evaluated for CIC by the FLC-RIA or Raji cell assay (Salinas *et al.*, 1981*b*). The results showed peak CIC sizes at 7–9 and 13–15 S for Group 1 sera, 10–12.5 and 16–18 S for Group 2, and 10–12.5 and 13–15 S for Group 3. An attempt to estimate the molecular ratio of antigen to antibody at each peak size was made. We considered a bivalent IgG antibody of $M_r \cong 150$ kd and a multivalent HOFA of $M_r \cong 15$ kd. Their tentative molecular ratio and the CIC size profiles of a representative set of patients' sera are depicted in Table VII. A summary of the kinetics of malignant melanoma patients' sera CIC size changes upon *in vitro* reaction with HOFA is given in Fig. 4. The CIC size changes observed are represented by

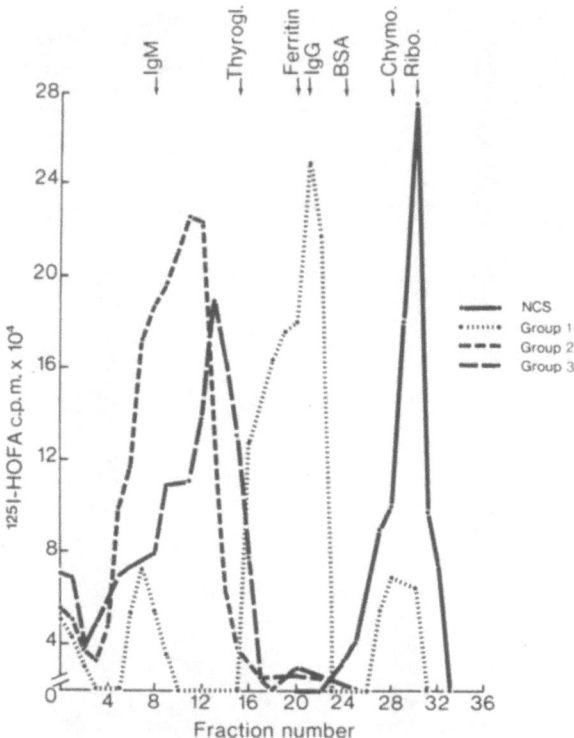

Figure 3. Sucrose gradient profiles after interaction of [^{125}I]-HOFA with malignant mela-noma patients' sera (50 μl 1:8 diluted) from Groups 1, and 2, and 3 and normal control serum. Each point represents the mean of triplicate determinations.

Table VII. Concentration and Size of Immune Complexes Formed *in Vitro* with HOFA

		CIC levels (FLC-RIA) (μg/ml)[a]							
IC size (SGF) (S)	Estimated molecular ratio	Group 1		Group 2		Group 3		Control normal sera	
		Pre	Post	Pre	Post	Pre	Post	Pre	Post
7–9	Ag$_2$ Ab$_1$	21	86	61	1	9	48	1	1
10–12.5	Ag$_4$ Ab$_2$	58	24	26	133	11	138	1	12
13–15	Ag$_6$ Ab$_3$	34	88	50	12	16	10	9	15
16–18	Ag$_{10}$ Ab$_5$	41	156	56	160	33	128	5	16
19–25	Ag$_{12}$ Ab$_6$	16	N.D.	40	26	88	11	10	1

[a]Each point represents the mean of triplicate determinations.

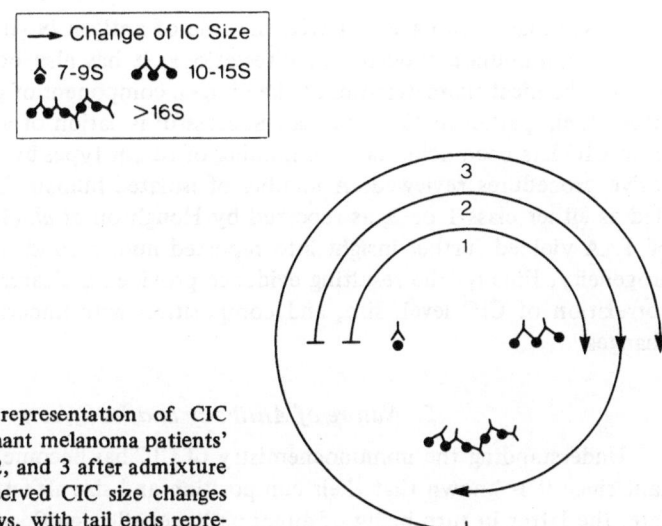

Figure 4. Schematic representation of CIC size changes of malignant melanoma patients' sera from Groups 1, 2, and 3 after admixture with HOFA. The observed CIC size changes are depicted by arrows, with tail ends representing initial and head ends final CIC sizes.

concentric lines to account for the origin of patients' sera. Arrows indicate the unidirectional changes of CIC sizes. This pattern of size changes resembled that of MAA autologous combinations. However, it was noted that in every case the resulting CIC peaks were qualitatively and quantitatively beyond those peak size changes observed with MAA. In fact, an estimation indicated that HOFA represented approximately 35–58%, and MAA 39–47% of the total antigen in CIC (Table VIII). These observations are in keeping with reported HOFA cross-reactivity with TAA (Salinas et al., 1978, 1980b, 1981b; Gupta and Morton, 1983; Hellström and Hellström, 1974). They also provided support for the antigenic heterogeneity of CIC observed in cancer patients (see Table II).

Table VIII. Estimated CIC Antigen Makeup in Cancer Patients' Sera

Malignant melanoma sera[a]	Antigenic occurrence in CIC (%)[b]		
	HOFA-associated	MAA-associated	Undetermined
Group 1	35.3	47.1	17.6
Group 2	58.5	39.9	1.6
Group 3	38.4	38.4	23.2

[a]Grouped according to tumor burden.
[b]Estimated antigenic concentration from HOFA interaction (Table VII and Fig. 1).

In summary, we have reviewed the role of antigen *in vivo* localization with regard to immunopathogenic manifestations. It has also been noted how the physicochemical characteristics of the antigen component of CIC may ultimately affect their pathogenetic potential. Successful isolation of antigen components from CIC has been achieved in a number of tumor types by the use of the innovative procedures reviewed. A number of isolated human TAA could be classified as either class 1 or 2, as reported by Houghton *et al.* (1983). The isolation of TAA yielded further insight into reported human solid tumor antigenic heterogeneity. Finally, the resulting evidence provided a clearer perspective on the correlation of CIC level, size, and composition with underlying tumor burden changes.

2. Nature of Antibody and Its Effects

Understanding the immunochemistry of CIC has become increasingly important since it is known that their composition and size affect their detection and fate, the latter in turn being of direct pathogenetic significance. A list of factors that influence the biological properties of CIC is given in Table IX. It includes characteristics relevant to antibody, antigen, CIC, host, and other factors. Increased levels of CIC are insufficient to explain how CIC leave the circulation to cause inflammation within the vessel wall (vasculitis) or within tissue parenchyma (systemic lupus erythematosus, nephritis). In addition, inconsistencies in relating CIC concentration to disease status can be explained by the nature of the bound antigen, immunoglobulin type and isotype, ability to bind complement and CIC size (Haakenstad and Mannik, 1977; Sinclair, 1979; Salinas and Wee, 1983). Antibody-related immunochemical and other factors that influence the formation, fate, and biological activity of CIC have been reviewed by Haakenstad and Mannik (1977), Barnett *et al.* (1979), R. C. Williams (1980), and Salinas *et al.* (1983*b*). Among the more prominent are the antibody isotope, class, valence, affinity, avidity, complement binding capacity, and molecular concentration (both relative and absolute) as determined by molecular combining ratio (Van Es *et al.*, 1979). Many of the characteristics of CIC-associated antibodies and their effects will be dealt with in Sections III.B and IV. Two selected specific effects of antibody influencing the functional biological properties of CIC are noted. The nature of antibody involved determines the intrinsic capacity of CIC to induce clearance *in vivo* or phagocytosis *in vitro*. At least two distinct mechanisms for the removal of IgA- and IgG-CIC are known (Finbloom *et al.*, 1980). The interaction of CIC with the classical and alternative complement pathways represents another effect of antibody on CIC properties. In fact, the classical complement pathway could be initiated by both IgG- or IgM-containing CIC. IgG_1 and IgG_3 isotypes and IgM-CIC are the most efficient initiators of the complement cascade, IgG_2 is less effective, and IgG_4 is inactive (Kaplan, 1981; Theofilopoulos and Dixon, 1979; Salinas and Wee, 1983).

Table IX. Factors Influencing Biological Properties
of Circulating Immune Complexes

1. Antigen-related
   Size
   Valence
   Steric topography of determinants
   Physicochemical properties

2. Antibody-related
   Size
   Valence
   Class and subclass
   Affinity
   Avidity
   Complement-binding capacity
   Number of antigen receptors

3. CIC-related
   Kinetics of lattice formation
   Minimum and maximum size
   Half-life, clearance, and deposition
   Kinetics of association/dissociation of reactants

4. Common factors
   Relative and absolute concentration
   Rate of synthesis or production
   Nonspecific interactions in the host: hydrophobic bonds,
      ionic charge, surface tension, van der Waals forces

5. Host-related
   Rate of production or synthesis
   Rate of nonimmune catabolisms
   Rate of removal by reticuloendothelial system
   Tissue deposition rate
   Rate of entry or exit from vascular to extravascular
      compartments

B. Composition of Immune Complexes

The nature and characteristics of both antigen and antibody determine to a great extent the biological characteristics of CIC. The molecular concentrations of antigen and antibody, both relative and absolute, as reflected by their molecular combining ratio, also play a prominent role (Van Es *et al.*, 1979; Salinas *et al.*, 1981c, 1983b). Antigen–antibody interactions are in principle reversible, and can act as the prototype model for interactions between macromolecules and ligands. The size and composition of CIC depend on factors that maintain the entire system in a dynamic steady state: Antigens and antibodies entering the circulation at varying rates establish equilibrium with CIC and each other.

Simultaneously, CIC are constantly being deposited in tissues, removed from circulation, or phagocytosed by the reticuloendothelial system.

An important concern in the field of CIC determination is the nature of immune complexes detected by antigen-nonspecific assays. Identification of associated antigens or antibodies in the reactive CIC will provide evidence of their occurrence and involvement in the pathogenetic manifestations associated with various malignancies. For almost a decade, with the exception of the antigen-specific detection reported by D'Amelio *et al.* (1981), it was not possible to prove that the material being detected in cancer patients was CIC. The fact that increased levels of CIC or CIC-like material have been detected in cancer patients does not necessarily imply that such material is composed of tumor antigens and antibodies (Agnello, 1981; Salinas *et al.*, 1983*b*); because aggregated IgG, polyamines, and bacterial lipopolysaccharides have been noted as contributors to putative CIC (Sobel *et al.*, 1975; Heier *et al.*, 1977; Cairns *et al.*, 1980; Agnello, 1981), although not as major constitutents. About five years elapsed between the first observations of CIC-associated tumor antigens in experimental animals (Price and Baldwin, 1977) and the establishment in some detail of the physical and immunochemical characteristics of CIC-derived in human malignancy. Given such a trend, the advent of antigen-specific methods to detect CIC—with emphasis on the functional role played by the heterogeneous molecular components of CIC in the pathogenesis of the underlying malignant disease—may be the next step. So far, efforts have been concentrated on the characterization of CIC detected by antigen-nonspecific methods based on methods for the concentration and isolation of CIC from serum.

1. Methods for Concentration of CIC

The relatively large size of CIC compared to their antigen or antibody components and other serum proteins has been successfully exploited in separation procedures. Commonly used CIC concentration procedures are listed in Table X.

2. Methods for Isolation of CIC

The majority of methods used for isolation have been derived from the detection capability of antigen-nonspecific assays. A summary of representative approaches is given in Table XI. (For a detailed review of the topic the reader is referred to Chapter 1.)

3. Dissociation of Isolated CIC

V. E. Jones and Orlans (1981) reviewed a number of methods now available to elute antigens or antibodies from solid matrix ligands. Regardless of the method selected the avidity of the antibodies encountered will be the determining

Table X. Methods Used for CIC Concentration

Method	References
1. Gel filtration chromatography	
Sephacryl S-300	Gupta *et al.* (1979)
Sephadex G-200	Salinas *et al.* (1984)
Sepharose 6B	Poulton *et al.* (1983)
Urogel AcA34	Hendrick *et al.* (1981)
2. Sucrose density gradient ultracentrifugation	Rossen *et al.* (1977)
(10–40%, 10–37%, 5–35% w/v)	Theofilopoulos *et al.* (1977)
	Salinas *et al.* (1981c, 1984)
	Phillips *et al.* (1981)
3. Polyethylene glycol precipitation (2.5–8% w/v)	Salinas *et al.* (1983b)
	Chia *et al.* (1979)
	Lahey *et al.* (1984)
4. Combinations of PEG precipitation and other methods	Male and Riott (1979)
	Maidment *et al.* (1981)

Table XI. Common CIC Isolation Methods

Method	References
1. Conglutinin binding	Casali and Lambert (1979)
	Chapter 1, this volume
2. Complement component binding	Scharfstein *et al.* (1979)
	Pereira *et al.* (1980)
	Phillips *et al.* (1982)
	Gupta *et al.* (1983a,b)
3. Antiglobulin binding	F. R. Jones *et al.* (1980)
	Gilead *et al.* (1981)
4. Cell-surface receptors	Theofilopoulos *et al.* (1977, 1978)
	Tucker *et al.* (1978)
	Salinas *et al.* (1984)
5. Anticomplement components	Pereira *et al.* (1980)
	Phillips *et al.* (1982)
	Kilgallon *et al.* (1983)
6. Staphylococcal protein A	Ray *et al.* (1982)
	Maidment *et al.* (1981)
	Tucker *et al.* (1978)
	Gupta *et al.* (1983a,b)
7. Dye–ligand chromatography	Quay *et al.* (1983)
8. Monoclonal antibody solid-phase immunoaffinity	Salinas *et al.* (1983a)

factor for dissociation. In addition, a number of common problems encountered during dissociation must be considered. These include the possibilities that the antigen or antibody could be modified in whole or in part by the removal agent, and that reassociation of antigen and antibody may occur once the agent is withdrawn, which in turn may result in reassociated immune complexes with altered molar ratios. CIC dissociation techniques—including treatment of isolated CIC with enzymes, chaotropic agents, and acid or alkaline buffers—have also been reviewed by Phillips *et al.* (1981). A brief description of useful considerations in selecting a particular method for the dissociation of isolated CIC has been given by V. E. Jones and Orlans (1981). These include (1) the relative affinity of the ligands used to isolate CIC (stronger agents are needed to elute CIC from high-affinity ligands); (2) emphasis on the recovery of intact immune complexes; (3) recovery of immunologically active antibody and antigen constituents; and (4) optimal recovery of antigen and/or antibody. A condensed description of successful CIC dissociation methods used in cancer patients has been assembled and is given in Table XII.

4. Detection of Immune Reactants

The usual approach for the detection of CIC constituents has been the identification of the antigen moiety from CIC. Ideally such identification, in cases where CIC are associated with active disease manifestations, should represent the best approach to document the relationship of CIC to the disease manifestations.

Although the presence of antigen and/or antibody in preformed CIC has been well documented, their identification in clinical material often encounters degrees of difficulties. The common explanations for such difficulties include loss of antigenic or antibody activity of the dissociated CIC components and inadequate separation of antigen and antibody, rendering recognition of CIC components extremely difficult. A summary of methods reported for detection of immune reactants in CIC is given in Table XIII (see also Section III.A.1). Others have noted how the molecular concentrations of antigen and antibody, both relative and absolute, play a role in establishing the moleculear combining ratio (Vans Es *et al.*, 1979; Salinas *et al.*, 1981*b*, 1983*b*). A number of factors contributing to antigen–antibody interactions influencing their biological characteristics are listed in Table IX.

5. Effect of Size and Number of CIC

The relationship of size and number of CIC to their effects on CIC clearance, deposition, and triggering of inflammatory reactions resulting in tissue damage is complex. Any attempt to isolate or identify these effects would be artificial and should be viewed as a didactic effort. There is a direct relationship between concentration and size in CIC. In fact, the effective management of patients with

Table XII. CIC Dissociation Methods Used in Human Cancer

Source of CIC	Method of CIC separation, dissociation, and recovery of reactants	Reference
Chronic lymphocytic leukemia	Acetate buffer (pH 3.5) and SGF (pH 8.3 or 3.5) for Ag and Ab recovery	Carpentier and Miescher (1983)
Malignant melanoma	Immobilized protein A and recovery by $MgCl_2$ (pH 6.8) elution, or by glycine-HCl buffer (pH 3.5)	Gupta et al. (1983a,b)
Malignant melanoma	Low-pH treatment and gel filtration on Urogel AcA34 using citrate–phosphate buffer as eluent	Hendrick et al. (1981)
Malignant melanoma	Acid and chaotropic ion dissociation	Phillips et al. (1981)
Breast carcinoma	Separation by Raji cell method; dissociation by SDS-PAGE, SGF, and isoelectrofocusing	Salinas et al. (1983a,b)
Breast carcinoma	Isolation by immunoaffinity (monoclonal-antibody-coated Sepharose beads); dissociation by SDS-PAGE and SGF	Salinas et al. (1983a)
Malignant melanoma	Low-pH treatment for separation and SGF (pH 2.9) for dissociation	Rossen and Morgan (1981)
Malignant melanoma	Isolation by Raji cell method and dissociation by SDS-PAGE and SGF	Salinas et al. (1984)
Ovarian carcinoma	Isolation by Raji cell method; dissociation by SDS-PAGE, SGF, and isoelectrofocusing	F. A. Salinas and K. H. Wee (unpublished results)
Breast carcinoma	Isolation by PEG fractionation, protein A, and isoelectrofocusing	Maidment et al. (1981)
Gestational trophoblastic neoplasia	Fractionation on Sephadex G-200 in acid buffer	Lahey et al. (1984)
Hodgkin's disease	Isolation by C1q-degalan, anti-C1q Sepharose, conglutinin (K)-degalan, and EDTA elution	Kilgallon et al. (1983)

Table XIII. Methods Used for Detection of Immune Reactants in CIC

Method	Reference
1. Indirect immunofluorescence	
Malignant melanoma	Theofilopoulos *et al.* (1977)
	Phillips *et al.* (1981, 1982)
2. Double countercurrent immunoelectrophoresis	
Malignant melanoma	Phillips *et al.* (1981)
3. Isoelectric focusing	
Breast carcinoma	Maidment *et al.* (1981)
	Salinas *et al.* (1982*b*)
Malignant melanoma	Salinas *et al.* (1981*c*, 1984)
4. Polyacrylamide gel electrophoresis	
Gross-virus-induced lymphoma	Tucker *et al.* (1978)
Malignant melanoma	Quay *et al.* (1983)
	Gupta *et al.* (1983*a*,*b*),
	Gupta and Morton (1984*c*)
	Salinas *et al.* (1981*c*, 1984)
Breast carcinoma	Salinas *et al.* (1982*b*, 1983*a*)
5. Radioimmunoassay	
Malignant melanoma	Theofilopoulos *et al.* (1977)
	Gupta *et al.* (1983*a*,*b*)
6. Antigen competition assay	
Malignant melanoma	Gupta and Morton (1984*a–c*)
7. Monoclonal antibody to tumor antigen	
Malignant melanoma	Morgan and McIntyre (1983)
Breast carcinoma	Salinas *et al.* (1983*a*,*b*), F. A.
	Salinas and K. H. Wee
	(unpublished results)
Ovarian carcinoma	Bhattacharya *et al.* (1982)

immune complex disease requires knowledge of both the number and size, of CIC together with a concomitant evaluation of interacting antigen and antibody (Salinas *et al.*, 1981*c*, 1983*b*).

Our results on malignant melanoma and breast and ovarian carcinoma single- and serial-sample CIC determinations, as well as their evaluation for CIC size and concentration, have shown that high CIC concentration led to immune complex size increase, effectively reducing CIC number (Salinas *et al.*, 1981*b*,*c*), and hence, elevated levels of CIC were observed in conjunction with small (7–9 S) CIC, while large (>19 S) CIC tended to be associated with reduced levels. Patients with intermediate-size (10–18 S) CIC presented moderate CIC levels (Salinas *et al.*, 1981*b–d*). These findings have direct implications for the clearance of CIC, and are in keeping with other reports (Theofilopoulos and Dixon, 1979; B. D.

Williams *et al.*, 1979). Normal clearance of CIC depends on many interacting factors, especially size. CIC must reach a critical size to be processed and cleared by the reticuloendothelial system. Thus, excess antigen or low-affinity antibody can result in small CIC with delayed clearance. Persistence of CIC may also reflect host immune status (Halpern, 1974; Salinas and Wee, 1983; Masson, 1978).

Our studies in generating and dissociating CIC by use of an *in vitro* model illustrated the kinetics of CIC size changes in relation to antigen/antibody concentrations. We used selected melanoma patients' sera mixed with MAA, and the analysis of the resulting CIC demonstrated that both the relative and absolute levels of reactants regulated the concentration, size, and composition of immune complexes (Salinas *et al.*, 1981c, 1984).

C. Fate of Immune Complexes

The ultimate fate of CIC depends on a multifactorial balance among synthesis, clearance, and deposition. Factors influencing this balance include lattice size, kinetics of association and dissociation, nature of antibody and antigen, interaction with complement, and status of the mononuclear phagocyte system, as listed in Table IX and reported earlier (Salinas and Wee, 1983; Lamers *et al.*, 1981). The fate and deposition of CIC and their relationship with the complement system will be discussed in detail in Section IV.

Both experimental and clinical results suggest variable requirements for the phagocytosis of CIC. Smaller complexes are processed by tissue phagocytes (e.g., Kupffer cells and splenic macrophages) but not by circulating phagocytic monocytes. Whether this is due to functional differences among such phagocytic cells or due to CIC aggregation at the clearance site is as yet unknown (Lammers, 1981). Overflow of CIC at sites unsuitable for elimination, (e.g., glomeruli, small blood vessels, and serous membrances) may result from overload, impaired function, or lack of macrophage interaction with antibodies owing to chemical modifications (Haakenstad and Mannik, 1974, 1977). Hemodynamic conditions such as blood flow and turbulence, blood pressure, vascular permeabiltity, C3 and Fc receptor density, and affinity of antigens for tissues are factors that have been reported to affect CIC localization (Haakenstad and Mannik, 1977; Lamers, 1981; Wilson and Dixon, 1981).

As discussed earlier, antiidiotypic antibodies are now recognized as components in the antigenic makeup of CIC. Their presence has been reported in bacterial infection (Waller *et al.*, 1968), associated with human malignancies (Catropia *et al.*, 1976), and in conjunction with the clearance of denatured immunoglobulins from the circulation (Hartmann, 1975). However, more recently anti-antibodies have been noted to contribute to CIC clearance by increasing CIC size, thus enhancing monocyte interaction and phagocytosis (Phillips *et al.*, Chapter 3, this volume). High-avidity antibodies to DNA leading to small CIC size have been reported to correlate with the pathogenesis of systemic lupus erythematosus-associated renal manifestations (Aarden, 1977; Haaskenstad and Mannik, 1977). Experimental evidence of the effects of cationized antibodies in preformed immune complex deposition and persistence in renal glomeruli has been reported. Whereas small CIC-cationized antibodies revealed initial deposition without persistence, large CIC-cationized antibodies showed rapid deposition and persistence in the glomeruli, particularly in the subendothelial area (Gauthier *et al.*, 1982). Reports of the harmful effects of different CIC size have varied, depending on the model used (Lamers, 1981; Pincus *et al.*, 1968). Whereas there is evidence that preformed large-latticed CIC ($>Ag_2 Ab_2$) are removed rapidly upon injection, small complexes are not (Lightfoot *et al.*, 1970; Mannik and Arend, 1971). Covalent IgG complexes of defined sizes were found to clear according to size. They fix complement *in vitro* in a size-dependent manner. While covalent complexes injected in small amounts remain stable (Brennan *et al.*, 1983), noncovalent complexes injected in antigen excess remain soluble, but their sizes change upon dissociation and reassociation (Mannik and Arend, 1971). The rate of removal of different oligomers seems directly related to size; the larger the complexes the faster their removal. The uptake of tetramers by the liver is maximal within 1–2 hr (Grace and Brennan, 1982). The *in vitro* rate-limiting step in phagocytosis for IgG-CIC is adherence to cells bearing Fc receptors, also known to be size-dependent. The liver has been reported to be the major organ involved in the uptake of IgA-CIC frequently observed in glomerulonephritis–cirrhosis nephropathy and Henoch–Schonlein purpura, and their clearance was directly related to lattice structure (Rifai and Mannik, 1984). Heavy polymers were localized mainly in the hepatic nonparenchymal cells. Evidence indicates that carbohydrate receptors recognize antigen in immune complex as an alternative to antibody Fc receptors in modulating the clearance and subsequent fate of CIC (Rifai *et al.*, 1982). The mechanism involved in IgA-CIC hepatobiliary transport, from blood to bile, represents a known and unique noninflammatory mechanism for antigen disposal (Brown *et al.*, 1982).

Macrophages discriminate complexes of different size and antibody class in the course of attachment, but not during processing (Segal and Hurwitz, 1977; Knutson *et al.*, 1977; Leslie, 1980). Studies on inhibitors of phagocytosis implied that complexes can be ingested via two mechanisms. The rapid phase of intake is probably associated with fluid-phase pinocytosis, which is inhibited by cytochalasin B, whereas the slower phase is associated with absorptive micropinocytosis (Leslie, 1980; Wills *et al.*, 1972; Silverstein *et al.*, 1977).

The risk of deposition of CIC outside the reticuloendothelial system is reduced by the increased solubility of complexes mediated by serum complement, and this may inhibit IgG-mediated clearance of antigen (Skogh and Stendahl, 1983). Protein A of *Staphylococcus aureus* significantly altered to clearance rate and tissue uptake of CIC containing murine leukemia virus p30 antigen.

Upon mixing CIC with protein A clearance from the liver was observed in 4 hr, and the amount localized in the spleen (sequestration) was reduced tenfold in 24 hr. Despite enhancement of whole-body elimination of CIC during the first 24 hr, protein A did not inhibit binding of antigen to antibody, but did inhibit CIC binding to lymphoid and phagocytic cells (Siag and Jones, 1982).

The pathogenetic role of low-affinity antibody in the induction of CIC disease is still not fully understood. However, in systemic lupus erythematosus and rheumatoid arthritis, as well as in experimental models, the disparity between high-affinity antibodies deposited as complexes and circulating low-affinity antibodies suggests a significant role of the former in tissue damage (Haakenstad and Mannik, 1977; Lookwood et al., 1979). This is consistent with the high complement-activating capacity and inefficient CIC elimination of the mononuclear phagocytic system (Rajnavolgki et al., 1978). While the reported harmful effects of small (10-15 S) and large (>19 S) CIC vary, depending on the models used (Salinas and Wee, 1983), analysis of CIC size in cancer patients (Salinas et al., 1983b), nephrotic conditions (Germuth and Rodriguez, 1973), and experimental models (Lightfoot et al., 1970; Brennan et al., 1983; Rifai and Mannik, 1984) provided evidence that CIC size is a primary factor in determining localization and ultimate pathological manifestations. For example, in renal disease, small CIC deposit in or on the epithelial side of the glomerular basement membrane, causing diffuse membranous glomerulonephritis. Slightly larger CIC (about 15 S) deposit in the subendothelial–mesangial region, resulting in a more proliferative type of glomerulonephritis, and large CIC deposit exclusively in the mesangial region (Germuth and Rodriguez, 1973; R. C. Williams, 1980).

Participation of macrophages and monocytes in experimental CIC glomerulonephritis has established that in acute serum sickness large numbers of macrophages occur in the glomeruli at a time of immune complex elimination, and proteinuria develops with maximal glomerular hypercellularity. The course of disease was related to the capacity of the host antibody response, which determined daily antigen dose, and consequently the levels of CIC. Marcrophage involvement was closely related to glomerular injury (Holdsworth et al., 1980). Despite the use of metabolically intact cell receptors, surface-bound CIC have been noted to cause inhibition of polymorphonuclear leukocyte locomotion. This in vivo phagocytic paralysis may be of relevance to macrophages and other cells bearing receptors for Fc when they come in close contact with antibody-coated target cells that they cannot ingest or with immobilized CIC such as those found on basal membrances (Rabinovitch et al., 1975; Dahlgren and Elwing, 1983). Conversely, both the percentage of phagocytic cells and the phagocytic rate were found to be increased among monocytes. Also, increased phagocytosis was found in 14 of 29 (48%) patients with localized malignancies and Hodgkin's disease, as compared to 2 of 24 (8%) control patients. The increased phagocytic response was related neither to age, sex, ABO blood group, Rh status, nor to number of circulating lymphocytes, monocytes, or granulocytes (Ruco *et al.*, 1980).

Antibody isotype and class are known to influence the induction of phagocytosis: IgG1 and IgG3 are effective, while IgG2, IgG4, and IgM are less effective or incapable of triggering phagocytosis (Salinas and Wee, 1983). The ultimate role of CIC will be the triggering of phagocytosis by mononuclear phagocytic cells and/or localization and deposition at specific tissue sites to cause subsequent pathogenetic manifestations. The several target organs at which CIC deposition commonly occurs include (1) kidney glomeruli, with ensuing nephrotic syndrome (Lewis *et al.*, 1971); (2) brain choroid plexus (Atkins *et al.*, 1972); (3) skin and lung capillary beds (Eagan *et al.*, 1979; Tan and Kunkle, 1966); and (4) eye retinal vessels and ciliary bodies (Andrews *et al.*, 1977).

IV. PATHOGENETIC EFFECTS OF CIC

Further studies on regulation of immunocompetent cells in the expression of normal immune functions, as a component of the overall regulatory effector and mediator mechanisms, have been among the more recent important developments in basic immunology (Fauci, 1981).

Investigation of the role of CIC in host immunoregulation has been one area in which important advances have occurred. Many of the CIC-related immunopathogenetic effects known to be associated with a variety of disease manifestations are also detected in cancer patients with variable frequency. The specific sequence of tissue damage is not always evident in conditions of chronic immune complex deposition such as in cancer. Leukocytes, platelet clotting factors, complement, cell and serum enzymes, and mechanical effects of CIC all contribute to tissue damage. Renal injury is a prominent consequence of CIC pathogenetic effects, but endo- and pericarditis, vasculitis, arteritis, serositis, pneumonitis, skin involvement (urticaria, vasculitis), central neuropathies, coagulopathies (fibrinolysis, infarct, thrombosis, platelet disorders), Arthus reaction, and fever are also encountered. In addition to the systemic manifestations listed, local immune complex manifestations have been described in clinical and experimental conditions such as thyroiditis and antigen-induced arthritis.

Renal injury has been extensively studied experimentally. The pathogenetic mechanisms involved in CIC-elicited disease manifestations have been reviewed in detail (Cochrane and Koffler, 1973; Germuth and Rodriguez, 1973; Weigle, 1961; Unanue and Dixon, 1967).

The association of cancer with systemic manifestations resembling several autoimmune diseases represents an area of interest that has attracted considerable attention. Although the mechanisms involved are not fully understood, several reports suggest these syndromes as early clues to malignant transformation (Greenberg *et al.*, 1964; Lee *et al.*, 1966; Friou, 1974; Salinas *et al.*, 1978; Zimmerman *et al.*, 1982). The association of cancer and nephrotic syndrome was noted as a representative example (Penn, 1981). Neoplastic diseases accompanied by nephrotic syndrome have been associated with renal amyloid involvement (Richmond *et al.*, 1962) or renal vein thrombosis (De Swiet and Wells, 1957). Nephrosis secondary to renal amyloidosis has been associated with Hodgkin's disease, multiple myeloma, lymphosarcoma, and carcinomas (Lee *et al.*, 1966).

A. Mechanical Effects

Anatomical sites with high blood flow per unit mass of tissue are high-risk areas for deposition of CIC and concomitant pathogenetic effects. Frequently affected sites include the synovium, skin, uveal tract, choroid plexus, glomerulus, capillary beds of skin and lungs, ciliary bodies, and retinal vessels (Phillips *et al.*, Chapter 3, this volume; Theofilopoulos and Dixon, 1979). It has been noted that CIC size is a primary factor in determining pathogenetic manifestations. The mechanical effects of CIC size in determining renal-associated pathological manifestations have been noted (see Section III.C). In brief, differing CIC size-dependent mechanically determined manifestations of glomerulonephritis have been observed (R. C. Williams, 1980).

The pathogenesis of tissue injury elicited by CIC has been related to their complement-activating capacity. CIC formed at equivalence are efficient complement activators and are eliminated efficiently. Those formed at antigen excess have weak complement-activating capacity and tend to be eliminated with difficulty. As a result chemotactic peptides responsible for infiltration of polymorphonuclear leukocytes (PMN) are released. CIC have been known to stimulate PMN to release lysosomal proteases, which participate in tissue damage by direct hydrolysis of susceptible substrates or indirectly by the generation of chemotactic peptides from C5 (Weiss and Ward, 1982). In addition, PMN exposed to CIC could mediate tissue damage via generation of cytotoxic oxygen metabolites (Petrone *et al.*, 1981; McCormick *et al.*, 1981). The magnitude and course of vascular responses observed during inflammation were not dependent on phagocytosis but were at least in part mediated by prostaglandins. Thus drug-induced inhibition of leukocyte infiltration was secondary to vascular response (Issekutz and Bhimji, 1982).

B. Inflammatory Effects

The occurrence of soluble immune complexes in the circulation is due either to the presence of antigen and the endogenous production of antibodies or to the passive introduction of CIC. Biological manifestations involving mechanical, inflammatory, and immunoregulatory effects that lead to damage of tissue are expressed in the form of local or systemic immune complex disease. The association between "hypersensitivity" or small vessel cutaneous vasculitis and a variety of neoplastic diseases is widely recognized. An interrelation between the pathophysiologies of the two disease processes, malignancy and vasculitis, has been noted (Cupps and Fauci, 1982).

Animal models, mostly rabbits and mice, have been used to study the pathogenetic events of immune complex disease. These models included: (1) spontaneous animal diseases in New Zealand mice, (2) injection of antigens to produce acute experimental serum sickness, and (3) injection of preformed immune complexes into New Zealand black mice.

The Arthus reaction is a basic model of experimental local immune complex disease induced actively or passively in immunized animals or humans by intradermal injection of antigen. The sequence of inflammatory events that ensues at the injection site is dependent on the formation of immune complexes in small vessel walls, mainly venules. Complement fixation, increased vascular permeability, influx of PMN and subsequent mononuclear cell infiltration, erythema, edema, vasulitis, fibrinolysis, and eventual phagocytosis leading to necrosis were observed (Cochrane and Weigle, 1958; Rother *et al.*, 1964; Ward and Cochrane, 1965; Haakenstad and Mannik, 1977; Steward and Devey, 1981). "Serum diseases" developed at a time when antigen was being eliminated from the circulation just prior to the appearance of free antibody (Von Pirquet, 1911; Longscope and Rackemann, 1918). Recently, Langone *et al.* (1984) have suggested that C3a, C4a, and C5a anaphylatoxins play a role in the physiological responses observed in protein A-treated cancer patients, but not in the tumoricidal or toxic activities of this mode of serotherapy.

C. Immunoregulatory Effects

The effect of CIC on the immune response has long been recognized and—because of the potential pathophysiological role that CIC may play in such disorders as autoimmune disease and particularly cancer—the nature of this relationship has been extensively reviewed (Rossen and Morgan, 1981; Salinas *et al.*, 1981*b*, 1983*b*; Sinclair, 1979; Theofilopoulos and Dixon, 1979). In these conditions, CIC occurrence has been documented in the context of CIC disease activity and manifestations (Abrass *et al.*, 1980; Cairns *et al.*, 1980; Gleicher and Siegel, 1981; Gupta and Morton, 1981, 1983; Gupta *et al.*, 1979; Kristensen *et al.*, 1980; Rajnavolgki *et al.*, 1978; Feldman and Diener, 1970, 1972; Diener and Feldman, 1970). The administration of CIC in antigen excess usually enhanced the antibody response, while in antibody excess suppression occurred. Further studies with soluble and particulate antigens demonstrated enhanced immune response when antigen was presented as an immune complex, but not when CIC were formed in excess IgG antibody (Laissue *et al.*, 1971; Dennert, 1971; Houston *et al.*, 1974). The precise mechanisms by which CIC regulate host cellular and humoral response are as yet not fully understood. However, in most instances these interactions were the result of either large- or small-latticed soluble CIC interacting with cells or cell products via surface receptors, the net result being either activation or inhibition of the cellular functions of a vast array of cell types (Salinas and Wee, 1983; Lamers *et al.*, 1981). A synopsis of the specific immunoregulatory effects of CIC in the immune response is given in the following section.

1. Specific and Nonspecific Immunoregulatory Effects of CIC

The regulatory role of CIC in the host immune response is well established. Both cellular and humoral responses against autologous tumors were either enhanced or inhibited depending on several conditions, particularly the size and composition of CIC. Historically, CIC and their constituents have been prominent as factors alleged to be capable of inhibiting cell-mediated immune responses in several cancer types (Giuliano *et al.*, 1979; Ninnemann, 1981). However, other evidence has implicated CIC as mediators of an enhanced host immune response (Salinas and Wee, 1983). *In vitro* inhibitory or blocking effects of cancer patients' serum CIC on lymphocyte effector mechanisms have been reported for several malignancies (Rossen and Morgan, 1981; Salinas *et al.*, 1981a,d; Theofilopoulos and Dixon, 1977; Williams, 1980), with tumor antigens included or excluded from such a role (Ninnemann, 1981; Tanaka *et al.*, 1979; Giuliano *et al.*, 1979; Hellstrom *et al.*, 1974, 1985). A modulation of *in vitro* lymphocyte reactivity was observed in malignant melanoma upon removal of CIC by plasmapheresis. In keeping with earlier reports (Hersey, 1976), and enhancing of *in vitro* lymphocyte reactivity in advanced malignant melanoma patients by plasmapheresis removal of CIC has been observed by us (Salinas *et al.*, 1981a,d) and others (Phillips *et al.*, Chapter 3, this volume). More recently, we reported an inverse relationship between natural killer (NK)-cell activity and CIC concentration in breast carcinoma patients. This relationship was further supported by *in vitro* addition of autologous serum containing high (85–145 µg/ml) and low (<1 µg/mL) CIC concentrations to the NK-cell assay (Silver *et al.*, 1983).

Another important aspect of CIC-mediated immune response suppression has been the stimulation of plasma cells to produce anti-antibodies, particularly antiidiotypic antibodies. These antiidiotypic antibodies may result in the production of idiotypic–antiidiotypic immune complexes; act as unbound components, suppressing interaction between specific antibodies and counterpart antigens; suppress antibody production at the cellular level; and/or regulate T-cell responses by interacting with lymphocyte receptors (Rose and Lambert, 1980; Phillips *et al.*, Chapter 3). Koprowski *et al.* (1984) have recently suggested that an alternative effector mechanism for monoclonal serotherapy of cancer patients might involve a network of interacting antiidiotypic T and B cells directed against the monoclonal antibody used.

Recently, studies on the role of CIC in suppressing resistance to an intracellular pathogen, and the extent to which CIC can contribute to immunosuppression, have been highlighted. The possible common path of the different mechanisms proposed for infections caused by pathogenic microorganisms appears more than coincidental to those mechanisms observed in cancer (Virgin and Unaune, 1984).

In summary: Clearance of CIC is a function of the reticuloendothelial system. Several factors responsible for defective clearance have been noted, including CIC size and composition, and impairment and/or overloading of the function of phagocytes. It was also noted that (1) the mononuclear phagocyte system is markedly affected by neoplastic disease, (2) cutaneous anergy frequently occurs in cancer patients, (3) impairment of inflammatory response is often associated with neoplastic disease, and (4) increased monocyte phagocytic activity is directly related to the mass of the tumor tissue but not to the extent of the disease.

V. ROLE OF CIC AS TUMOR MARKERS

Identification of tumor markers by immunological means holds considerable promise for diagnostic applications because of the high degree of specificity and sensitivity involved. However, the majority of techniques presently available to quantitate CIC are by definition of no direct value for the clinical screening or diagnosis of cancer patients owing to their nonspecific nature (Salinas *et al.*, 1983*b*). In fact, similar conclusions were reported in several studies on CIC and human breast cancer. None of six assays evaluated has sufficient discriminatory capacity for diagnostic use (Herberman *et al.*, 1981), nor does the simultaneous use of three different assays in breast carcinoma and malignant melanoma appear practical for tumor screening (Krapf *et al.*, 1983). Despite the above arguments [reviewed by Salinas *et al.* (1983*b*)] C1q binding determination of CIC levels allowed for the differential diagnosis of benign and malignant breast disease (Papsidero *et al.*, 1979; Rossen *et al.*, 1977; Baldwin and Robins, 1980). A report of 211 melanoma patients tested for CIC suggested limited diagnostic value when two different assays were used (Ruel *et al.*, 1982). A collaborative evaluation of 19 different assays for detection of CIC in patients with lung cancer showed that, in 12 out of 19 assays, significantly higher CIC levels were detected in cancer patients than in controls. Assays based on CIC interaction with Fc receptors of different cells discriminated CIC occurrence in cancer and control sera. Accurate classification of individuals tested was achieved by discriminant analysis of three selected assays. However, correlations of results of individual sera obtained by different assays were poor (Fust *et al.*, 1981).

Our initial experience with single- and serial-sample CIC determinations demonstrated that, for effective management of patients with immune-complex-associated diseases, knowledge of not only the number of CIC, but also of their composition and size was required (Salinas and Wee, 1983; Salinas et al., 1980b). In addition, the need for measurement of more than one reactant in cancer patients was highlighted. Analysis of serum anti-xenogeneic oncofetal antigen activity in relation to tumor burden in both single- and serial-sample studies suggested a complex interrelationship of antigen, antibody, and immune complex. The resulting immune stimulation or inhibition is better evaluated by the examination of more than one reactant (Salinas et al., 1980b).

Regardless of the value of tumor markers for diagnosis, they deserve greater or at least equal merit for the assessment of prognosis, or as monitors of tumor burden for following disease recurrence, detection of early recurrence, or postsurgical follow-up—applications in which markers need not be tumor-specific. Indeed, tumor markers with relatively broader specificity need to be identified and evaluated for use in human cancer, and CIC represent one such class of marker (Silver et al., 1979; Salinas et al., 1983b).

In view of recent reports that provide evidence of association of CIC with an unfavorable disease course, and the impact that these new developments may have on the clinical management of cancer patients' treatment, the significance of CIC as a tumor marker in the following clinical circumstances will be discussed: (1) assessment of clinical prognosis, (2) detection of early recurrence, (3) postsurgical follow-up, and (4) monitoring of tumor burden changes.

A. Prognosis

Any attempt to evaluate the significance of CIC for the assessment of clinical status and prognosis in cancer patients is confronted with reported inconsistencies in relating these variables (Baldwin and Robins, 1980; Herberman et al., 1981; Rossen and Morgan, 1981; Ruel et al., 1982; Salinas et al., 1983b). Some of these inconsistencies may be explained by the nature of reacted antigen, immunoglobulin isotype, relative and absolute concentrations of reactants, and CIC size (Salinas and Wee, 1983). Other contributing factors that merit attention are the lack of an integrated evaluation of all immune reactants involved in the host response to tumors resulting in a less than ideal assessment of CIC; the fact that quantitation of one component may not be a sufficiently predictable monitor of clinical prognosis; and the relative concentration of free to bound antigen, a key factor in the dynamic balance of CIC formation, deposition, and breakdown (Ray et al., 1982). Decreased C1q binding was observed in patients with disease-free intervals of at least a year, whereas in those breast cancer patients with poor prognosis CIC remained elevated (Baldwin and Robins, 1980). Similar findings were observed in a large study that compared pre- and posttreatment CIC levels with clinical outcome a year posttreatment (Hoffken *et al.*, 1977). In ovarian carcinoma patients, CIC were elevated only in those cases where tumor had recurred (Poulton *et al.*, 1978).

In acute myeloid leukemia, acute lymphatic leukemia, and chronic myeloid leukemia there was an association of CIC with the acute phase of disease, and this was more distinct when CIC were measured serially. In 13 cases CIC became undetectable upon induction of complete remission. The detection of CIC appeared to be of prognostic signficance in patients in complete remission for more than one year and whose serum was negative during several months in early remission (Carpentier and Miescher, 1983). The relationship between the presence of CIC and the histological type of the tumor with poor prognosis has been reported in Hodgkin's disease (Amlot *et al.*, 1978). Prognostic value of CIC levels in malignant skin melanoma has been demonstrated by a correlation between CIC activity, as measured by two assays, and relapse of stage I and II patients (Kristensen *et al.*, 1980).

A synopsis of pertinent studies concerning the assessment of prognosis from CIC determination is listed in Table XIV. The single most important observation emerging from the experimental clinical evidence reviewed is the correlation of poor prognosis or unfavorable course of disease with increased levels of CIC in cancer patients.

B. Early Recurrence

A tumor marker that will identify patients at high risk of recurrence will be an extremely useful monitor in the management of cancer patients. Interestingly, in one report of increased CIC levels in dogs with benign and malignant breast disease, CIC levels returned to normal in all dogs with benign disease but in only a fraction (33%) of those with breast carcinoma. Those with persistent elevation of CIC were at greater risk of developing recurrent metastasis (Gordon *et al.*, 1980). Similar findings in 86 children with Hodgkin's disease showed that prior to therapy 81% of the children had elevated CIC levels. During treatment 33% were still positive, and a year posttreatment 37% remained above normal levels. At relapse, 63% had higher CIC levels than at earlier periods (Brandeis *et al.*, 1978). In a sequential study, 9 of 14 patients with leukemia showed CIC occurrence 3 weeks to 5.5 months prior to relapse (Carpentier and Miescher, 1983). Our studies on malignant melanoma patients demonstrated that changes in CIC levels frequently antedated other objective clinical evidence of relapse by up to 4.5 months (Salinas *et al.*, 1980b,c), an observation that has been subsequently confirmed by others (Ruel *et al.*, 1982). In addition, a retrospective study of breast cancer patients showed that CIC levels correlated with the clinicopathological prognosis of the tumor and that CIC determinations could be useful for estimating prognosis and for identification of patients with residual tumor (Hoffken *et al.*, 1977).

Table XIV. CIC in the Assessment of Prognosis

Disease	Finding	Reference
Breast carcinoma	Increased CIC reflect poor prognosis	Hoffken et al. (1977), Salinas et al. (1982b)
	Decreased CIC associated with disease-free interval; elevated CIC reflect poor prognosis.	Baldwin and Robins (1980)
	Eighty percent of postsurgery patients with reduced CIC were disease-free 1 year later.	Horvath et al. (1982)
	22/24 increased CIC decreased postmastectomy; CIC reduction correlated with mastectomy.	Israel et al. (1977)
Malignant breast disease in dogs	Persistent CIC-elevated subjects were at high risk of recurrence.	Gordon et al. (1980)
Ovarian carcinoma	CIC was elevated only in cases of recurrence.	Poulton et al. (1978)
Acute lymphatic, chronic myeloid, and acute myeloid leukemia	Association of CIC with acute phase of disease. CIC appear to be of prognostic significance for subjects in complete remission. Median survival time (5 years) was significantly lower in patients with CIC.	Carpentier and Miescher (1983)
Hodgkin's disease	CIC occurrence and poor prognosis.	Amlot et al. (1978)
Malignant melanoma	Correlation of CIC activity with relapse in stages I and II.	Kristensen et al. (1980)
Bronchial carcinoma	Patients with increased first-test CIC associated with rapid growth of recurrent tumor.	Rossen et al. (1977)
Lung carcinoma	CIC levels correlated with survival time; better prognostic indicator than performance status.	Poskitt and Poskitt (1979)

C. Postsurgical Follow-up

The clinical signficance of CIC levels as a tumor marker during postsurgical follow-up has not been the subject of a systematic study; however, pieces of scattered evidence have been consistently reported. Decreased C1q binding was observed in a large study in which pre- and postoperative CIC levels were compared with clinical outcome two year's postmastectomy, and those patients that remained CIC-elevated had a poor prognosis. In patients without lymph node involvement of surgery, CIC returned to normal levels within a year of primary tumor removal. Conversely, patients with lymph node involvement, and those with recurrent disease or fatal outcome within two years postsurgery, remained CIC-elevated (Baldwin and Robins, 1980; Hoffken *et al.*, 1977). A study of 16 breast carcinomas using the complement consumption test showed that in 12 of 15 patients (80%) having reduced CIC levels after surgery, no tumor could be detected one year postmastectomy (Horvath *et al.*, 1982). Combined applications of CIC in detection of early recurrence, postsurgical follow-up, prognosis, and monitoring of tumor burden are often reported; for example, carcinoembryonic antigen (CEA)-CIC levels were markers with regard to tumor burden and prognosis in gastrointestinal carcinoma (Staab *et al.*, 1980). The occurrence of CEA-CIC during postsurgical follow-up appeared as an indicator of recurrence in 32 out of 55 relapse cases, all of whom developed metastatic spread of the disease (Staab *et al.*, 1980).

D. Monitoring of Tumor Burden

A consistent clinical pattern of decreased survival in those cancer patients with persistently elevated CIC has been observed (Crane *et al.*, 1984). This observation accounts for the renewed surge of interest in the relevance of CIC levels for monitoring therapy and their relationship to tumor burden. An earlier and still common approach consisted of correlating CIC levels to disease stages in cancer patients. There has been a great deal of variation among individual patients' results, even among those in the same disease stage (Dorval and Pross, 1983). The degree of inconsistency observed with this approach is best reflected by the contradicting reports of both significant and negative correlations between CIC levels and disease stages among cancer patients (Gupta *et al.*, 1979; Ruel *et al.*, 1982; Rossen and Morgan, 1981; Dorval and Pross, 1983). It has thus become evident that CIC analysis may not be fully applicable to the clinical staging of cancer patients. In a number of these patients, serum samples were obtained after surgical excision of tumor, effectively reducing their tumor burden to a possible minimal tumor load not reflected in their initial staging. These results, as well as a simultaneous reevaluation of CIC analysis on the basis of tumor burden, have demonstrated that incidence of CIC correlates with tumor burden rather than clinical stage of disease. Any attempt to study the relationship between CIC and tumor burden requires careful consideration, to include only those patients having objectively evaluable tumor burden and histopathological confirmation of diagnosis (Salinas *et al.*, 1981b). The specific details of such groupings may vary according to the tumor types involved, and our reported groupings for malignant melanoma have been earlier noted (Salinas *et al.*, 1980b) (see also

Section III.A). Similar groupings have been reported for breast (Silver *et al.*, 1981a) and ovarian (Silver *et al.*, 1981*b*) carcinoma patients.

Contrary to prevailing reports that indicated significantly lower CIC levels among cancer patients with no evidence of disease than in those with metastatic disease (Theofilopoulos *et al.*, 1977; Theopoulos and Dixon, 1979), our earlier report suggested a slightly different picture for malignant melanoma. Patients with no evidence of disease (Group I) and patients with advanced disease (Group III) had significantly lower CIC levels than patients who had intermediate tumor burden (Group II), as measured by FLC-RIA (Salinas *et al.*, 1981*b*). The relationship between CIC level and tumor burden was not linear, and simultaneous evaluation of tumor-associated antibodies and CIC levels more clearly reflected patients' tumor burden (Salinas *et al.*, 1980*b*). These results emphasize the dynamic relationship of tumor burden to antigen concentration, antibody activity, and CIC levels. The higher incidence of CIC levels in Group II patients with moderate tumor burden was an expression of antigen and antibody molecular ratios close to equivalence. Patients with low tumor burden (Group I) had immune complexes in antibody excess, and those with high tumor burden (Group III) had immune complexes in antigen excess. Subsequent support and confirming evidence came from our own group as well as independent groups using different assays (Gupta *et al.*, 1979; Gupta and Morton, 1981; Gauci *et al.*, 1981; Kristensen *et al.*, 1980).

Since the relationship between CIC and tumor burden was not linear in malignant melanoma sera, we analyzed tumor burden and its relationship to antigen concentration, size, and composition of CIC in serum samples of selected melanoma patients. SGF and PAGE analyses were used to determine the size of CIC Serum samples of patients from Group I with no evidence of disease contained medium (10–15 S)-size CIC; Group II patients had small (7–9 S), medium, and large (>16 S) CIC, and Group III patients with advanced disease had small and large CIC (Salinas *et al.*, 1981*c*). Subsequent studies on the kinetics of immune complex formation and breakdown were carried out *in vitro* and have been discussed in Section III.A. Gupta *et al.* (1979; Gupta and Morton, 1981) had provided similar evidence by the use of a different approach, which led support to our interpretation that the fluctuating CIC levels observed in cancer patients could be due to changes in tumor burden or changes in the dynamic equilibrium of immune reactants, which are frequently observed after therapeutic interventions (Salinas *et al.*, 1983*b*). Further supporting evidence has recently become available through studies on human T-cell lymphoma and malignant melanoma. CIC-associated viral antigens have been reported to be related not only to stage of disease but also to number of tumor cells in patients with human T-cell leukemia/lymphoma (Schupbach *et al.*, 1984). Morgan *et al.* (1984) suggest that measurement of MAA in patients' sera may be useful for monitoring tumor burden.

With few exceptions, no systematic approach has been undertaken to assess the influence of therapeutic interventions on CIC levels in cancer patients. A report on 67 neuroblastoma patients noted close correlation of CIC levels with stage of disease and treatment. Increased CIC were often observed in samples taken "before treatment," with decreasing CIC noted over the course of treatment (Brandeis *et al.*, 1978). A report on 87 children with Hodgkin's disease noted the correlation of CIC levels with clinical stage, histological type, sex, age, and treatment. Significant were the changes of CIC levels during disease activity and following treatment. Prior to therapy, 81% of children had elevated CIC levels, which were still elevated in 33% during treatment. A year after treatment 37% remained CIC levels elevated, and at relapse 63% had CIC that were higher than at other periods (Brandeis *et al.*, 1978). In ovarian carcinoma CIC were found only in cases of tumor recurrence (Poulton *et al.*, 1978). The association of CIC with the acute phase of disease was particularly evident when CIC were measured serially in chronic myeloid leukemia (Carpentier and Miescher, 1983). A recent study on lung cancer patients noted a marked correlation of CIC levels with survival time, suggesting CIC levels as a better prognostic factor than performance status at the time of diagnosis. Serial CIC levels decreased concomitantly with response to therapy, and often increased prior to objective clinical evidence of disease progression (Poskitt and Poskitt, 1979). When CIC levels in malignant lymphoma were examined in relation to both the extent of the disease and the presence of general symptoms, it appeared that CIC detection was more often related to dissemination of the disease than to systemic symptoms (Carpentier and Miescher, 1983).

Reported inconsistencies in correlating CIC levels with tumor burden in cancer patients most likely stem from a number of related factors which may be summarized as follows: (1) Expression of immune response complexity, (2) heterogeneity of TAA involved, (3) different metastatic behavior as well as growth of malignant cellular populations, (4) intrinsic characteristics of immune complexes, and (5) less than optimal tumor burden grouping.

An overview of clinical studies on CIC levels and their relation to tumor burden and disease stages showed that, with but few exceptions, there has been a lack of systematic approaches to this important question. In addition, in those studies where extra efforts were made to evaluate patients' tumor load objectively, useful clinical correlations of CIC levels with the extent of tumor burden were observed (Salinas *et al.*, 1984; Gupta and Morton, 1981). Similar clinical correlations of CIC levels not only to stage of disease but also to number of tumor cells (Schupbach *et al.*, 1984) and to antigen concentration (Salinas *et al.*, 1983b) have been established. Although a considerable number of useful clinical correlations with CIC levels have recently been reported (Carpentier and Miescher, 1983), plenty of ground remains to be explored.

VI. THERAPEUTIC ROLE OF IMMUNE COMPLEXES

A. Rationale and Major Findings

Some strains of *Staphylococcus aureus* contain protein A as a cell wall component. Protein A was found to bind Fc receptor for IgG from most mammalian species (Forsgren and Sjöquist, 1966) and CIC (Kessler, 1975). The potential role of protein A in cancer therapy has been derived from its use for the removal of specific and nonspecific immune blocking factors. Many approaches to remove blocking factors from patients' sera have been directed toward removal of CIC. Plasmapheresis (Isbister *et al.*, 1975; Salinas *et al.*, 1981a; Serrou and Rosenfeld, 1981) and/or extracorporeal immunoadsorption have resulted in subjective and objective clinical response in tumor-bearing patients and experimental animals. These attempts subsequently stimulated clinical trials for cancer therapy in animals (Terman *et al.*, 1980; Ray *et al.*, 1981; F. R. Jones *et al.*, 1980; Holohan *et al.*, 1982) and in humans (Bansal *et al.*, 1978; Ray *et al.*, 1982; Terman *et al.*, 1981; Bensinger *et al.*, 1982; MacKintosh *et al.*, 1983; Masserschmidt *et al.*, 1982) with advanced carcinomas of the breast, colon, and lung and other tumor types. Overall toxic effects evaluated by phase I studies ranged from lethal (Masserschmidt *et al.*, 1982) to severe but manageable (Terman *et al.*, 1981; Ray *et al.*, 1982) to moderate (MacKintosh *et al.*, 1983). More frequently noted toxic effects included fever, chills, hypotension, tachycardia, and bronchospasm. Although it is not realistic to assess response rates in phase I studies, reported response rates ranged from 0% (Masserschmidt *et al.*, 1982) to 60% (Terman *et al.*, 1981) in series involving five or more patients.

A considerable amount of data has been generated in this area by several groups of investigators, and relevant clinical and technical implications can be drawn from this avalanche of information. Some reported developments included the following: (1) Materials used for *ex vivo* perfusions of plasma over protein A varied from heat-killed or formalin-stabilized *S. aureus* Cowan I alone (Bansal *et al.*, 1978; Ray *et al.*, 1982) to protein A adsorbed onto collodion charcoal (Terman *et al.*, 1981) or protein A covalently linked to an inert silica matrix (Bensinger *et al.*, 1982) or agarose (MacKintosh *et al.*, 1983). (2) The volumes of plasma infused ranged from attempted total exchange to volumes as low as 20 ml. (3) The quantities of protein A used varied from few milliliters to no more than necessary to remove IgG from 20% of the patient's plasma in the most aggressive protocols. (4) The efficacy of these manipulations, the techniques for relating the best reagents to use, and the mechanisms of action involved are all largely unclear. (5) Information concerning the immunologic basis of these treatments is limited.

Most approaches have been aimed toward removal of CIC. Yet the efficiency of these procedures in the removal of CIC—as well as other specific or nonspecific factors (T-cell-derived suppressor factors) that could interfere with the patient's immune response—remains to be elucidated. More interesting is the possibility, generally accepted, that the observed effects may be secondary to activation of unknown factors or even to leaching of various components of the immuno-adsorbing columns used. Also, other staphylococcal toxins that may be involved in the reported effects of protein A have not been excluded. Despite the impressive tumor regression noted in a high proportion of subjects in animal studies (Terman *et al.*, 1980; Holohan *et al.*, 1982), the results in patients with advanced cancer demonstrated modest but definitive objective response rates (11%) without complete remission in all the trials reported at a recent NCI (USA) symposium on immunoadsorption therapy (Oldham, 1984). Until now, the disparity between results from preclinical and human trials has not been successfully explained by the available data.

B. Experience with Plasma Exchange and Plasmapheresis

One of the earlier therapeutic approaches directed toward the physical removal or reduction of specific and nonspecific blocking factors interfering with the patient's immune response was the use of plasma exchange. Plasmapheresis is a powerful means for modifying the intravascular compartment; however, as a result of the body's homeostatic mechanisms, the ensuing effects are often unpredictable (Salinas *et al.*, 1983b). Although there have been encouraging reports on the effects of multiple plasma exchange regimens as single- or multimodality therapies for patients with disseminated cancer, their sucess in cancer has not been as dramatic as that of similar regimens reported for collagen–vascular diseases and glomerulonephritis (Salinas *et al.*, 1983b). Partial response to repeated plasma exchanges has been reported in 8 of 23 and 1 of 4 cancer patients treated (Israel *et al.*, 1977; Hersey *et al.*, 1976). The efficacy of plasmapheresis alone or in combination with extracorporeal immunoadsorption or other treatment modalities has since been tested by several groups (Salinas *et al.*, 1983b). However, the overall limited patient response has not encouraged extensive pursuit of this modality.

C. Experience with Protein A Immunoadsorption

The technique of selectively removing CIC and/or other factors from plasma by use of a ligand has been aimed at reducing factors that are likely to block the host immune response to tumors. Although the concept is not new (Hellström and Hellström, 1974), it achieved renewed interest in recent years with the advent of immunoadsorption therapy. The considerable amount of data generated by several investigators lent support to the concept of a humoral effect dependent on interaction of patients' sera with protein A as an alternative component responsible for clinically observed tumoricidal effects. However, evidence supporting a tumoricidal or toxic activity role of protein A-generated anaphylatoxins has been reported (Langone *et al.*, 1984). For a detailed account of experimental and clinical idiosyncracies the reader is referred to Chapters 5–8 of this volume.

1. Experimental Results

The earlier findings of Steele *et al.* (1974) provided a rationale for subsequent development of immunoperfusion procedures using protein A to remove plasma CIC by an extracorporeal technique. Capitalizing on these observations, Terman *et al.* (1980) reported partial tumor regression upon protein A immunoadsorbent treatment in several dogs with spontaneous mammary carcinoma. In those dogs receiving a similar immunoadsorption regime, but followed by cystosine arabinose, a dramatic tumor-necrotizing response was reported. These results suggested a synergistic effect of the treatment components. Conversely, no beneficial results were achieved by use of protein A-deficient *S. aureus* Wood 46. On-line plasma adsorption of dogs with a transplantable canine venereal tumor led to impressive tumor regression—tumor volume attritions from 24 to 99% (Ray *et al.*, 1981). There was induction of partial response in five of ten dogs with spontaneous mammary carcinoma upon immunoadsorption of autologous plasma with protein A. No complete regression was noted, and the response appeared to depend on the site of tumor. CIC were more effectively removed from the "responder group" (67% removal) than from the "nonresponders" (10% removal) (Holohan *et al.*, 1982). F. R. Jones *et al.* (1980) used immunoadsorption in an attempt to remove CIC in leukemic cats, and observed reversal of feline leukemia viremia with reduction in circulating lymphoblasts. Clinical improvement was noted in three of five cats that had been spontaneously infected with feline leukemia virus and then perfused over heat-killed and formalin-fixed protein A.

2. Clinical Results

The single most prominent characteristic of the serotherapeutic studies has been the diversity of procedures and reagents used.

The pioneering report of Bansal *et al.* (1978) described a metastatic colon carcinoma patient with peritoneal carcinomatosis perfused 20 times over an on-line continuous flow system over *S. aureus* paste. Tumoricidal response, tumor regression, and histologic evidence of tumor response were observed. Terman *et al.* (1981) reported a series of five breast carcinoma patients treated with a cartridge system containing protein A immobilized over a charcoal collodion matrix. Toxicity was similar to that noted by Bansal *et al.*, and symptoms included chills, fever, hypotension, tachycardia, nausea, and vomiting. Four patients had reduction in tumor size, viz. three partial and one minimal response. However, the role played by earlier therapies received by the patients was not fully clear, nor was it clear whether the effects observed were due to removal or to leaching. Bensinger *et al.* (1982) studied five breast carcinoma patients treated with large quantities of purified protein A covalently coupled in inert silica matrix as the immunoadsorbent. By means of extracorporeal procedures, they observed a partial remission in three patients.

MacKintosh *et al.* (1983) have reported on 14 patients receiving autologous plasma treatments using off-line perfusion over protein A bound to Sepharose-4B. Objective tumor regressions have been observed in 2 of 12 evaluable patients, while an additional 5 patients had stabilization of disease for 4–12 weeks. Currently, this group has 44 patients in phase I trials who have received approximately 600 infusions of protein A-treated autologous plasma (see Chapter 7 in this volume) with no unmanageable toxicity associated with therapy. Ray *et al.* (1981, 1982) have reported perfusion in several patients using immunoadsorption with intact protein A-containing nonviable *S. aureus*. Clinical improvement was reported in two of these treated patients: in one multiple myeloma patient and one patient with chronic lymphocytic leukemia (see also Chapter 5 in this volume). Purified protein A covalently linked to polyacrylamide-coated glass beads has been used in an *ex vivo* immunoadsorption treatment of 11 patients with solid tumors and three patients with thrombotic thrombocytopenic purpura (Korec *et al.*, 1984). A modest response rate has been reported; three patients showed partial tumor regression that lasted 3–6 months. Protein A charcoal matrix has been used in an *ex vivo* immunoadsorption study in six patients with advanced breast or brain cancer. A strong mitogenic response of perfused patients' plasma to normal lymphocytes was reported (Bertram *et al.*, 1984).

Two trials at NCI (USA) have attempted to reproduce the rather impressive antitumor effects reported earlier by Terman *et al.* (1981). The initial trial, a test in dogs with mammary carcinoma, involved the use of formalin-killed protein A in the perfusion system. Thereafter five patients were treated, with approximately 20–60% of total plasma volume perfused over protein A (Masserschmidt *et al.*, 1982). No antitumor response was observed, but there was formidable toxicity. Cardiorespiratory failure was felt to be the contributory cause of death in two patients. The trial was stopped after five patients, owing to the severe toxicity observed. These results were in contrast to the earlier studies reported by the Baylor group. Since the observed discrepancies may have been due to differing technical procedures, a second trial was initiated at NCI (USA). This time special consideration was given to ensuring reproduction of conditions and patient population. Extensive immunological monitoring was performed. No significant tumor response was observed in the first four patients after twelve treatments. In the absence of toxicity, the dose was increased. Neither toxicity nor antitumor effects were noted. However, discrepancies in the production of protein A by the manufacturer may have subtracted bioactive components that were found in earlier preparations (Fer *et al.*, 1984; see also Chapter 8).

In summary, the removal of CIC and other factors that inhibit antitumor immunity appears to be an apparently straightforward approach to cancer therapy. Several groups have documented *in vitro* and *in vivo* tumor response to protein A-bearing material in a variety of experimental and clinical approaches. However, plasma immunoadsorption in clinical human cancer patients has thus far not achieved the beneficial effects noted in animal studies. Data from feline leukemia studies had provided a clear-cut correlation between decreased CIC levels and clinical response. Although some provocative results have been documented in humans, the value of this form of therapy still remains to be validated.

VII. OVERVIEW AND CONCLUDING REMARKS

Despite the expression of TAA and its frequent recognition by the host to induce tumor rejection, tumor growth and its concomitant manifestations invariably threaten host survival. Circulating tumor antigens alone or in the form of CIC interfere with the development of an effective immune response. Although the specific mechanisms of this inhibition have not been fully defined, CIC, including those containing oncofetal and idiotypic antigens, have been implicated as important immune response modulators.

The occurrence and increased incidence CIC in cancer patients have been established. Despite assay idiosyncracies and discrepancies in the interpretation of results, CIC have been frequently detected at increased levels in cancer patients. A variety of characteristics of CIC appear to contribute to their immuno-regulatory activity, including size, concentration, and nature of the component antigen and antibody. In addition to direct immunoregulation, CIC play a significant pathogenetic role in human neoplasia. This is often expressed as local or systemic injury, largely mediated by the kinin, complement, or coagulation systems. Injuries result from mechanical, inflammatory, and immune blocking or enhancing by specific and nonspecific factors or cells.

The most immediate potential clinical application of immune complex technology is in the monitoring of cancer patients. CIC concentrations have been clearly related to overall prognosis. Further study with special attention to immune complex size and composition may permit more specific monitoring for prognosis, early recurrence, or evaluation of tumor burden changes.

The therapeutic benefit of reducing CIC and other blocking factors in the tumor-bearing host is to reinstate an effective tumor immunity otherwise inhibited as a result of suppressor cell response to circulating mediator factors. The physical removal of CIC and other specific and nonspecific factors has been effected through plasma exchange or plasmapheresis; overall low response rates have discouraged further intensive investigation. An alternative approach using *S. aureus* protein A as a ligand to remove CIC and other factors selectively has been developed; and is aimed at reducing factors likely to block an otherwise effective immune response to tumors. Protein A, purified or otherwise, has been used alone or immobilized on bacteria, collodion charcoal, Sepharose, or inert silica matrix in several serotherapeutic protocols to treat cancer in humans or experimental animals. The exact mechanisms involved and the efficiency of the perfusion procedures used have yet to be fully determined. The disparity between results from preclinical and clinical trials has not yet been successfully explained by available data. Whether the demonstrated *in vitro* or *in vivo* tumor responses are to the effects of the protein A materials used in the immunoadsorption procedures, to removal of CIC blocking factors, to tumor site complement activation, or to leaching of noncovalent materials or bioreacting components remains to be determined. While any of the above noted alternatives could be responsible for the observed beneficial effects, a combined, synergistic, or bioreactive mechanism may be operative in different settings. Although immunoadsorption with protein A has resulted in demonstrable tumor necrosis and some provocative results have been reported in man, detailed information on mechanisms of action is required before this therapeutic modality can be established as an effective cancer treatment.

ACKNOWLEDGMENTS

This work has been supported in part by a grant from the National Cancer Institute of Canada. We thank Linda Wood for her secretrial expertise. Figures 1, 3, and 4 reprinted with permission from Salinas *et al.* (1984, 1985), copyright Pergamon Press.

VIII. REFERENCES

Aarden, L. A., 1977, Pathogenesis of immune complexes, in: *Non-articular Forms of Rheumatoid Arthritis* (T. A. N. Feltkamp, ed.), pp. 15–36, Stafleu, Leiden.

Abrass, C. K., Nies, K. M., Louie, J. S., Border, W. A., and Glassock, R. J., 1980, Correlation and predictive accuracy of circulating immune complexes with disease activity in patients with systemic lupus erythematosus, *Arthritis Rheum.* 23:273.

Agnello, V., 1981, Immune complex assays: The first ten years (editorial), *Ann. Int. Med.* 94:266.

Amlot, P. L., Pussel, D., Slaney, J. M., and Williams, B. D., 1978, Correlation between immune complexes and prognostic factors in Hodgkin's disease, *Clin. Exp. Immunol.* 31:166.

Andrews, B. S., McIntosh, J., Petts, V., and Penny, R., 1977, Circulating immune complexes in retinal vasculitis, *Clin. Exp. Immunol.* 29:23.

Atkins, C. J., Kondon, J. J., Quismorio, F. P., and Friou, G. J., 1972, The choroid plexus in systemic lupus erythematosus, *Ann. Int. Med.* 76:65.

Baldwin, R. W., and Robins, R. A., 1980, Circulating immune complexes in cancer, in: *Cancer Markers* (S. Sell, ed.), pp. 507–531, Humana Press, Clifton, New Jersey.

Bansal, S. C., Bansal, B. R., Thomas, H. L., Siegel, P. D., Rhoads, J. E., Cooper, D. R., Terman, D. S., and Mark, R., 1978, *Ex vivo* removal of serum IgG in a patient with colon carcinoma, *Cancer* 42:1.

Barnett, E. V., Knutson, D. W., Abrass, C. K., Chia, D. S., Young, L. S., and Liebling, M. R., 1979, Circulating immune complexes: Their immunohistochemistry, detection and importance, *Ann. Intern. Med.* 91:430.

Benacerraf, B., Sebestyen, M., and Cooper, N. S., 1959, The clearance of antigen–antibody complexes from the blood by the reticuloendothelial system, *J. Immunol.* 82:131.

Bensinger, W. I., Kinet, J. B., Hennen, G., Franckenne, F., Schaus, C., Saint-Remy, M., Hoyoux, P., and Mahieu, P., 1982, Plasma perfused over immobilized protein A for breast cancer, *N. Engl. J. Med.* 306:935.

Bertram, J. H., Hengst, C. D., and Mitchell, M. S., 1984, Staphylococcal protein A immuno-adsorptive column induces mitogenicity in perfused plasma, *J. Biol. Resp. Modif.* 3:235.

Berzofsky, J. A., and Berkower, I. J., 1984, Antigen–antibody interaction, in: *Fundamental Immunology* (W. E. Paul, ed.), pp. 595–644, Raven Press, New York.

Bhattacharya, M., Chatterjee, S. K., Barlow, J. J., and Fuji, H., 1982, Monoclonal antibodies recognizing tumor-associated antigen of human ovarian mucinous cystadenocarcinomas, *Cancer Res.* 42:1650.

Brandeis, W. E., Welson, L., Wang, Y., Good, R. A., and Day, N. K., 1978, Circulating immune complexes in sera of children with neuroblastoma, *Clin. Invest.* 62:1201.

Brennan, F. M., Grace, S. A., and Elson, C. J., 1983, Preparation of covalent IgG complexes of defined size and their clearance from the circulation of mice, *J. Immunol. Methods* 56:149.

Brown, T. S., Russel, M. W., and Mestecky, J., 1982, Hepatobiliary transport of IgA immune complexes: Molecular and cellular aspects, *J. Immunol.* 128:2183.

Cairns, S. A., London, A., and Mallick, N. P., 1980, The value of three immune complex assays in the management of systemic lupus erythematosus: An assessment of immune complex level, size and immunochemical properties in relation to disease activity and manifestations, *Clin. Exp. Immunol.* 40:273.

Carpentier, N. A., and Miescher, P. A., 1983, The clinical relevance of circulating immune complexes in cancer, kidney transplantation and pregnancy, in: *Immunobiology of Transplantation, Cancer and Pregnancy* (P. K. Ray, ed.), pp. 375–408, Pergamon Press, New York.

Casali, P., and Lambert, P. H., 1979, Purification of soluble immune complexes using poly-methylmethacrylate beads coated with conglutinin or C1q, *Clin. Exp. Immunol.* 37:295.

Catropia, J. P., Gutterman, J. V., Hersh, E. M., Granatek, C. H., and Mavligit, G. M., 1976, Antigen expression and cell surface properties of human leukemia blasts, *Ann. N.Y. Acad. Sci.* 276:146.

Ceriani, R. L., Sasaki, M., Sussman, H., Wara, W. M., and Blank, E. W., 1982, Circulating human mammary epithelial antigens in breast cancer, *Proc. Natl. Acad. Sci. USA* 79:5420.

Chee, D. O., Gupta, R. B., and Morton, D. L., 1983, Humoral response of melanoma patients to two different tumor-associated antigens, *J. Surg. Oncol.* 23:228.

Chia, D., Barnett, E. V., Yamagata, J., Knutson, D., Restivo, C., and Furst, D., 1979, Quantitation and characterization of soluble immune complexes precipitated from sera by polyethylene glycol (PEG), *Clin. Exp. Immunol.* 60:399.

Chu, T. M., Maidment, B. M., Koestler, T. P., Papsidero, L. D., Inaji, H., Creghan, G., Killian, C. S., Loor, R. M., Douglas, H. O., Berjian, R., and Nemoto, T., 1983, Immune complexes and cancer, in: *Immunodiagnosis* (R. Alosi and J. Hyun, eds.), pp. 259–268, Alan R. Liss, New York.

Cochrane, C. G., and Koffler, D., 1973, Immune complex disease in experimental animals and man, *Adv. Immunol.* 16:185.

Cochrane, C. G., and Weigle, W. O., 1958, The cutaneous reaction to soluble antigen–antibody complexes: A comparison with the Arthus phenomenon, *J. Exp. Med.* 108:591.

Crane, M. M., Rossen, R. D., McCredie, K. B., and Trujillo, J. M., 1984, Association of circulating immune complexes with cytogenetic abnormalities but not with prognosis in acute nonlymphocytic leukemia, *Cancer Res.* 44:3125.

Cronin, W. J., Dorsett, B. H., and Ioachim, H. L., 1982, Isolation of lung carcinoma-associated antibodies from immune complexes and production of heterologous antisera, *Cancer Res.* 42:292.

Cupps, T. R., and Fauci, A. S., 1982, Neoplasm and systemic vasculitis: A case report, *Arthritis Rheum.* 25:475.

Currie, A., 1973, Circulating antigen as inhibitor of tumor immunity in man, *Br. J. Cancer* (Suppl. 1) 28:153.

Dahlgren, C., and Elwing, H., 1983, Inhibition of polymorphonuclear leukocyte locomotion by surface bound antigen–antibody complex, *Immunology* 49:329.

D'Amelio, R., Brighouse, G., Barnet, M., and Lambert, P. H., 1981, Antigen-specific detection of soluble immune complexes in conglutinin binding assays, *Clin. Exp. Immunol.* 45:283.

Day, N. K., Winfield, J. B., Gee, T., Winchester, R. J., Teshima, H., and Kunkel, H. G., 1976, Evidence for immune complexes involved in antilymphocyte antibodies associated with hypocomplementemia in chronic lymphocytic leukemia (CLL), *Clin. Exp. Immunol.* 26:189.

Delire, M., Cambiaso, C. L., and Masson, P. L., 1978, Circulating immune complexes in infants fed on cow's milk, *Nature* 272:632.

Dennert, G., 1971, The mechanism of antibody-induced stimulation and inhibition of the immune response, *J. Immunol.* 106:951.

De Swiet, J., and Wells, A. L., 1957, Nephrotic syndrome associated with renal venous thrombosis and bronchial carcinoma, *Br. Med. J.* 5031:1341.

Diener, E., and Feldman, M., 1970, Antibody-mediated suppression of the immune response *in vitro*. II. A new approach to the phenomenon of immunological tolerance, *J. Exp. Med.* 132:31.

Dixon, F. J., Vasquez, J. J., Weigle, W. O., and Cochrane, C. G., 1958, Pathogenesis of serum sickness, *Arch. Pathol.* 65:18.

Dixon, F. J., Feldman, J. D., and Vasquez, J. J., 1961, Experimental glomerulonephritis, *J. Exp. Med.* 113:899.

Dorval, G., and Pross, H., 1983, Immune complexes in cancer, in: *Circulating Immune Complexes* (L. Espinoza and C. Osterland, eds.), pp. 161–171, Futura, New York.

Eagan, J. W., Roberts, J. L., Schwartz, M. M., and Lewis, E. J., 1979, The composition of pulmonary immune deposits in systemic lupus erythematosus, *Clin. Immunol. Immunopathol.* 12:204.

Fauci, A. S., 1981, The revolution in clinical immunology, *J. Am. Med. Assoc.* 246:2567.

Feldman, M., and Diener, E., 1970, Antibody-mediated suppression of the immune response *in vitro*, *J. Exp. Med.* 131:247.

Feldman, M., and Diener, E., 1972, Antibody mediated suppression of the immune response *in vitro*. IV. The effect of antibody fragments, *J. Immunol.* 108:93.

Fer, M. F., Beman, J., Stevenson, H. C., Maluish, A., Moratz, C., Delawter, T., Foon, K., Herberman, R. B., Oldham, R. K., Terman, D. S., Young, J. B., and Daskal, Y., 1984, A trial of autologous plasma perfusion over protein A in patients with breast cancer, *J. Biol. Resp. Modif.* 3:352.

Finbloom, D. S., Abeles, D., Rifai, A., and Plotz, P. H., 1980, The specificity of uptake of model immune complexes and other protein aggregates by the murine reticuloendothelial system, *J. Immunol.* 125:1060.

Forsgren, A., and Sjöquist, J., 1966, Protein A from *Staphylococcus aureus*. I. Pseudo immune reaction with human globulin, *J. Immunol.* 97:822.

Friou, G. J., 1974, Current knowledge and concepts of the relationship of malignancy, autoimmunity and immunologic disease, *Ann. N.Y. Acad. Sci.* 230:23.

Frost, P., and Kerbel, R. S., 1983, Immunology of metastasis. Can the immune response cope with disseminated tumor? *Cancer Metastasis Reviews* 2:239.

Fust, G., Fekete, B., Angyal, I., Jakab, A., Pal, A., Meretey, K., Falus, A., Torok, K., Szegedi, Gy., Kavai, M., Puskas, E., Cseci-Nagy, M., Szabo, T., Lenkey, A., and Misz, M., 1981, Evaluation of different methods for detecting circulating immune complexes: Studies in patients with lung cancer, *J. Immunol. Methods* 46:259.

Gauci, L., Caraux, J., and Serrou, B., 1981, Immune complexes in the context of the immune response in cancer patients, in: *Immune Complexes and Plasma Exchanges in Cancer Patients* (B. Serrou and C. Rosenfeld, eds.), pp. 37–98, Elsevier/North-Holland, Amsterdam.

Gauthier, V. J., Mannik, M., and Striker, G. E., 1982, Effect of cationized antibodies in preformed immune complexes on deposition and persistence in renal glomeruli, *J. Exp. Med.* 156:766.

Germuth, F. G., Jr., and Rodriguez, E., 1973, *Immunopathology of the Renal Glomerulus*, Little, Brown, Boston.

Germuth, F. G., Jr., Flanagan, C., and Montenegro, M. R., 1957, The relationship between the chemical nature of the antigen, antigen dosage rate of antibody synthesis and the occurrence of arteritis and glomerulonephritis in experimental hypersensitivity, *Johns Hopkins Med. J.* 101:149.

Gilead, Z., Troy, F. A., and Sulitzeanu, D., 1981, Isolation and electrophoretic analysis of immune complexes from patients with breast cancer, *Eur. J. Cancer Clin. Oncol.* 17:1165.

Giuliano, A. E., Rangel, D., Golub, S. H., Holmes, E. C., and Morton, D. L., 1979, Serummediated immunosuppression in lung cancer, *Cancer* 43:917.

Gleicher, N., and Siegel, I., 1981, Common denominators of pregnancy and malignancy, in: *Reproductive Immunology* (N. Gleicher, ed.), pp. 339–353, Alan R. Liss, New York.

Gordon, B. R., Moroff, S., Hurvitz, A. I., Matus, R. E., MacEwen, E. G., Good, R. A., and Day, N. K., 1980, Circulating immune complexes in sera of dogs with benign and malignant breast disease, *Cancer Res.* 40:3627.

Grace, S. A., and Brennan, F. M., 1982, Clearance and localization of immunoglobulin oligomers in mice with chronic circulating endogenous complexes, *Immunology* 47:221.

Grandeis, W. E., Tan, C., Yang, Y., Good, R. A., and Day, N. K., 1980, Circulating immune complexes, complement and complement component levels in childhood Hodgkin's disease, *Clin. Exp. Immunol.* 39:551.

Greenberg, E., Divertie, M. B., and Woolner, L. B., 1964, A review of unusual systemic manifestations associated with carcinoma, *Am. J. Med.* 36:106.

Gupta, R. K., and Morton, D. L., 1981, Possible clinical significance of circulating immune complexes in melanoma patients, in: *Fundamental Mechanisms in Human Cancer Immunology* (J. P. Sanders, J. Daniels, B. Serrou, D. Rosenfeld, and C. Denney, eds.), pp. 305–320, Elsevier/North Holland, Amsterdam.

Gupta, R. K., and Morton, D. L., 1983, Immunochemical characterization of fetal antigen isolated from spent culture medium of a human melanoma cell line, *J. Natl. Cancer Inst.* 70:993.

Gupta, R. K., and Morton, D. L., 1984a, Studies of a melanoma tumor-associated antigen detected in spent culture medium of a human melanoma cell line by allogeneic antibody. I. Purification and development of a radioimmunoassay, *J. Natl. Cancer Inst.* 72:67.

Gupta, R. K., and Morton, D. L., 1984b, Studies of a melanoma tumor-associated antigen detected in spent culture medium of a human melanoma cell line by allogeneic antibody. II. Immunobiological characterization, *J. Natl. Cancer Inst.* **72**:75.

Gupta, R. K., and Morton, D. L., 1984c, Studies of a melanoma tumor-associated antigen detected in spent culture medium of a human melanoma cell line by allogeneic antibody. III. Physicochemical properties, *J. Natl. Cancer Inst.* **72**:83.

Gupta, R. K., Golub, S. H., and Morton, D. L., 1979, Correlation between tumor burden and anticomplementary activity in sera from cancer patients, *Cancer Immunol. Immunother.* **6**:63.

Gupta, R. K., Leitch, A. M., and Morton, D. L., 1983a, Detection of tumor-associated antigen in eluates from protein-A columns used for *ex-vivo* immunoadsorption of plasma from melanoma patients by radioimmunoassay, *Clin. Exp. Immunol.* **53**:589.

Gupta, R. K., Leitch, A. M., and Morton, 1983b, Nature of antigens and antibodies in immune complexes isolated by staphylococcal protein A from plasma of melanoma patients, *Cancer Immunol. Immunother.* **16**:40.

Haakenstad, A. O., and Mannik, M., 1974, Saturation of the reticuloendothelial system with soluble immune complexes, *J. Immunol.* **112**:1939.

Haakenstad, A. O., and Mannik, M., 1977, The biology of immune complexes, in: *Autoimmunity* (N. Talal, ed.), pp. 277–360, Academic Press, New York.

Halpern, B., 1974, Role of the reticuloendothelial system in the clearance of macromolecules, in: *Enzyme Therapy in Lysosomal Storage Disease* (J. M. Tager, G. J. M. Hooghwinkel, and Th. W. Daems, eds.), pp. 111–123, North Holland, Amsterdam.

Hartmann, D. P., 1975, The identification and role of anti-immunoglobulin in human malignancy, Ph.D. thesis, McGill University, Montreal, Canada.

Hay, F. C., Lynn, J., Roitt, N., and Roitt, I. M., 1976, Routine assay for the detection of immune complexes of known immunoglobulin class using solid phase C1q, *Clin. Exp. Immunol.* **24**:396.

Heier, H. E., Carpentier, N., Lange, G., Lambert, P. H., and Godal, T., 1977, Circulating immune complexes in patients with malignant lymphoma and solid tumors, *Int. J. Cancer* **20**:887.

Heimer, R., and Per, S., 1982, Pitfalls in the methodology for detection of immune complexes, *Surv. Immunol. Res.* **1**:109.

Hellström, K. E., and Hellström, I., 1974, Lymphocyte-mediated cytotoxicity and blocking serum activity to tumor antigen, *Adv. Immunol.* **18**:209.

Hendrick, J. C., Zangerle, P. F., Franchimonk, P., Samak, R., and Israel, L., 1981, Isolation of immune complexes from cancerous patients and antigen characterization, in: *Immune Complexes and Plasma Exchanges in Cancer Patients* (B. Serrou and G. C. Rosenfeld, eds.), pp. 29–36, Elsevier/North-Holland, Amsterdam.

Herberman, R. B., 1982, Immunological approach to the biochemical markers for cancer, in: *Biochemical Markers for Cancer* (T. Ming Chu, ed.), pp. 1–23, Marcel Dekker, New York.

Herberman, R. B., Bordes, M., Lambert, P. H., Luthra, H. S., Robins, R. A., Sizaret, P., and Theofilopoulos, A., 1981, Report on international comparative evaluation of possible value of assays for immune complexes for diagnosis of human breast cancer, *Int. J. Cancer* **27**:569.

Hersey, P., Edward, A., Adams, E., Ibister, J. P. Murrey, E., Biggs, J. C., and Milton, S. W., 1976, Antibody-dependent cell-mediated cytotoxicity against melanoma cells induced by plasmapheresis, *Lancet* **1**:825.

Higgens, M. R., Randall, R. E., and Still, W. J. S., 1974, Nephrotic syndrome with oat-cell carcinoma, *Br. Med. J.* **3**:450.

Hoffken, K., Meredith, I. D., Robins, R. A., Baldwin, R. W., Davis, C. J., and Blamery, R. W., 1977, Circulating immune complexes in patients with breast cancer, *Br. Med. J.* **2**:218.

Holdsworth, S. R., Neale, T. J., and Wilson, C. B., 1980, The participation of macrophages and monocytes in experimental immune complex glomerulonephritis, *Clin. Immunol. Immunopathol.* **15**:510.

Holohan, T. V., Philips, T. M., Bowles, C., and Deisseroth, A., 1982, Regression of canine mammary carcinoma after immunoadsorption therapy, *Cancer Res.* **42**:3663.

Horvath, M., Fekete, B., and Rahoty, P., 1982, Investigation of circulating immune complexes in patients with breast cancer, *Oncology* **39**:20.

Houghton, A. N., Brooks, H., Cote, P. J., Taormina, M. C., Oettgen, H. F., and Old, L. J., 1983, Detection of cell surface and intracellular antigens by human monoclonal antibodies: Hybrid cell lines derived from lymphocytes of patients with malignant melanoma, *J. Exp. Med.* **158**:53.

Houston, W. E., Pedersen, C. E., Jr., Cole, F. E., Jr., and Spertzel, R. O., 1974, Effects of antigen–antibody complexes in the primary immune response in Rhesus monkeys, *Infect. Immun.* **10**:437.

Isbister, W. H., Noonan, F. P., Halliday, W. J., and Clunie, G., 1975, Human thoracic duct cannulation: Manipulation of tumor-specific blocking factors in a patient with malignant melanoma, *Cancer* **35**:1465.

Israel, L., Edelstein, R., Mannoni, P., Rodot, E., and Greenspan, E. M., 1977, Plasmapheresis in patients with disseminated cancer: Clinical results and correlations with changes in serum protein. The concept of nonspecific blocking factors, *Cancer* **40**:3146.

Issekutz, A. C., and Bhimji, S., 1982, Effect of nonsteroid anti-inflammatory agents on immune complex and chemotactic factor-induced inflammation, *Immunopharmacology* **4**:253.

Jaffers, G. J., Colvin, R. B., Cosini, A. B., Giorgi, J. V., Goldstein, G., Fuller, T. C., Kurnick, J. T., Lillehie, C., and Russell, P. S., 1983, Immunological monitoring of diabetic and nondiabetic recipients of renal allografts, *Transplant. Proc.* **15**:646.

Jones, F. R., Yoshida, L. H., Ladiges, W. C., and Kennedy, M. A., 1980, Treatment of feline leukemia and reversal of FeLV by *ex vivo* removal of IgG: A preliminary report, *Cancer* **46**:675.

Jones, V. E., and Orlans, E., 1981, Isolation of immune complexes and characterization of their constituent antigens and antibodies in some human diseases: A review, *J. Immunol. Methods* **44**:249.

Kabat, E. A., 1980, Basic principles of antigen–antibody reactions, *Methods Enzymol.* **70A**:3.

Kaplan, A. P., 1981, Immune complexes and connective tissue disease, *Bull. N.Y. Acad. Med.* **57**:638.

Kessler, S. W., 1975, Rapid isolation of antigen from cells with a staphylococcal protein A antibody adsorbent: Parameters of the interaction of antibody–antigen complexes, *J. Immunol.* **115**:1617.

Kilgallon, W., Amlot, P. L., and Williams, B. D., 1983, Immune complexes in Hodgkin's disease: Isolation, immunochemical and physiochemical analysis, *Clin. Exp. Immunol.* **53**:308.

Knutson, D. W., Kylstra, A., and Van Es, L. A., 1977, Association and dissociation of aggregated IgA from rat peritoneal macrophases, *J. Exp. Med.* **145**:1368.

Koprowski, H., Herlyn, D., Lubeck, M., DeFreitas, E., and Sears, H. F., 1984, Human anti-idiotype antibodies in cancer patients: Is the modulation of the immune response beneficial for the patient? *Proc. Natl. Acad. Sci. USA* **81**:216.

Korec, S., Smith, F. P., Schein, P. S., and Phillips, T. M., 1984, Clinical experiences with extracorporeal immunoperfusion of plasma from cancer patients, *J. Biol. Resp. Modif.* **3**:330.

Krapf, F., Renger, D., Schedel, I., Fricke, M., Kemper, A., and Deicher, H., 1983, Circulating immune complexes in malignant diseases: Increased detection rate by simultaneous use of three assay methods, *Cancer Immunol. Immunother.* 15:138.

Kristensen, E., Brandslund, I., Nielsen, H., and Svehag, S. E., 1980, Prognostic value of assays for circulating immune complexes and natural cytotoxicity in malignant skin melanoma (stages I and II), *Cancer Immunol. Immunother.* 9:31.

Lachmann, P. J., Macanovic, M., Harkiss, G. D., Oldroyd, R. G., and Habicht, J., 1981, The isolation of the antibody moieties of immune complexes from serum by the pepsin digestion of conglutinin–anti-conglutinin complexes, *Clin. Exp. Immunol.* 46:250.

Lahey, S. J., Steele, G., Jr., Rodrick, M. L., Berkowitz, R., Goldstein, D. P., Ross, D. S., Ravikumar, T. S., Wilson, R. E., Byrn, R., Thomas, P., and Zamcheck, N., 1984, Characterization of antigenic components from circulating immune complexes in patients with gestational trophoblastic neoplasia, *Cancer* 53:1316.

Laissue, J., Cottier, H., Hess, M. W., and Stoner, R. D., 1971, Early and enhanced germinal centre formation and antibody responses in mice after primary stimulation with antigen-isologous antibody complexes as compared with antigen alone, *J. Immunol.* 107:822.

Lambert, P. H., Dixon, F. J., Zubler, R. H., Agnello, V., Cambiaso, C., Casali, P., Clarke, J., Cowdery, J. S., McDuffie, F. C., Hay, F. C., MacLennan, I. C. M., Masson, P., Muller-Eberhard, H. J., Penttinen, K., Smith, M., Tappeiner, G., Theofilopoulos, A. N., and Verroust, P., 1978, A WHO collaborative study for the evaluation of eighteen methods for detecting immune complexes in serum, *J. Clin. Lab. Immunol.* 1:1.

Lamers, M. C., 1981, Factors influencing the development of immune complex diseases, *Allergy* 36:527.

Lamers, M. C., DeGroot, E. R., and Roos, D., 1981, Phagocytosis and degradation of DNA-anti-DNA complexes by human phagocytes. I. Assays, conditions, quantitative aspects and differences between human blood monocytes and neutrophils, *Eur. J. Immunol.* 11:757.

Langone, J. J., Das, C., Bennett, D., and Terman, D. S., 1984, Generation of human C3a, C4a, and C5a anaphylatoxins by protein A of *Staphylococcus aureus* and immobilized protein A reagents used in serotherapy of cancer, *J. Immunol.* 133(2):1057.

Lee, J. C., Yamauchi, H., and Hopper, J., 1966, The association of cancer and the nephrotic syndrome, *Ann. Intern. Med.* 64:41.

Leslie, R. G. Q., 1980, Macrophage handling of soluble immune complexes: Use of specific inhibitors to study the biochemical events involved in complex catabolism, *Eur. J. Immunol.* 10:799.

Lewis, M. G., and Pelgrum, G. D., 1978, Autoimmune antibodies in chronic lymphatic leukemia, *Br. J. Haematol.* 38:75.

Lewis, M. G., Loughridge, L. W., and Phillips, T. M., 1971, Immunological studies on a patient with the nephrotic syndrome associated with malignancy of non-renal origin, *Lancet* 2:134.

Lightfoot, R. W., Drusin, R. E., and Christian, C. L., 1970, Properties of soluble immune complexes, *J. Immunol.* 105:1493.

Longscope, W. T., and Rackemann, F. M., 1918, The relation of circulating antibodies to serum disease, *J. Exp. Med.* 27:341.

Lookwood, C. M., Worlledge, S., Nicholas, A., Cotton, C., and Peters, D. K., 1979, Reversal of impaired splenic function by plasma exchange, *N. Engl. J. Med.* 300:524.

McCormick, J. R., Harkin, M. M., Johnson, K. J., and Ward, P. A., 1981, Suppression of superoxide dismutase of immune-complex-induced pulmonary alveolitis and dermal inflammation, *Am. J. Pathol.* 102:55.

MacKintosh, F. R., Bennet, K., Schiff, S., and Hall, S. W., 1983, Treatment of advanced malignancy with plasma perfused over staphylococcal protein A, *West. J. Med.* 139:36.

Maidment, B. W., Papsidero, L. D., Nemoto, T., and Chu, T. M., 1981, Recovery of immunologically reactive antibodies and antigens from breast cancer immune complexes by preparative isoelectric focusing, *Cancer Res.* **41**:795.

Male, D., and Roitt, I. M., 1979, Analysis of the components of immune complexes, *J. Mol. Immunol.* **16**:197.

Mannik, M., and Arend, W. P., 1971, Fate of preformed immune complexes in rabbits and rhesus monkeys, *J. Exp. Med.* **134**:195.

Masserschmidt, G., Bowles, C., Dean, D., Parker, M., Lester, R., Dowling, R., Holohan, T., Osborn, L., Schaff, B. F., McCormack, K., Corbitt, R., Phillips, T., Glasstein, E., and Diesseroth, A., 1982, Phase II trial of *S. aureus* Cowan I immunoperfusion, *Cancer Treat. Rep.* **66**:2027.

Masson, P., 1978, Are circulating immune complexes the key to immunopathology? in: *Protides of the Biological Fluids* (H. Peeters, ed.), Vol. 25, pp. 3-7, Pergamon Press, New York.

Morgan, A. C., and McIntyre, R. F., 1983, Monoclonal antibodies to human melanoma-associated antigens: An amplified enzyme-linked immunoadsorbent assay for the detection of antigen, antibody and immune complexes, *Cancer Res.* **43**:3155-3159.

Morgan, A. C., Jr., Crane, M. M., and Rossen, R. D., 1984, Measurement of a monoclonal antibody-defined, melanoma-associated antigen in human sera: Correlation of circulating antigen levels with tumor burden, *J. Natl. Cancer Inst.* **72**:243.

Ninnemann, J. L., 1981, Tumor associated immunosuppressive serum proteins, in: *The Handbook of Cancer Immunology* (H. Waters, ed.), pp. 376-406, Garland STPM Press, New York.

Nydegger, U. E., Kazatchkine, M. D., Lambert, P. H., and Miescher, P. A., 1983, Immunopathology of immune complex disease, in: *The Reticuloendothelial System: A Comprehensive Treatise*, Vol. 4: *Immunopathology* (N. R. Rose and B. V. Siegel, eds.), pp. 371-390, Plenum Press, New York.

Oldham, R. K., 1984, Introduction, *J. Biol. Resp. Modif.* **3**:229-230.

Ozawa, T., Pluss, R., Lacher, J., Boedecker, E., Guggenheim, S., Hammond, W., and McIntosh, R., 1971, Endogenous immune complex nephropathy associated with malignancy. I. Studies of the nature and immunopathogenic significance of glomerular bound antigen and antibody isolation and characterization of tumor specific antigen and antibody and circulating immune complexes, *Q. J. Med.* **44**:523.

Paganelli, R., Levinsky, R. J., Brosstoff, J., and Wraith, D. G., 1979, Immune complexes containing food proteins in normal and atopic subjects after oral challenge and effect of sodium chromoglycate on antigen absorption, *Lancet* **1**:1270.

Papsidero, L. D., Nemoto, T., Snyderman, M. C., and Chu, T. M., 1979, Immune complexes in breast cancer patients as detected by C1q binding, *Cancer* **44**:1636.

Peeters, H. (ed.), 1979, *Protides of the Biological Fluids*, Vol. 26, Pergamon Press, London.

Penn, I., 1981, Depressed immunity and the development of cancer, *Clin. Exp. Immunol.* **46**:459.

Pereira, A. B., Theofilopoulos, A. N., and Dixon, F. J., 1980, Detection and partial characterization of circulating immune complexes with solid-phase anti-C3, *J. Immunol.* **1025**:763.

Petrone, W. F., English, D. K., Wong, K., and McCord, J. M., 1981, Free radicals and inflammation: The superoxide dependent activation of a neutrophil chemotactic factor in plasma, *Proc. Natl. Acad. Sci. USA* **77**:1159.

Phillips, T. M., MacDonald, J. S., and Lewis, M. G., 1981, Towards tumour antibody isolation and characterization in immune complexes, in: *Immune Complexes and Plasma Exchanges in Cancer Patients* (B. Serrou and C. Rosenfeld, eds.), pp. 3-28, Elsevier/North-Holland, Amsterdam.

Phillips, T. M., Queen, W. D., and Lewis, M. G., 1982, The significance of circulating immune complexes in patients with malignant melanoma, in: *Melanoma Antigens and Antibodies* (R. A. Reisfeld and S. Ferrone, eds.), pp. 289–316, Plenum Press, New York.

Pincus, T., Haberkern, R., and Christian, C. L., 1968, Experimental chronic glomerulitis, *J. Exp. Med.* 127:819.

Poskitt, P. K., and Poskitt, T. R., 1979, The L1210 assay for immune complexes: Application in cancer patients and correlation with disease progress, *Int. J. Cancer* 24:560.

Poulton, T. A., Crowther, M. E., Hay, F. C., and Nineham, L. J., 1978, Immune complexes in ovarian cancer, *Lancet* 2:72.

Poulton, T. A., Mooney, N. A., Nineham, L. J., and Hay, F. C., 1983, Characteristics of immune complexes detectable by two independent assays in gynaecological malignancies, *Clin. Exp. Immunol.* 53:573.

Price, M. R., and Baldwin, R. W., 1977, Shedding of tumor cell surface antigens, in: *Dynamic Aspects of Cell Surface Organization* (G. Poste and G. Nicolson, eds.), pp. 423–471, Elsevier/North-Holland, New York.

Puskas, E., Fust, G., Angyal, I., Phi, N. C., and Gergely, J., 1982, Serial measurement of circulating immune complexes in healthy subjects, *Immunol. Lett.* 4:223.

Quay, S. C., Murphy, G. F., and Mihm, M. C., Jr., 1983, Biochemical studies of immune complexes. II. Purification of immune complexes from sera of patients with malignant melanoma, *Clin. Immunol. Immunopathol.* 26:318.

Rabinovitch, M., Manejias, R. E., and Nussenzweig, V., 1975, Selective phagocytic paralysis induced by immobilized immune complexes, *J. Exp. Med.* 142:827.

Rajnavolgki, E., Fust, G., Kulics, J., Ember, J., Medgyesi, G. A., and Gergely, J., 1978, The effect of immune complex composition on complement activation and complement dependent complex disease, *Immunochemistry* 15:887.

Ray, P. K., McClaughlin, D., Mohammed, J., Idiculla, A., Rhoads, J. E., Jr., Mark, R., Bassett, J. G., and Cooper, D. R., 1981, *Ex vivo* immunoadsorption of IgG or its complexes—A new modality of cancer treatment, in: *Immune Complexes and Plasma Exchanges in Cancer Patients* (B. Serrou and C. Rosenfeld, eds.), pp. 197–220, Elsevier/North-Holland, Amsterdam.

Ray, P. K., Idiculla, A., Mark, R., Rhoads, J. E., Jr., Thomas, H., Bassett, J. G., and Cooper, D. R., 1982, Extracorporeal immunoadsorption of plasma from a metastatic colon carcinoma patient by protein A-containing nonviable *S. aureus*, *Cancer* 49:1800.

Richmond, J., Sherman, R. S., Diamond, H. D., and Craver, L. F., 1962, Renal lesions associated with malignant lymphomas, *Am. J. Med.* 32:184.

Rifai, A., and Mannik, M., 1984, Clearance kinetics and fate of mouse IgA immune complexes prepared with monomeric or dimeric IgA, *J. Immunol.* 130:1826.

Rifai, A., Finbloom, D. S., Magilavy, D. B., and Plotz, P. H., 1982, Modulation of the circulation and hepatic uptake of immune complexes by carbohydrate recognition systems, *J. Immunol.* 128:2269.

Rose, L., and Lambert, P. H., 1980, The natural occurrence of circulating idiotype anti-idiotype complexes during a secondary immune response to phosphorylcholine, *Clin. Immunol. Immunopathol.* 15:481.

Rossen, R. D., and Barnes, B. C., 1978, Measuring serum immune complexes in cancer (editorial), *Ann. Int. Med.* 88:570.

Rossen, R. D., and Morgan, A. C., 1981, Blockage of the humoral immune response: Immune complexes in cancer, in: *The Handbook of Cancer Immunology*, Vol. 9 (H. Waters, ed.), pp. 209–280, Garland STPM Press, New York.

Rossen, R. D., Reisberg, M. A., Hersh, E. M., and Gutterman, J. V., 1977, The C1q binding test for soluble immune complexes: Clinical correlations obtained in patients with cancer, *J. Natl. Cancer Inst.* 58:1205.

Rother, K., Rother, U., and Schindera, F., 1964, Passive Arthus-reaktion bei komplement-defekten Kanirchen, Z. Immun. Allergieforsch. 126:473.

Ruco, L. P., Procopio, A., Uccini, S., and Baroni, C. D., 1980, Increased monocyte phago-cytosis in cancer patients, Eur. J. Cancer 16:1315.

Ruel, P., Murray, E., McCarthy, W. H., and Hersey, P., 1982, Evaluation of assays to detect immune complexes as an immunodiagnostic aid in patients with melanoma, Oncodev. Biol. Med. 3:1.

Salinas, F. A., and Wee, K. H., 1983, Immune complexes and human neoplasia. I., Biomed. Pharmacother. 36:119.

Salinas, F. A., Sheikh, K. H., and Chandor, S. B., 1978, Serological reactivity in cancer pa-tients to human and mouse fetal liver cells, Cancer Res. 38:401.

Salinas, F. A., Silver, H. K. B., Weir, E. R., and Swenerton, K., 1980a, Circulating immune complexes (CIC) in ovarian carcinoma, Proc. Am. Soc. Clin. Oncol. 21:162.

Salinas, F. A., Wee, K. H., and Silver, H. K. B., 1980b, Detection and characterization of antibodies to xenogeneic oncofetal antigen (XOFA) in human neoplasia, in: Serologic Analysis of Human Cancer Antigens (S. A. Rosenberg, ed.), pp. 539-568 and 665-667, Academic Press, New York.

Salinas, F. A., Wee, K. H., and Silver, H. K. B., 1980c, Xenogenic oncofetal antigen (XOFA) and its relation with tumor burden in malignant melanoma (MM) patients, Proc. Am. Assoc. Cancer Res. 21:225.

Salinas, F. A., Silver, H. K. B., Grossman, L., and Thomas, J. W., 1981a, Plasmapheresis: A new approach in the management of advanced malignant melanoma, in: Immune Com-plexes and Plasma Exchanges in Cancer Patients (B. Serrou and C. Rosenfeld, eds.), pp. 253-270, Elsevier/North-Holland. Amsterdam.

Salinas, F. A., Wee, K. H., and Silver, H. K. B., 1981b, Immune complexes and human neo-plasia: Detection and quantitation of circulating immune complexes by the fetal liver cell assay, Cancer Immunol. Immunother. 12:11.

Salinas, F. A., Wee, K. H., and Silver, H. K. B., 1981c, Malignant melanoma tumor burden and its relationship to antigen concentration, size and composition of circulating immune complexes, Proc. Am. Assoc. Cancer Res. 20:181.

Salinas, F. A., Wee, K. H., and Silver, H. K. B., 1981d, Modulation of lymphocyte activation by plasmapheresis in advanced malignant melanoma, in: Mechanisms of Lymphocyte Activation (K. Resch, ed.), pp. 4790-4791, Elsevier/North-Holland, Amsterdam.

Salinas, F. A., Wee, K. H., and Silver, H. K. B., 1982a, Xenogeneic oncofetal antigen (XOFA) immunoregulation in malignant melanoma, Proc. Int. Cancer Cong. 13:309.

Salinas, F. A., Wee, K. H., Silver, H. K. B., and Ragaz, J., 1982b, Circulating immune com-plexes and associated antigen in breast carcinoma, Proc. Am. Assoc. Cancer Res. 23:250.

Salinas, F. A., Wee, K. H., and Silver, H. K. B., 1983a, Detection of epithelial breast car-cinoma associated antigen (BCAA) by monoclonal antibodies, Proc. Am. Soc. Clin. Oncol. 2:103.

Salinas, F. A., Wee, K. H., and Silver, H. K. B., 1983b, Immune complexes and human neo-plasia: Review II, Biomed. Pharmacother. 37:211.

Salinas, F. A., Wee, K. H., and Silver, H. K. B., 1984, Tumor burden and its relationship to antigen, size and composition of immune complexes, in: Protides of the Biological Fluids (H. Peeters, ed.), Vol. 31, pp. 749-752, Pergamon Press, Oxford.

Salinas, F. A., Wee, K. H., and Silver, H. K. B., 1985, Clinical relevance of human oncofetal antigen (HOFA) as a marker of tumor burden, in: Protides of the Biological Fluids (H. Peeters, ed.), Vol. 32, pp. 779-782, Pergamon Press, Oxford.

Scharfstein, J., Correa, E. B., Gallo, G. R., and Nussenzwieg, V., 1979, Human C4-binding protein: Association with immune complexes in-vitro and in-vivo, J. Clin. Invest. 63:437.

Schupbach, J., Kalyanaraman, V. S., Sarngadharan, M. G., Gunn, P. A., Blayney, D. W., and

Gallo, R. C., 1984, Demonstration of viral antigen p24 in circulating immune complexes of two patients with human T-cell leukemia/lymphoma virus (HTLV) positive lymphoma, *Lancet* 1:302.

Segal, D. M., and Hurwitz, E., 1977, Binding of affinity cross-linked oligomers of IgG to cells bearing Fc receptors, *J. Immunol.* 118:1338.

Sela, M., 1969, Antigenicity: Some molecular aspects, *Science* 166:1365.

Serrou, B., and Rosenfeld, C. (eds.), 1981, *Immune Complexes and Plasma Exchanges in Cancer Patients,* Elsevier/North-Holland, Amsterdam.

Siag, W. M., and Jones, J. M., 1982, Alteration by protein A of the distribution of immune complexes containing antigen of retrovirus, *Clin. Immunol. Immunopathol.* 24:186.

Silver, H. K. B., Karim, K. A., Archibald, E. L., and Salinas, F. A., 1979, Serum sialic acid and sialyltransferase as monitors of tumor burden in malignant melanoma patients, *Cancer Res.* 39:5036.

Silver, H. K. B., Karim, K., Gray, M. J., and Salinas, F. A., 1981*a*, High performance liquid chromatography quantitation of N-acetylneuraminic acid in malignant melanoma and breast carcinoma, *J. Chromatogr. (Biomed. Appl.)* 224:381.

Silver, H. K. B., Karim, K., Salinas, F. A., and Swenerton, K. D., 1981*b*, Significance of sialic acid and carcinoembryonic antigen as monitors of tumor burden among patients with carcinoma of the ovary, *J. Surg. Gynecol. Obstet.* 153:209.

Silver, H. K. B., Connors, J. M., Karim, K. A., Kong, S., Spinelli, J. J., de Jong, G., McLean, D. M., and Salinas, F. A., 1983, Effect of lymphoblastoid interferon on lymphocyte subsets in cancer patients, *J. Biol. Resp. Mod.* 2:428.

Silverstein, S. C., Steinman, R. M., and Cohn, Z. A., 1977, Endocytosis, *Annu. Rev. Biochem.* 46:669.

Sinclair, StC. N. R., 1979, Modulation of immunity by antibody antigen–antibody complexes and antigen, *Pharmacol. Ther.* 4:355.

Skogh, T., and Stendahl, O., 1983, Complement-mediated delay in immune complex clearance from the blood owing to reduced deposition outside the reticuloendothelial system, *Immunology* 49:53.

Sobel, A. T., Botish, J. A., and Muller-Eberhart, H. J., 1975, C1Q deviation test for the detection of immune complexes, aggregates of IgG and bacterial products in human serum, *J. Exp. Med.* 142:130.

Spremulli, E. N., and Dexter, D. L., 1983, Human tumor cell heterogeneity and metastasis, *J. Clin. Oncol.* 1:496.

Staab, H. J., Anderer, F. A., Stumpf, E., and Fisher, R., 1980, Are CEA immune complexes a prognostic marker in patients with carcinoma at the gastrointestinal tract? *Br. J. Cancer* 42:26.

Steele, G., Ankerst, J., and Sjögren, H. O., 1974, Alteration of *in vitro* activity of tumor bearer sera by adsorption with *Staphylococcus aureus* Cowan I, *Int. J. Cancer* 14:83.

Steward, M. W., and Devey, M. E., 1981, Antigen–antibody complexes: Their nature and role in animal models of antigen–antibody complex disease, in: *Immunological Aspects of Rheumatology* (W. C. Dick, ed.), pp. 63–91, Elsevier/North-Holland, London.

Tan, E. M., and Kunkle, H. G., 1966, An immunofluorescent study of the skin lesions in systemic lupus erythematosus, *Arthritis Rheum.* 2:37.

Tanaka, F., Yonemoto, R. H., and Waldman, S. R., 1979, Blocking factors in sera of breast cancer patients, *Cancer* 43:838.

Terman, D. S., Yamamoto, T., Mattioli, M., Cook, G., Tillquist, R., Henry, J., Poser, M. R., and Daskal, Y., 1980, Extensive necrosis of spontaneous canine mammary adenocarcinoma after extracorporeal perfusion over *Staphylococcus aureus* Cowan I, *J. Immunol.* 124:795.

Terman, D. S., Young, J. B., Shearer, W. T., Ayus, C., Mattioli, C., Lehane, D., Espada, R., Howell, J. F., Yamamoto, T., Zeleski, H. I., Henry, J. F., Feldman, L., Miller, L., Frommer, P., Tillquist, R., Cook, G., and Daskal, Y., 1981, Preliminary observations of the effects on breast carcinoma of plasma perfused over immobilized protein A, *N. Engl. J. Med.* **305**:1195.

Theofilopoulos, A. N., and Dixon, F. J., 1979, The biology and detection of immune complexes, *Adv. Immunol.* **28**:89.

Theofilopoulos, A. N., Andrews, B. S., Urist, M. M., Morton, D. L., and Dixon, F. J., 1977, The nature of immune complexes in human cancer sera, *J. Immunol.* **119**:657.

Theofilopoulos, A. N., Eisenberg, R. A., and Dixon, F. J., 1978, Isolation of circulating immune complexes using Raji cells: Separation of antigen from immune complexes and production of antiserum, *J. Clin. Invest.* **61**:1570.

Tucker, D. F., Begent, R. H., and Hogg, N. M., 1978, Characterization of immune complexes in serum by absorption on staphylococcal protein A: Model studies and application to sera of rats bearing a Gross virus-induced lymphoma, *J. Immunol.* **121**:1644.

Unanue, E. R., and Dixon, F. J., 1967, Experimental allergic glomerulonephritis induced in the rabbit with heterologous renal antigens, *J. Exp. Med.* **125**:149.

Van Es, L. A., Knutson, D. W., Kayser, B. S., and Glassock, R. J., 1979, Soluble oligovalent antigen–antibody complexes. I. The effect of antigen valence and combining ratio on the composition of fluorescein-carrier antifluorescein complexes, *Immunology* **37**:485.

Virgin, H. W., IV, and Unanue, E. R., 1984, Suppression of the immune response to *Listeria monocytogenes*. I. Immune complexes inhibit resistance, *J. Immunol.* **133**:104.

Von Pirquet, C. E., 1911, Allergy, *Arch. Intern. Med.* **7**:259.

Waller, M., Curry, S., and Richard, A., 1968, Serological specificity of IgG and IgM antiglobulin antibodies in anti-gm (a) antisera, *Exp. Immunol.* **3**:631.

Ward, P. A., and Cochrane, C. G., 1965, Bound complement and immunologic injury of blood vessels, *J. Exp. Med.* **121**:215.

Weigle, W. O., 1961, The immune response of rabbits tolerant to bovine serum albumin, *J. Exp. Med.* **114**:111.

Weiss, S. J., and Ward, P. A., 1982, Immune complex induced generation of oxygen metabolites by human neutrophils, *J. Immunol.* **129**:309.

Williams, B. D., Pussel, B. A., Lookwood, C. M., and Cotton, C., 1979, Defective reticuloendothelial system function in rheumatoid arthritis, *Lancet* **1**:1311.

Williams, R. C., Jr., 1980, *Immune Complexes in Clinical and Experimental Medicine*, Harvard University Press, Cambridge, Massachusetts.

Wills, E. J., Davies, P., Allison, A. C., and Haswell, A. D., 1972, Cytochalasin B fails to inhibit pinocytosis by macrophages, *Nature* **240**:58.

Wilson, C. B., and Dixon, F. J., 1981, The renal response to immunological injury, in: *The Kidney*, 2nd ed. (M. Bairy, B. M. Brenner, and F. C. Rector, eds.), pp. 1237–1350, Saunders, Philadelphia.

Winchester, R. J., 1983, Foreword, in: *Circulating Immune Complexes* (L. Espinoza and C. Osterland, eds.), pp. vii–ix, Futura, New York.

World Health Organization, 1977, The role of immune complexes in disease, Technical report series 606, WHO, Geneva.

Zimmerman, S. E., Smith, F. P., Phillips, T. M., Coffey, R. J., and Schein, P. S., 1982, Gastric carcinoma and thrombotic thrombocytopenic purpura: Association with plasma immune complex concentrations, *Br. Med. J.* **284**:1432.

Zubler, R. H., and Lambert, P. H., 1977, Immune complexes in clinical investigation, in: *Recent Advances in Clinical Immunology* (R. A. Thomson, ed.), pp. 125–143, Churchill Livingstone, New York.

Zubler, R. H., Lange, G., Lambert, P. H., and Meischer, P. A., 1976, Detection of immune complexes in unheated sera by modified ^{125}I-C1q binding test: Effect on the binding of C1q by immune complexes and application of the test to systemic lupus erythematosus, *J. Immunol.* **116**:232.

Chapter 3

The Pathophysiology of Circulating Immune Complexes: Their Role in Host–Tumor Interactions and Removal by Immunoadsorption Therapy

Terence M. Phillips

Immunochemistry Laboratory
George Washington University Medical Center
Washington, D.C. 20037

Thomas V. Holohan

Food and Drug Administration   and *Immunochemistry Laboratory*
United States Public Health Service   *George Washington University*
Rockville, Maryland 20857   *Medical Center*
                                     Washington, D.C. 20037

Stefan Korac

Medical Oncology Division
Georgetown University Hospital
Washington, D.C. 20007

and

Newton S. More and William D. Queen

Immunochemistry Laboratory
George Washington University Medical Center
Washington, D.C. 20037

I. INTRODUCTION

Circulating immune complexes (CIC) have received much attention during the past few years, and many different techniques have been devised to measure and

111

isolate them. As our knowledge of immunology has expanded, so has our understanding of these entities, which in reality are aggregates of floating immunological debris, having the potential not only to cause damage to a number of different organs but also to play a role in immune regulation.

Our knowledge has progressed from cataloging every disease in which these entities may be detected (Theofilopoulos and Dixon, 1980) to attempting to study the consequences of their presence. Initially, most of the pathophysiological data came from experimental models of serum sickness (Germuth, 1953; Dixon, 1963; Von Pirquet and Schick, 1905) and kidney disease (Dixon *et al.*, 1961; Cochrane *et al.*, 1973, 1976). Later it was noted that immune complexes arise wherever a humoral immune response is elicited (Jewell and MacLennan, 1973), and it was the tumor immunologists who further contributed to our knowledge of the role of immune complexes in the deregulation of the immunological host defences against the growing neoplasm.

The existence of an immunological response to tumors has been documented by many investigators (Southam, 1967; Fairley, 1969; Piessons, 1970; Klein, 1971, 1975; Ferrone and Pellegrino, 1978; Phillips and Lewis, 1976; Old *et al.*, 1968; Morton *et al.*, 1968; Lewis *et al.*, 1969; Mastrangelo *et al.*, 1974; Aoki *et al.*, 1976; Shiku *et al.*, 1976; Pesce *et al.*, 1980). However, the effectiveness of this response may be impaired by circulating factors that seem to possess the ability to interdict such antitumor activity. *In vitro* studies have indicated that cell-mediated cytotoxicity may be ineffective in the presence of sera obtained from the tumor-bearing host, but active in normal sera, thus implying the presence of soluble immunosuppressive substances (I. Hellström and Hellström, 1969; Jose and Seshada, 1974; Robins and Baldwin, 1978; Bansal and Sjögren, 1971, 1976; Browne *et al.*, 1976; Jerry *et al.*, 1976). These "blocking factors" appear to develop in the early stages of tumor growth and have been demonstrated in the sera of animals and humans with growing tumors, but are absent following tumor extirpation. (I. Hellström and Hellström, 1969). Blocking activity has been variously ascribed to free tumor antigen, tumor-directed antibodies, and CIC (I. Hellström and Hellström, 1969; Jose and Seshada, 1974; Huber and Lucas, 1978; Bansal and Sjögren, 1971, 1976; Langvad *et al.*, 1975; Hersey *et al.*, 1976).

Other evidence demonstrated that patients with an active immunological defence against their tumors suffered from other non-tumor-related diseases, such as nephrotic syndrome (Lewis *et al.*, 1971; Olsen *et al.*, 1979; Dosa *et al.*, 1983), anemia (Kremer and Laszlo, 1974), and thrombotic thrombocytopenic purpura (TTP) (S. E. Zimmerman *et al.*, 1982; Cantrell *et al.*, 1982). All of these diseases point to pathological problems arising from the presence of CIC.

In addition, anti-antibodies and antibody/anti-antibody immune complexes have been described in various tumor systems (Hartmann, 1976; Lewis *et al.*, 1976, 1979; Twomey *et al.*, 1976) in which it has been noted that an immune derangement rather than a blockade is in progress (Jerry *et al.*, 1976; Lewis *et al.*,

1979). Experimental work on the regulation and particularly the shutdown of an immune response has shown that the action of certain anti-antibodies plays an important central role (Rowley *et al.*, 1973; Beatty *et al.*, 1976). This is particularly true of antiidiotypic antibodies, but evidence is also accumulating that rheumatoid-factor-like anti-antibodies play a role, via reprocessing of immune complex antigens, in the induction of such regulatory anti-antibodies.

In this chapter we will attempt to outline some of the pathophysiology of CIC and relate clinical experiences with techniques designed to remove such complexes from the circulation of cancer patients in an attempt to restore immunological control of their tumor.

II. ANTIIMMUNOGLOBULINS AND THEIR EFFECT ON THE VARIETY OF CIC FORMED IN THE PLASMA OF CANCER PATIENTS

A. Types of Immune Complexes

It must be remembered that at any given time, several different immunological responses will be active in any given individual, and in the cases where antibody activity is involved, the resulting immunological debris will enter the circulation as CIC. These complexes may take many different forms and—depending on their composition, size, complement-binding ability, and charge—will affect the host in several different ways. In addition, the composition of each individual complex may be very different, in terms of both the ratio of antigen to antibody and the composition of the material that is considered antigenic. The ratio of antigen to antibody will affect the fate of the complex and will influence the nature of its interactions with other cells in the host body.

In addition to generally accepted concepts of what is considered antigenic, the immune system also considers autologous antibodies as antigens. Several different types of anti-antibodies have been described, many of which can be detected in the plasma of cancer patients during the progression of their disease (Hartmann, 1976; Jerry *et al.*, 1976, Phillips *et al.*, 1982). These anti-antibodies can also attach to existing immune complexes, thus giving rise to a new form of large complex: the antigen/antibody/anti-antibody immune complex. Table I outlines a simplistic overview of the possible types of immune complex that may exist either simultaneously or metachronously during the period that the host mounts an immunological attack on the growing neoplasm.

Antigen/antibody complexes may be formed in varying ratios, the three most important ratios being equivalence, antigen excess, and antibody excess. The two latter ratios are the most common forms found in the circulation and often give rise to many different interactions between the CIC and both cellular

Table I. Different Types of Immune Complexes Found in Human Sera

Antigen (excess)/antibody
Antigen/antibody (equilibrium)
Antigen/antibody (excess)
Antibody/anti-antibody (anti-Fc)
Antibody/anti-antibody (antihinge)
Antibody/anti-antibody (antiallotype)
Antibody/anti-antibody (antiidiotype)
Antigen/antibody/anti-antibody

and molecular components of the immune and other body systems. These interactions will be discussed in greater detail in later sections in this chapter.

B. Antibody/Anti-Antibody Immune Complexes

The immunoglobulin G (IgG) molecule is a target for several different anti-antibodies, of which the anti-Fc or rheumatoid factor is the best known (Waaler, 1940; Bartfield, 1969; Osterland *et al.*, 1963; Nisenoff *et al.*, 1975). However, there are also antibodies directed against the hinge region of the target IgG (Waller *et al.*, 1968) and against both the allotypic and idiotypic epitopes of the antigen receptor region (Fig. 1). These anti-antibodies have several different functions, the least exciting of which is aiding in the clearance of damaged immunoglobulins and immune complexes.

Recent studies, performed at the Immunochemistry Laboratory at George Washington University Medical Center, have shown that rheumatoid factor may have an immunoregulatory role, in that it can induce the formation of suppressive antiidiotypic antibodies *in vivo* in a murine model (Phillips *et al.*, 1985). Idiotypic antibodies complexed with naturally occurring rheumatoid factor, in antigen excess, were shown to be reprocessed by macrophages, with the resulting production of antiidiotypic suppressive anti-antibodies. These suppressive antibodies could also shut down the production of the initial idiotypic antibody at the cellular level (Fig. 2). In our past studies of malignant melanoma, we often demonstrated the presence of rheumatoid factor in patients' plasma prior to a suppression or loss of their antitumor responses. In these patients the presence of antibody/anti-antibody immune complexes was a common finding (Table II) (Lewis *et al.*, 1979; Phillips *et al.*, 1982). The presence of such regulatory mechanisms would naturally act as a suppressive arm of the immune control system, especially in patients who have had a long-standing, active humoral response to their tumor. However, this shutdown would also be detrimental in that it would remove one branch of the host's defensive mechanism.

The action of antiidiotypic and antiallotypic anti-antibodies would cause the

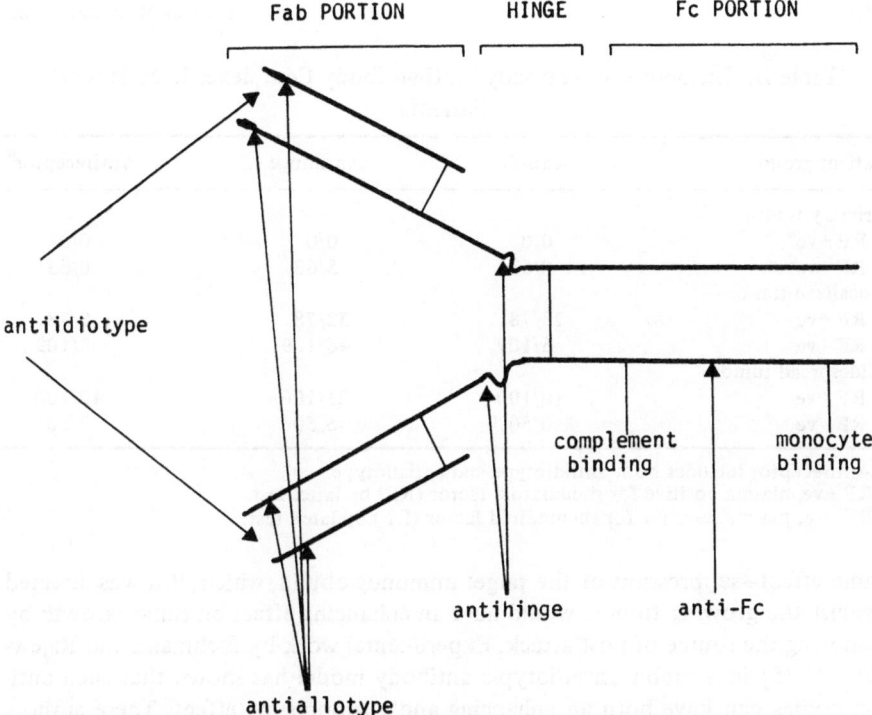

Figure 1. Schematic diagram of an IgG molecule, showing the general area to which different types of anti-antibodies are directed.

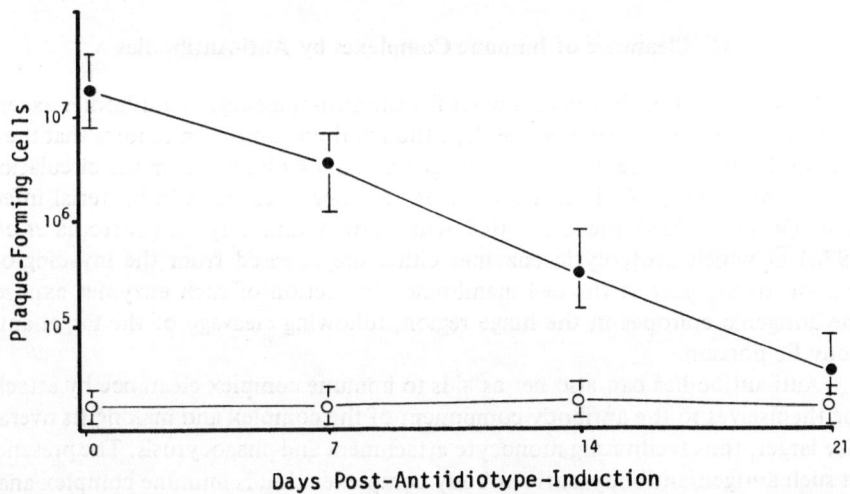

Figure 2. The suppressive action of antiidiotypic antibodies at the cellular level. ●, Decline in idiotype-producing cells, as measured by the Jerne plaque technique, over 21 days after antiidiotype induction. ○, Reactivity of control cells from unimmunized mice of the same strain who were also given the same idiotype induction regime.

Table II. Incidence of Antibody/Anti-antibody Complexes in Melanoma Patients

Patient group	Anti-Fc	Antihinge	Antireceptor[a]
Primary tumor			
RF +ve[b]	0/0	0/0	0/0
RF −ve[c]	0/63	5/63	0/63
Localized tumor			
RF +ve	23/78	32/78	8/78
RF −ve	5/109	46/109	7/109
Widespread tumor			
RF +ve	10/100	21/100	42/100
RF −ve	0/50	5/50	3/50

[a] Antireceptor includes both antiidiotype and antiallotype.
[b] RF +ve, plasma positive for rheumatoid factor (RF) by latex test.
[c] RF −ve, plasma negative for rheumatoid factor (RF) by latex test.

same effect—suppression of the target immunoglobulin, which, if it was directed against the growing tumor, would have an enhancing effect on tumor growth by removing the source of host attack. Experimental work by Eichmann and Rajewsky (1975) in a rabbit antiidiotypic antibody model has shown that such anti-antibodies can have both an enhancing and a suppressing effect. These authors conclude that antiidiotypic antibodies can act as immune regulatory molecules at the clonal level.

C. Clearance of Immune Complexes by Anti-Antibodies

No real function has been shown for the anti-hinge-region antibodies except as immune complex clearance agents, although there have been reports that these anti-antibodies also help to clear damaged immunoglobulins from the circulation (Hartmann, 1976). Such anti-antibodies have been described in bacterial infections (Waller, 1968) and associated with certain tumor types (Cotropia *et al.*, 1976) in which proteolytic enzymes either are released from the invading organisms or are part of the cell membrane. The action of such enzymes exposes the antigenic epitopes in the hinge region, following cleavage of the target antibody Fc portion.

Anti-antibodies can also act as aids to immune complex clearance by attaching themselves to the antibody component of the complex and making its overall size larger, thus facilitating monocyte attachment and phagocytosis. The presence of such antigen/antibody/anti-antibody complexes clouds immune complex analysis and even in defined systems is probably responsible for the strange results obtained during dissociation and analysis of complexed antibody activity. Recovery of the anti-antibody rather than the complexed antibody will result in a failure to demonstrate the expected specificity. This situation is true in human tumor systems in which the antibody recovered from an isolated immune complex may demonstrate no reactivity against the tumor of any of its internal components. In such a case, it is wise to test such antibodies for rheumatoid or other anti-antibody activity.

It is clear that multiple combinations are possible for the composition of immune complexes and that no one assay will distinguish whether the complexes detected are the same, different, or even related to the host tumor interactions. In the future, it is hoped that analytical techniques for immune complex isolation and characterization will be developed and that specific immune complexes will be examined for their relationship to the course of the patient's disease.

III. INTERACTION OF CIC AND COMPLEMENT WITH THE CLOTTING, KININ, AND FIBRINOLYTIC SYSTEMS

It must always be borne in mind that the components of the immune system are biochemically integrated with elements of the fibrinolytic, kinin, complement, and coagulation systems by many different interactions at both the cellular and molecular levels. Important to the activation of many of these interactions is the attachment of CIC to platelets and red blood cells.

A. Interaction of CIC with the Clotting, Kinin, and Fibrinolytic Systems

There also exist biochemical pathways in which direct interactions between CIC and components of the clotting, kinin, and fibrinolytic systems may take place (Fig. 3). Central to many of these interactions is the Hageman factor, which can participate in pathways that activate both the intrinsic and the extrinsic co-

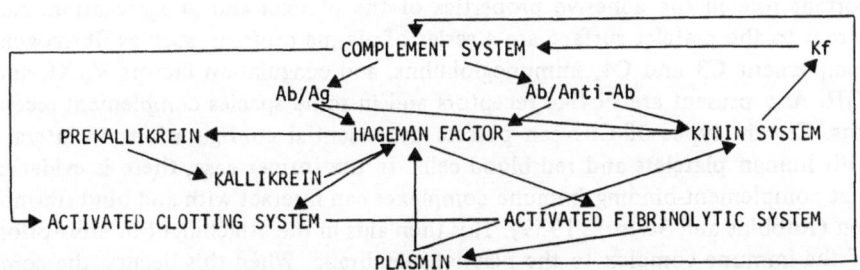

Figure 3. Schematic diagram of the interactions between CIC and the clotting, kinin, and fibrinolytic systems.

agulation systems as well as complement. There is also evidence that immune complexes can act as kinin activators (Davies and Lowe, 1960; Eisen and Smith, 1963), especially complexes that contain IgM and IgG anti-antibody components. In this case, the complex may participate in the release of kinin from plasma in the presence of activated Hageman factor (Eisen and Smith, 1963). It has also been shown that an IgM/IgG complex may even activate Hageman factor *in vitro* (Kaplan *et al.*, 1971). Activated Hageman factor can in turn activate prekallikrein, which then converts to kallikrein, which can act as an activator of more Hageman factor (Margaretten and McKay, 1971). Therefore, this interaction gives rise to a continuing cyclic interaction among the complexes and the clotting and kinin cascades.

B. Interaction of Complement with the Clotting, Kinin, and Fibrinolytic Systems

In addition, it is known that complement possesses components that have the potential to interact with the coagulation systems. Activation of the kinin system by Hageman factor can lead to the generation of a kinin fragment, Kf, which can effect the binding of C4 and C2 to the activated C1 complex. This reaction results in the activation of a more efficient pathway to C3 convertase formation (Gigli *et al.*, 1971). Plasmin has also been shown to activate C1 (Ratnoff and Naff, 1967), cleave C3a anaphylatoxin from C3 (Taylor and Ward, 1967), and activate the C567 complex (Muller-Eberhard, 1976).

IV. INTERACTION OF CIC WITH PLATELETS AND RED BLOOD CELLS

A. Interaction with Platelets

The human platelet is a disk-shaped cell with a membrane rich in acidic mucopolysaccharides and glycoproteins. These surface molecules play an important role in the adhesive properties of the platelet and in aggregation. Adherent to the platelet surface are a series of plasma proteins, such as fibrinogen, complement C3 and C4, immunoglobulins, and coagulation factors V, XI, and XIII. Also present are Fc-like receptors and in some species complement receptors. Certain types of CIC can possess the essential configurations to interact with human platelets and red blood cells. In the former case, there is evidence that complement-binding immune complexes can interact with and bind fibrinogen (Robbins and Stetson, 1959). This then aids in the attachment or adsorption of the immune complex to the platelet membrane. When this occurs, the complement lyses the platelet, thus releasing some vasoactive substances and allowing the complex to deposit on the surrounding vessel wall. This deposition is aided by the increased flow of vascular fluid through the altered permeability

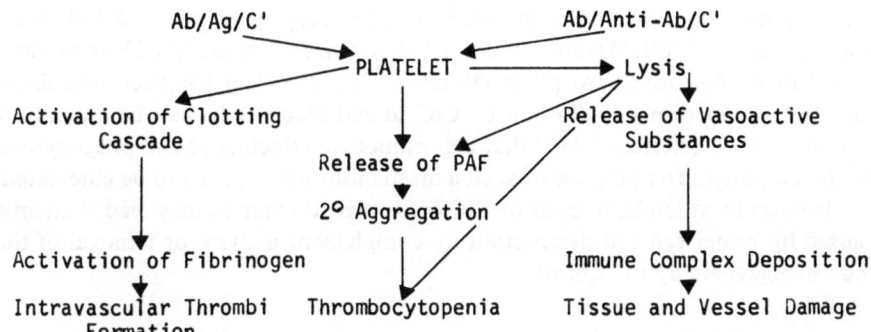

Figure 4. Schematic diagram of the interactions between CIC and platelets. The pathways show the involvement of platelets in immune complex deposition (right-hand side) and either the formation of a thrombocytopenic state (center) or activation of the clotting cascade and formation of intravascular thrombi (left-hand side).

of the affected vessel (Humphrey and Jaques, 1955). However, in some cases the attached complex does not lyse the platelet but induces it to release platelet-aggregating factor, which in turn causes other "innocent bystander" platelets to adhere and undergo primary aggregation. If the stimulus is great enough, then the primary aggregation will progress to secondary aggregation and the formation of occluding thrombi (Fig. 4).

It is known that platelets passively absorb IgG onto their membranes and that in certain species, e.g., the rabbit, platelets contain receptors for C3 and C3b (T. S. Zimmerman, 1974; Theofilopoulos and Dixon, 1980). With their readiness to adhere to immune complexes it is easy to postulate that platelets have a function in the clearance of complexes. They adhere to certain charged complexes, thus forming a loose aggregate that in turn will release chemotactic chemicals that recruit monocytes. In this way, platelets assist in wrapping up a potentially dangerous immune complex and make it easier for the monocytes to locate and remove it. When this system becomes overactive or the immune complex contains enough platelet-activating substance to tip the adherence into the aggregation phase, then a pathological stage may arise in which platelets are destroyed, circulating microthrombi are formed, vessels become occluded, and a general state of thrombocytopenia often associated with purpura is induced. Once in the state, the patient is at risk of death by vital organ ischemia owing to vessel blockage or a bleeding disorder.

B. Interaction with Red Blood Cells

Red blood cells can also interact with CIC and often form weakly interacting rosettes around the complexes. There is some evidence that this rossette formation is caused either by an interaction between bound complement in the immune complex and a low-affinity C3b receptor on the red cell membrane (Fearon, 1980; Aikawa *et al.*, 1979; Cornacoff *et al.*, 1981) or by non-complement-mediated adsorption (Virella *et al.*, 1983). It has been postulated that this interaction or adhesion of CIC to red blood cells may be a complex clearing system (Nelson, 1953) that aids monocyte attachment and phagocytosis of the complex. The purpose of such a mechanism still remains to be elucidated, but in cases in which high levels of CIC exist, this attachment may lead to anemia caused by either red cell destruction by complement activity or removal of the red cell aggregate by the spleen.

V. THE ROLE OF CIC IN LYMPHOCYTE FUNCTION

The interaction between CIC and lymphocytes can have both a suppressive and an enhancing effect on the host's immune system. Complexes have been reported as the "blocking factors" responsible for suppressing lymphocyte reactions against tumor cells (Baldwin and Robins, 1975; Sjögren *et al.*, 1971; K. E. Hellström *et al.*, 1977) yet there is also experimental evidence that complexes may have enhancing effects on both T- and B-cell function (Uhr and Phillips, 1966; Yoshida and Andersson, 1972; Vansnick *et al.*, 1978; Thoman *et al.*, 1981). Table III summarizes the possible effects that CIC may exert on lymphocyte immune functions.

Table III. Effects of CIC on Lymphocyte Immune Functions

Suppression
    Enhance production of T suppressor cells
    Block macrophage/T-cell cooperation
    Block delayed hypersensitivity reactions
    Block cell-mediated cytotoxicity reactions
    Block antibody-dependent cytotoxicity reactions
    Block T/B-cell cooperation
    Block B-cell activation by antigen masking
    Block B-cell activation by reactions with Fc and antigen receptors
    Induction of suppressive antiidiotypic antibodies

Enhancement
    Enhance macrophage processing of antigen
    Stimulate T helper cells
    Stimulate B-cell differentiation
    Enhance T/B cooperation by acting as antigen presenter
    Stimulate T and B cells by induction of enhancing antiidiotypic antibodies

A. Suppressive Effects on T and B Cells

CIC may have an effect on any cell that expresses an Fc, complement, or antigen receptor. It is via these receptors that the complexes may exert their effects, especially on lymphocytes. The suppressive or enhancing effect will be determined by the makeup of the complex and the type of receptor to which it is attached. At the T-cell level, CIC can affect the traffic of lymphocytes and block both delayed hypersensitivity (Gauci et al., 1981) and cell-mediated cytotoxicity reactions (Jose and Seshada, 1974; Panay et al., 1977) by binding to specific antigen receptors. In addition, they can enhance the production of suppressor T cells and affect macrophage/T-cell antigen processing (Klaus, 1979; Gauci et al., 1980).

At the B-cell level CIC can block the interactions between T and B cells and can suppress B-cell activity by either antigen masking or interaction with specific antigen and Fc receptors (Sinclair and Chan, 1971; Kolsch et al., 1980). Interaction with specific antigen receptors may also induce the release of suppressor factors.

B. Enhancing Effects on T and B Cells

On the other hand, immune complexes have been shown to enhance both T- and B-cell responses by enhancing macrophage processing of antigen, stimulating T helper cells, aiding in stimulation of B-cell differentiation, and acting as bridging agents in T/B-cell cooperative interactions (Uhr and Phillips, 1966).

C. Effects of CIC Interactions with Lymphocytes in Cancer Patients

In cancer patients, the immune complex acts as a tumor growth promoter by affecting the immune response either at the effector stage or by interactions at the lymphocyte activation stage. At the effector level, B-cell activity is reduced following membrane interaction with immune complexes either via Fc receptors or through antigen receptors (Kolsch et al., 1980). There can be selective suppression of T-cell activity following contact of the primed lymphocyte with complexed antigen.

Experimental evidence has shown that immune complexes are both immunogens and adjuvants all in one (Uhr and Phillips, 1966) and that they can induce the formation of anti-antibodies, which have another effect on the immune system. Antiidiotypic antibodies directed against antigen receptors on T cells will act as both masking agents and suppressive factors. An antiidiotypic antibody reaction with either a membrane idiotype or its corresponding antigen receptor will induce a suppressive effect on the target T cell (Eichmann, 1978). In addition, such antiidiotypes will also interact with circulating antibody and neutralize its activity at the molecular level and its production at the clonal level.

VI. CLINICAL SIGNIFICANCE OF CIC IN CANCER PATIENTS

The detection and measurement of CIC in cancer patients has shown both good and poor correlation with the progression of the disease. The best example of prognostic value comes from the excellent work of Carpentier and co-workers (1982), who have shown a correlation between immune complex levels and the prognosis of acute nonlymphocytic leukemia. However, many other workers have demonstrated only partial correlations (Amlot *et al.*, 1976; Chollet *et al.*, 1980; Hubbard *et al.*, 1981; Phillips *et al.*, 1982) or no correlation (Minden *et al.*, 1980; Pesce *et al.*, 1980; Williams *et al.*, 1983) with the course of neoplastic disease.

However, there are other reasons for monitoring the presence of immune complexes and analyzing both their components and their pathophysiological roles. Detection of immune complexes is important in assessing the immunological status of the patient. The presence of complexes will indicate (1) that a humoral response is in progress, (2) that there is a potential interaction between the CIC and the cellular or molecular components of other systems, and (3) that there is a danger that pathological lesions may arise from immune complex deposition. Analysis of such pathophysiological roles of CIC as cryoprecipitation, lymphocyte blocking, platelet and erythrocyte aggregation, and anti-antibody activity can give important information on the course of the patient's disease (Table IV).

Table IV. Pathological Conditions Arising from the Presence of CIC

Condition	Cause
Glomerulonephritis	Immune complex deposition in kidneys
Vasculitis	Immune complex deposition in vessels
Purpura	Immune complex deposition in skin
Retinal vasculitis	Immune complex deposition in retinal blood vessels
Thrombocytopenia	Immune complex interaction with platelets
Anemia	Immune complex interaction with erythrocytes
Intravascular coagulation	Immune complex interaction with the clotting, kinin, and fibrinolytic systems
Anergy	Immune complex interaction with lymphocytes

A. Immune Complex Deposition in Tissues

There are several important target organs for immune complex deposition. The most easily recognized process is deposition in the kidney glomeruli, with resulting nephrotic syndrome (Lewis *et al.*, 1971; L. W. Jones *et al.*, 1975; Pascal *et al.*, 1976; Olsen *et al.*, 1979; Dosa *et al.*, 1983). Complex deposition can also take place in the choroid plexus of the brain (Atkins *et al.*, 1972) in the capillary beds of skin and lungs (Tan and Kunkle, 1966; Schroeter *et al.*, 1976; Eagan *et al.*, 1979), and in the ciliary body and retinal vessels of the eye (Andrews *et al.*, 1977).

B. Effects on the Host Coagulation System

In addition, the presence of platelet-activating immune complexes may lead to *in vivo* platelet aggregation and thrombocytopenia. In several patients treated with mitomycin C as part of their treatment regime for colonic and gastric cancer, TTP arose as a result of platelet-activating immune complexes (S. E. Zimmerman *et al.*, 1982; Cantrell *et al.*, 1982). These complexes arose following a host response against the tumor, and in some cases the thrombocytopenia was the primary cause of death. Although evidence of intravascular coagulation and thrombi could be found at autopsy, the residual tumor mass was minimal. Removal of the complexes by plasmapheresis resulted in a return to reasonably good health in half of the patients. Interaction of CIC with other components of the coagulation system may lead to intravascular coagulation, mediated through complex-bound complement interaction with fibrinogen and Hageman factor.

C. Effects on the Host Immune System

The effect of complexes on the functions of primed lymphocytes is an important aspect to monitor. The suppression or masking of cell-mediated responses to the tumor results in a promotion of tumor growth. In addition, the effects of immune complexes on the suppression of B-cell responses will lead to a shutdown of cytotoxic antibody production, and again a situation of potential tumor growth promotion.

However, the most important aspect of immune-complex-mediated suppression will be the stimulation of plasma cells to produce anti-antibodies, especially antiidiotypes. These anti-antibodies can suppress not only the interaction of specific antibodies with their respective antigens but also their production at the cellular level. Antiidiotypes can also suppress and regulate T-cell responses by interaction with idiotypic receptors on the lymphocyte membrane (Klaus, 1979). The full potential of antibody regulation, especially the suppressive aspect, has not been fully characterized to date, but daily experimental work is proving that this regulatory feedback mechanism is as powerful as it was originally described to be by Jerne (1974). Detection of such initiating factors as antitumor antibody/anti-antibody complexes may prove to be of great value in assessing the future immune status of the cancer patient and could play a vital role in treatment management.

VII. CLINICAL TREATMENT MODALITIES FOR THE REMOVAL OF CIC

A. Experience with Plasma Exchange and Plasmapheresis

Following the work of Hersey *et al.* (1976), in which it was shown that cellular immunity could be restored in melanoma patients following removal of CIC by plasmapheresis, we treated ten cancer patients (five colon, two gastric, one nasopharyngeal, one sarcoma, and one melanoma) at the Georgetown University School of Medicine with first plasma exchange and then continuous-flow plasmapheresis. Although we succeeded in reducing the levels of immune complexes detectable by C1q (Zubler *et al.*, 1976) and Raji cell (Theofilopoulos *et al.*, 1976) assays, this reduction did not improve the immunological defense against the tumors in six of the ten patients studied. The four patients who responded to the treatment showed a marked improvement in their cell-mediated immune response to their tumors, although none showed any clinical improvement. The findings from this study are summarized in Table V. However, the materials obtained from the removed immune complexes were valuable in establishing assays for further monitoring of the patients response to the complexed antigen.

B. Experience with Protein A Immunotherapy

Protein A, found in the cell wall of the Cowan I strain of *Staphylococcus aureus* (SAC), possesses the characteristics of binding to IgG via the Fc portion of the molecule (Kessler, 1975; Forsgren and Sjoquist, 1966; Kronval *et al.*, 1977). Furthermore, it has been shown that IgG complexed with antigen binds more avidly than, and is not displaced by, free IgG (Kessler, 1975). These findings would imply that passage of plasma over SAC or immobilized protein A might be an effective method for removing CIC, which in turn may decrease the blocking activity in tumor hosts and influence the immunological environment in a beneficial fashion. Indeed, early studies in a single human by Bansal *et al.* (1978*a*,*b*) and in dogs with mammary carcinoma by Terman (1979) and Terman

Table V. Effects of Plasmapheresis on Blocking of Cell-Mediated Immunity

Patients	C1q assay[a]		Raji cell assay[b]		Cell-mediated immunity[c]	
	Pre	Post	Pre	Post	Pre	Post
Colon						
1	23	19	234	157	5	12
2	18	9	206	107	9	35
3	19	12	184	133	11	17
4	21	7	115	59	18	49
5	17	13	215	146	3	10
Gastric						
1	14	6	183	47	3	31
2	25	15	218	160	10	18
Nasopharyngeal	23	17	175	109	14	20
Melanoma	16	5	139	51	21	52
Sarcoma	21	12	208	56	5	14

[a] C1q assay values are expressed as percent inhibition.
[b] Raji cell assay values are expressed as μg AHGG (aggregated human gamma globulin)/ml.
[c] Cell-mediated cytotoxicity expressed as percent kill of autologous tumor cells at a lymphocyte/target cell ratio of 300:1.

et al. (1980) indicated that plasma passage over SAC could result in tumor regression in the absence of other intervention. These studies, however, did not employ a separate concurrent control group, nor evaluate the potential effects of materials that might be eluted from SAC and enter the circulation.

1. Laboratory Experience with Protein A Immunoadsorbents

Immunoperfusion over columns containing agarose-immobilized protein A was performed on the plasma from eight additional patients with various cancers (four melanoma, two colon, one eosphageal, and one testicular) who were undergoing plasmapheresis therapy. Levels of immune complexes were measured pre- and posttreatment by C1q and Raji cell assays. The treatment was shown to be more effective than straight plasmapheresis, the levels of the immune complexes being reduced significantly ($P < 0.001$ by paired t-test) in seven of the eight subjects (Fig. 5). Perfusion over plain agarose did not demonstrate such removal. However, it was found that at least two to three perfusions, over fresh agarose/ protein A columns, were required before complete removal of CIC could be achieved (Fig. 6).

2. Animal Studies on Immunoperfusion Therapy

To elucidate further the observations reported by Bansal *et al.* (1976) and Terman *et al.* (1980), we studied a series of 20 dogs with spontaneous mammary

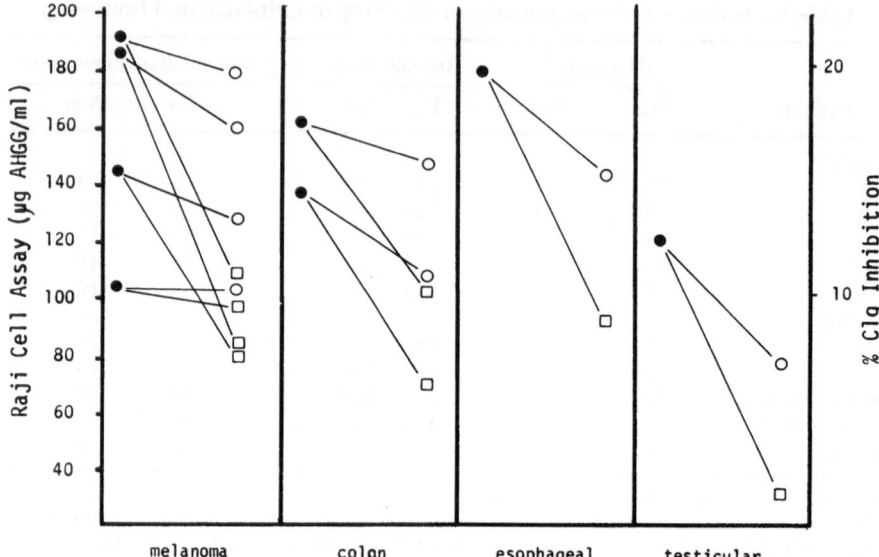

Figure 5. Comparison between plasmapheresis and protein A treatment for the removal of CIC in cancer patients. ●, Pretreatment levels of complexes, as measured by the Raji cell assay. ○, Immune complex levels following plasmapheresis. □, Pretreatment plasma that was perfused over agarose-immobilized protein A. In seven of eight patients, the protein A treatment was more efficient than straight plasmapheresis in removing the complexes.

carcinomas at the National Cancer Institute, National Institutes of Health (NCI, NIH). Ten animals were treated by passage of plasma over a SAC suspension by use of a cell separator in line with 0.2-μm filters loaded with 0.2 g SAC/kg body weight ("treatment" group), and five with passage of plasma through filters filled with only normal saline ("control" group). In order to assess the potential effect of leaching of materials from the SAC suspension, five dogs were treated with intravenous infusion of pooled normal dog plasma that had been passed through filters loaded with SAC suspension ("infusion" group) (Holohan *et al.*, 1982). We observed a 50% or greater reduction of measureable chest wall tumor in five of the ten treatment group animals (responders). None of the five control animals and none of the five infusion group animals exhibited tumor regression and these were considered nonresponders (Holohan *et al.*, 1982).

Immune complex detection and analysis were carried out on the pre- and postimmunoadsorption plasma of the treatment group dogs. Immune complexes capable of blocking cell-mediated cytotoxicity *in vitro* were more effectively removed in responder animals (67% removal) than in nonresponders (10% removal) (Table VI), but these differences did not achieve statistical significance. IgG levels were unaffected by the immunoadsorption procedures, and no significant toxicity was observed. The predicted benefit of immunoperfusion over SAC was the re-

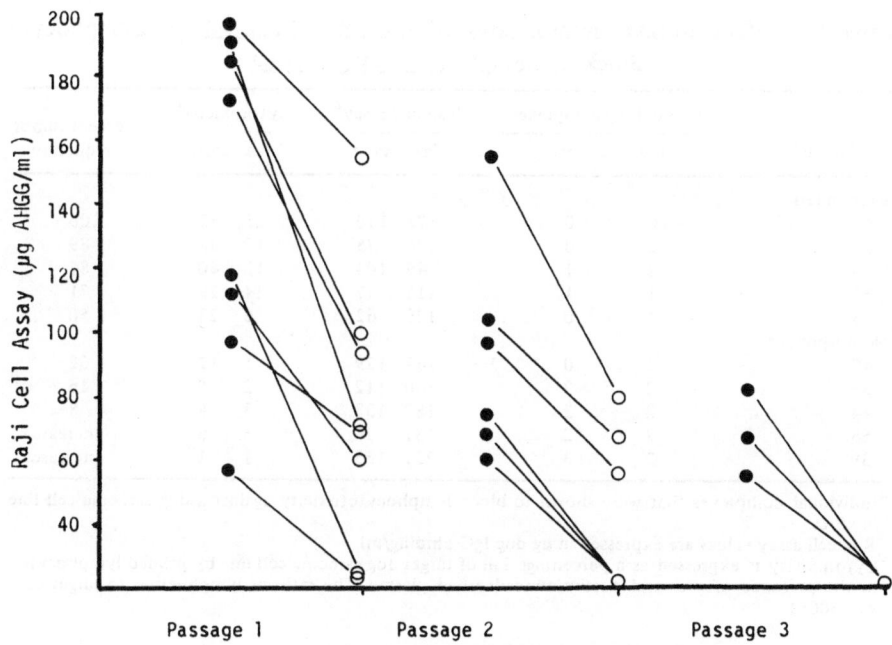

Passage over Agarose - Protein A

Figure 6. Agarose-immobilized protein A removal of CIC. ●, Pretreatment levels of immune complexes, as measured by the Raji cell assay. ○, Posttreatment levels. In six of eight plasma samples, a second passage over fresh protein A was required to further diminish the immune complex levels, and in three of six a third passage over fresh protein A was required before the immune complexes were completely cleared.

moval of immunosuppressive material—particularly, given the binding properties of protein A, the removal of CIC. Such immune complexes have been demonstrated in the sera of dogs with mammary carcinoma (Terman, 1979; Terman et al., 1980; Gordon et al., 1980), and persistence after surgical removal of the tumor was associated with a high likelihood of recurrence (Gordon et al., 1980). The lack of response to SAC-treated, normal pooled dog plasma implied that the observed tumor reduction was not due to the leaching of some eluate of the SAC, but rather required an interaction of the bacterial suspension with autologous plasma.

3. Clinical Experience with Immunoadsorption Therapy

a. NCI, NIH Experience. We concluded that plasma immunoadsorption with material able to remove CIC was capable of producing partial regression in soft tissue primary and metastatic tumor in a preclinical canine model, although

Table VI. Effects of SAC Immunoadsorption on the Removal of Lymphocyte Blocking Complexes in a Dog Model

Animal	No. blocking complexes[a]		Raji cell assay[b]		Cytotoxicity[c]		Percent tumor reduction
	Pre	Post	Pre	Post	Pre	Post	
Responders							
42	0	0	172	110	25	53	100
24	2	0	126	75	17	38	89
34	2	1	149	103	12	40	84
36	1	1	115	97	14	29	71
43	1	0	129	62	8	23	50
Nonresponders							
40	2	0	167	129	5	12	32
35	2	2	100	112	2	10	16
44	2	2	189	133	3	8	8
55	2	2	161	120	5	5	Increase
39	2	3	237	133	1	1	Increase

[a]Individual complexes that were shown to block lymphocytotoxicity against a dog sarcoma cell line *in vitro*.
[b]Raji cell assay values are expressed in μg dog IgG binding/ml.
[c]Cytotoxicity is expressed as a percentage kill of target dog sarcoma cell line by primed lymphocytes, in the presence of pre- and postimmunoadsorbed plasma. The ratio of lymphocytes to target cells was 300:1.

we were unable to demonstrate a quantitative relationship between immune complex levels and tumor reduction. Consequently, a phase I trial in humans was begun at the Clinical Center, NCI, NIH. The materials and equipment were essentially the same as previously described (Holohan *et al.*, 1982), except that patients were successively treated with increasing quantities of SAC, comprising 0.1, 0.2, 0.4, 0.8, and 1.0 g SAC/kg body weight, respectively, for patients one through five (Deisseroth and Holohan, 1980). Patients selected were those for whom no standard therapy was effective; no restrictions were placed on tumor type, previous treatment, nor performance status of these five study patients (two esophageal carcinomas and one each colon carcinoma, synovial cell sarcoma, and melanoma). All were classified as poor performance status (3 or 4 on Eastern Cooperative Oncology Group Scale).

CIC were measured pre- and posttreatment by C1q and Raji cell assays and isolated by polyethylene glycol and sucrose gradient centrifugation (Phillips *et al.*, 1982), and each individual complex was evaluated for its ability to aggregate platelets. Immunoadsorption was effective in reducing the quantity of immune complexes to an average of approximately one-half of their pretreatment values (Table VII). Adsorbed materials were acid-eluted from the SAC filters; these were shown by Raji cell assay and polyethylene glycol density gradient analysis to consist nearly completely of immune complexes (Phillips and Lewis, 1980; Phillips *et al.*, 1982), and were maximal in the first few filters of each run; later

Table VII.   Effect of SAC Immunoadsorption in Cancer Patients: Removal of
Platelet-Aggregating Complexes

	Pretreatment	Posttreatment
C1q assay ($\bar{x}$)	23.8%	11.6%
Raji cell assay ($\bar{x}$)	232.8 μg/ml	138.8 μg/ml
Percent positive platelet-aggregating factor	84.6	27.0

filters eluted little or no absorbed material, even though elevated immune complex levels were present in the majority of postadsorption plasma samples (Fig. 7). The reason for this observation was not clear but it was felt to be due to dilution effects of the cell separator procedures.* In addition, other complications such as filter plugging and systemic toxicity resulted in only 25–60% of the planned plasma volume being processed. Removal of CIC was slightly less effective than in the preclinical canine studies, in part owing to increased technical problems with filter plugging. However, in contrast to the animal studies, no significant tumor regression was observed in the five humans treated. Pain at the site of the tumor was reported in approximately half of the perfusion procedures, but unlike the case reported by Bansal *et al.* (1976), tumor necrosis did not follow treatment.

Excessive toxicity was incurred by the immunoadsorption procedure in this group of patients. The major clinical problems were cardiorespiratory in nature, consisting of hypotension in the face of increased cardiac output and a marked increase in the alveolar–arterial gradient. This required fluid administration and vasopressors as well as oxygen administration in the majority of procedures. These hemodynamic and respiratory complications were felt to be a contributory cause of death in two patients. The hemodynamic changes were quite closely related temporarily to the reinfusion of adsorbed plasma. These side effects occurred at a treatment level far below that employed in the canine studies, and were quite similar to, though more marked than, those later reported by Young *et al.* (1983) using pure protein A immobilized in a solid charcoal matrix.

b. Georgetown Experience. In later studies of plasma immunoadsorption conducted at the Lombardi Cancer Center at the Georgetown University School of Medicine, pure protein A was employed rather than SAC and was covalently linked to polyacrylamide-coated glass beads (Korac *et al.*, 1984). Plastic cylinder filters were packed with beads containing 60 mg of protein A per treatment.

*Plasmapheresis kinetics are described by the equation $X = e^{-p}$, where X is the proportion of unexchanged plasma remaining and p is the proportion of exchanged plasma, assuming the intravascular volume to be a closed space.

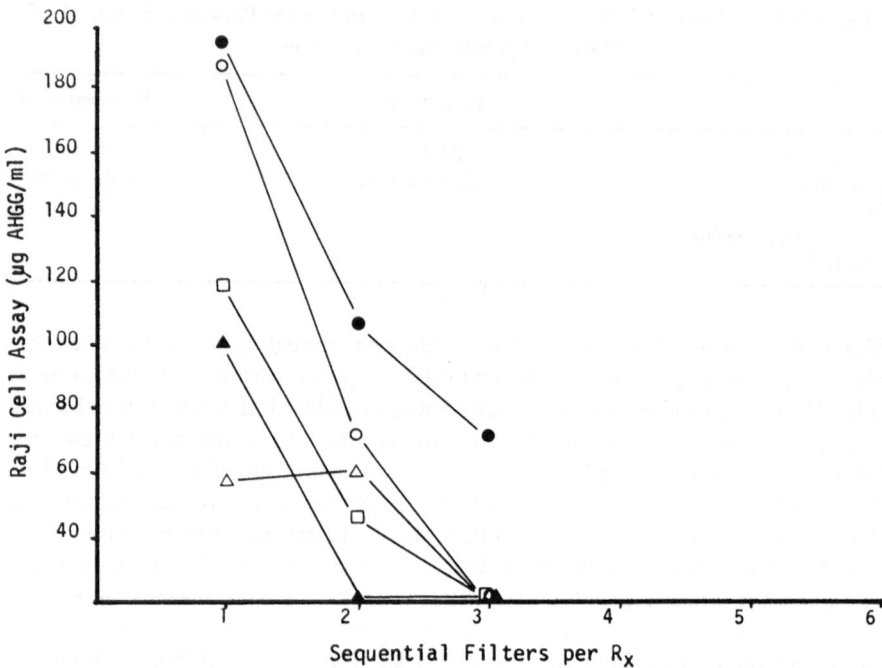

Figure 7. Levels of CIC recovered from sequential SAC filters in the five NCI, NIH phase I patients, showing little or no material retained following the third filter. ●, One of the esophageal carcinoma patients; ○, the other esophageal carcinoma patient; □, the colon carcinoma patient; △, the synovial cell sarcoma patient; ▲, the melanoma patient.

This therapy was applied to 11 patients with solid tumors (five colon, two ovarian, two melanomas, one prostate, and one breast carcinoma) who were not eligible for conventional treatment, and to three patients with TTP occurring after therapy with mitomycin C for gastric and colonic cancer. Antitumor effects were observed, but were modest in degree: Three patients showed partial tumor regression lasting from 3 to 6 months. Table VIII summarizes the results found in these 11 patients. Two of the TTP patients evidenced dramatic clinical improvement, with two- to fivefold increases in platelet count and approximately 50% increases in hematocrit. However, this treatment did not appear to affect their tumors, and they were discharged from the study after four and five immunoadsorptions, respectively. Diminution in treatment toxicity from the NCI phase I trials were achieved; in contrast to the NCI study (employing SAC), which engendered significant cardiorespiratory compromise, a fall in blood pressure greater than 35 mm Hg was observed in less than 5% of the treatments, and bronchial construction was observed only once, in patient with known asthma. Chills and fever occurred in more than one-fifth of the procedures.

Table VIII.   Effects of Immobilized Protein A Immunoadsorption[a]

Patient No.	Tumor size			Raji cell assay[b]		Clq assay[c]	
	Pre	Post	Response	Pre	Post	Pre	Post
Colon							
1	S	S	+	135	78	14	6
2	L	L	+	259	140	27	18
3	L	L	–	NT	NT	NT	NT
4	L	L	–	145	73	12	10
5	S	S	–	205	177	20	14
Melanoma							
1	L	L	–	169	100	18	9
2	–	–	–	NT	NT	NT	NT
Ovary	S	S	+	104	62	10	4
Prostate	L	L	–	163	101	20	12
Breast	L	L	–	152	98	17	10

[a] *Abbreviations:* followable tumor mass: S, small tumor mass (<5 cm); L, large tumor mass
(>5 cm). +, Positive response to immunoadsorption; –, negative response to immunoadsorption; NT, not tested.
[b] Raji cell assay values are expressed in μg AHGG/ml.
[c] Clq values are expressed in percent inhibition.

C. Conclusions

Plasma immunoadsorption with either SAC or purified protein A in human
tumor patients has thus far not achieved the success reported for animal studies,
notwithstanding the more optimistic report of Terman *et al.* (1981) of five
breast cancer patients treated with protein A immunoadsorption. At a recent
NCI symposium on immunoadsorption therapy, the overall response rate of all
reported trials was approximately 11%, with no complete remissions reported.
Despite these modest benefits in human trials, animal studies in canine mammary carcinoma (Terman, 1979; Terman *et al.*, 1980; Holohan *et al.*, 1982) and
feline leukemia (F. R. Jones *et al.*, 1980; Snyder *et al.*, 1982) uniformly document impressive tumor regression in a high proportion of subjects. As yet, the
data do not permit an explanation for the disparity between preclinical and
human studies. Indeed, although many tentative explanations regarding mechanisms of tumor necrosis induction have been offered, we do not feel that there
is sufficient evidence to rule out any of the more common explanations, including, among others, "blocking factor" removal, complement activation at the
tumor site, the "escape" of minute amounts of protein A into the circulation
(Langone *et al.*, 1983), and lymphocyte activation. Further clinical progress will
depend upon a painstaking experimental evaluation of the multiple possible
alternatives, employing rigorous controls.

VIII. REFERENCES

Aikawa, T., Mitamura, T., Tanimoto, K., and Horiudri, Y., 1979, Detection of circulating immune complexes by using human red blood cells, *J. Lab. Clin. Med.* **94**:902.

Amlot, P. L., Pussell, B., Slaney, J. M., and Williams, B. D., 1976, Correlation between immune complexes and prognostic factors in Hodgkin's disease, *Clin. Exp. Immunol.* **31**:166.

Andrews, B. S., McIntosh, J., Petts, V., and Penny, R., 1977, Circulating immune complexes in retinal vasculitis, *Clin. Exp. Immunol.* **29**:23.

Aoki, T., Walling, M. J., Bushar, G. S., Liu, M., and Hsu, K. C., 1976, Natural antibodies in sera from healthy humans to antigens on surfaces of type C RNA viruses and cells from primates, *Proc. Natl. Acad. Sci. USA* **73**:2491.

Atkins, C. J., Kondon, J. J., Quismorio, F. P., and Friou, G. J., 1972, The choroid plexus in systemic lupus erythematosus, *Ann. Intern. Med.* **76**:65.

Baldwin, R. W., and Robins, R. A., 1975, Humoral factors abrogating cell-mediated immunity in the tumour-bearing host, *Curr. Topics Microbiol. Immunol.* **72**:21.

Bansal, S. C., and Sjögren, H. O., 1971, Unblocking serum activity *in-vitro* in the polyoma system may correlate with antitumor effects of antiserum *in-vivo*, *Nature New Biol.* **233**:76.

Bansal, S. C., Bansal, B. R., and Boland, J. P., 1976, Blocking and unblocking serum factors in neoplasia, *Curr. Topics Microbiol. Immunol.* **75**:45.

Bansal, S. C., Bansal, B. R., Rhoads, J. E., Cooper, D. R., Boland, J. P., and Mark, E., 1978*a*, Ex-vivo removal of mammalian immunoglobulin G: Method and immunological alterations, *Int. J. Artif. Organs* **1**:94.

Bansal, S. C., Bansal, B. R., Thomas, H. L., Siegel, P. D., Rhoads, J. E., Cooper, D. R., Terman, D. S., and Mark, E., 1978*b*, Ex-vivo removal of serum IgG in a patient with colon carcinoma, *Cancer* **42**:1.

Bartfield, H., 1969, Distribution of rheumatoid factor activity in nonrheumatoid states, *Ann. N. Y. Acad. Sci.* **168**:126.

Beatty, P. G., Kim, B. S., Rowley, D. A., and Coppleston, L. W., 1976, Antibody against the antigen receptor of a plasmacytoma prolongs survival of mice bearing the tumor, *J. Immunol.* **116**:1391.

Browne, O., Bell, J., Holland, P., and Thornes, R., 1976, Plasmapheresis and immunostimulation, *Lancet* **2**:96.

Cantrell, J. E., Phillips, T. M., Smith, F. P., and Schein, P. S., 1982, Immune complex analysis and plasmapheresis in cancer related thrombotic thrombocytopenic purpura (TTP)/hemolytic uremic syndrome (HUS), *Blood* **60**:185a.

Carpentier, N. A., Fiere, D. M., Schuh, D., Lange, G. T., and Lambert, P. H., 1982, Circulating immune complexes and the prognosis of acute myeloid leukemia, *N. Engl. J. Med.* **307**:1174.

Chollet, P., Carpentier, N., Chassagne, G., Betail, J. M., Bidet, P. H., Lambert, P. H., and Plagne, R., 1980, Clinical relevance of circulating immune complexes in breast cancer, in: *International Symposium on New Trends in Human Immunology and Cancer Immunotherapy* (B. Serrou and C. Rosenfeld, eds.), pp. 496–503, Dion/Saunders, Paris.

Cochrane, C. G., and Dixon, F. J., 1976, Antigen–antibody complex induced disease, in: *Textbook of Immunopathology* (P. A. Miescher and H. J. Muller-Eberhard, eds.), pp. 137–156, Grune and Stratton, New York.

Cochrane, C. G., and Koffler, D., 1973, Immune complex disease in experimental animals and man, *Adv. Immunol.* **16**:185.

Cornacoff, J. B., Zager, R. A., and Herbert, L. A., 1981, Mechanisms of binding of immune complexes to human erythrocytes, *Clin. Res.* **29**:364A.

Cotropia, J. P., Gutterman, J. U., Hersh, E. M., Granatek, C. H., and Mavligit, G. M., 1976, Antigen expression and cell surface properties of human leukemia blasts, *Ann. N. Y. Acad. Sci.* 276:146.

Davies, G. E., and Lowe, J. S., 1960, A permeability factor released from guinea pig serum by antigen-antibody precipitates, *Br. J. Exp. Pathol.* 41:335.

Deisseroth, A., and Holohan, T. V., 1980, Extracorporeal immunoadsorption of plasma in cancer patients employing Cowan I *S. aureus*, Initial Proposal of Clinical Research Project Protocol, COP, DCT, National Cancer Institute, National Institutes of Health, Bethesda, Maryland.

Dixon, F. J., 1963, The role of antigen-antibody complexes in disease, *Harvey Lect.* 58:21.

Dixon, F. J., Feldman, J. D., and Vazquez, J. J., 1961, Experimental glomerulonephritis: The pathogenesis of a laboratory model resembling the spectrum of human glomerulo-nephritis, *J. Exp. Med.* 113:899.

Dosa, S., Phillips, T. M., Segal, A., Guha, A., and Thompson, A. M., 1983, Acute myeloblastic leukemia associated with nephrotic syndrome: An immunochemical study, *Nephron* 34:125.

Eagan, J. W., Roberts, J. L., Schwartz, M. M., and Lewis, E. J., 1979, The composition of pulmonary immune deposits in systemic lupus erythematosus, *Clin. Immunol. Immuno-pathol.* 12:204.

Eichmann, K., 1978, Expression and function of idiotypes on lymphocytes, *Adv. Immunol.* 26:195.

Eichmann, K., and Rajewsky, K., 1975, Induction of T and B cell immunity by anti-idiotypic antibody, *Eur. J. Immunol.* 5:661.

Eisen, V., and Smith, H. G., 1963, Plasma kinin formation by complexes of aggregated gamma globulin and serum proteins, *Br. J. Exp. Pathol.* 51:328.

Fairley, G. H., 1969, Immunity to malignant disease, *Br. Med. J.* 1:467.

Fearon, D. T., 1980, Identification of the membrane glycoprotein that is the C3b receptor of the human erythrocytes, polymorphonuclear leucocytes, B lymphocytes and mono-cytes, *J. Exp. Med.* 152:20.

Ferrone, S., and Pellegrino, M. A., 1978, Antigens and antibodies in malignant melanoma, in: *The Handbook of Cancer Immunology* (H. Waters, ed.), pp. 291-328, Garland STPM Press, New York.

Forsgren, A., and Sjoquist, J., 1966, Pseudo-immune reaction with human gamma globulin, *J. Immunol.* 97:822.

Gauci, L., Caraux, J., Cupissol, D., and Serrou, B., 1980, The relationship between circulating immune complexes and cellular immunity in cancer patients, in: *International Symposium on New Trends in Human Immunology and Cancer Immunotherapy* (B. Serrou and C. Rosenfeld, eds.), pp. 504-520, Dion/Saunders, Paris.

Gauci, L., Caraux, J., and Serrou, B., 1981, Immune complexes in the context of the immune response in cancer patients, in *Human Cancer Immunology: Immune Complexes and Plasma Exchanges in Cancer Patients* (B. Serrou and C. Rosenfeld, eds.), Vol. 1, pp. 37-98, Elsevier/North-Holland, Amsterdam.

Germuth, F. G., 1953, A comparative histologic and immunologic study in rabbits of induced hypersensitivity of the serum sickness type, *J. Exp. Med.* 97:257.

Gigli, I., Kaplan, A. P., and Austen, K. F., 1971, Modulation of function of the activated first component of complement by a fragment derived from serum, *J. Exp. Med.* 134:1466.

Gordon, B. R., Moroff, S., Hurvitz, A. T., Matas, R. E., MacEwen, E. G., Good, R. A., and Day, N. K., 1980, Circulating immune complexes in sera of dogs with benign and malig-nant breast disease, *Cancer. Res.* 40:3627.

Hartmann, D. P., 1976, The identification and role of anti-immunoglobulin in human malignancy, Ph.D. Thesis, McGill University, Montreal, Canada.

Hellström, I., and Hellström, K. E., 1969, Colony-inhibition studies on blocking and nonblocking serum effects on cellular immunity in Moloney sarcoma, *Int. J. Cancer* 5:159.

Hellström, K. E., Hellström, I., and Nepom, J. T., 1977, Specific blocking factors–Are they important? *Biochem. Biophys. Acta Rev. Cancer* 473:121.

Hersey, P., Edwards, A., Adams, E., Isbister, J. P., Murrey, E., Biggs, J. C., and Milton, G.W., 1976, Antibody-dependent cell-mediated cytotoxicity against melanoma cells induced by plasmapheresis, *Lancet* 1:825.

Holohan, T. V., Phillips, T. M., Bowles, C., and Deisseroth, A., 1982, Regression of canine mammary carcinoma after immunoadsorption therapy, *Cancer Res.* 42:3663.

Hubbard, R. A., Aggio, M. C., Lozzio, B. B., and Wust, D. J., 1981, Correlation of circulating immune complexes and disease status in patients with leukemia, *Clin. Exp. Immunol.* 43:46.

Huber, S., and Lucas, Z., 1978, Immune response to a mammary adenocarcinoma. V. Sera from tumor-bearing rats contain multiple factors blocking cell-mediated immunity, *J. Immunol.* 121:2485.

Humphrey, J. H., and Jaques, R., 1955, The release of histamine and 5-HT (serotonin) from platelets by antigen–antibody reactions (in vitro), *J. Physiol.* 128:9.

Jerne, N. K., 1974, Immune regulation in a lymphocyte network, in: *Cellular Selection and Regulation in the Immune Response* (G. M. Edelman, ed.), pp. 39–45, Raven Press, New York.

Jerry, L. M., Rowden, G., Cano, P. O., Phillips, T. M., Deutsch, G. F., Capek, A., Hartmann, D., and Lewis, M. G., 1976, Immune complexes in human melanoma: A consequence of deranged immune regulation, *Scand. J. Immunol.* 5:845.

Jewell, D. P., and MacLennan, I. C. M., 1973, Circulating immune complexes in inflammatory bowel disease, *Clin. Exp. Immunol.* 14:219.

Jones, F. R., Yoshida, L. H., Ladiges, W. C., and Kenny, M. A., 1980, Treatment of feline leukemia and reversal of FeLV by ex-vivo removal of IgG: A preliminary report, *Cancer* 46:675.

Jones, L. W., Levin, A., and Fudenberg, H. H., 1975, Glomerular antigen complexes associated with transitional cell carcinoma, *Surg. Gynecol. Obstet.* 140:896.

Jose, D. G., and Seshada, R., 1974, Circulating immune complexes in human neuroblastoma: Direct assay and role in blocking specific cellular immunity, *Int. J. Cancer* 13:824.

Kaplan, A. P., Spragg, J., and Austen, K. F., 1971, The bradykinin forming system of man, in: *Biochemistry of the Acute Allergic Reaction* (K. F. Austem and E. L. Becker, eds.), pp. 279–302, Blackwell, Oxford.

Kessler, S. W., 1975, Rapid isolation of antigens from cells with a staphylococcal protein A antibody adsorbent: Parameters of the interaction of antibody–antigen complexes with protein A, *J. Immunol.* 115:1617.

Klaus, G. G. B., 1979, Cooperation between antigen-reactive T cells and anti-idiotypic responses to antigen–antibody complexes, *Nature* 278:354.

Klein, G., 1971, Immunological studies on human tumors: Dilemmas of the experimentalist, *Isr. J. Med. Sci.* 7:111.

Klein, G., 1984, Induction, expression, and manipulation of immunity to tumors: A summary, in: *Progress in Immunology*, Vol. 5 (Y. Yamamura and T. Tada, eds.), pp. 1269–1275, Academic Press, New York.

Kolsch, E., Oberbarnscheidt, J., Bruner, K., and Heure, J., 1980, The Fc-receptor: Its role in the transmission of differentiation signals, *Immunol. Rev.* 49:61.

Korac, S., Smith, F. P., Schein, P. S., and Phillips, T. M., 1984, Clinical experience with extra-corporeal immunoperfusion of plasma from cancer patients, *J. Biol. Resp. Modif.* 3:330.

Kremer, W. B., and Laszlo, A., 1974, Hematologic effects of cancer, in: *Cancer Medicine* (J. Holland and E. Freii, eds.), pp. 1085–1090, Lea and Febiger, Philadelphia.

Kronval, T., Applebaum, E., Popovic, D., Gill, L., Sisson, G., Wood, G., and Anderson, B., 1977, Demonstration of immunoglobulin in tumor and marginal tissues of squamous cell carcinomas of the head and neck, *J. Natl. Cancer Inst.* 59:1089.

Langone, J. J., Das, C., Bennett, D., and Terman, D. S., 1983, Radioimmunoassays for protein A of *Staphylococcus aureus, J. Immunol. Methods* 63:145.

Langvad, E., Hyden, H., Wolf, H., and Kroeigaard, N., 1975, Extracorporeal immunoadsorption of circulating specific serum factors in cancer patients, *Br. J. Cancer* 32:680.

Lewis, M. G., Ikonopisov, R. L., Nairn, R. C., Phillips, T. M., Hamilton Fairley, G., Bodenham, D. C., and Alexander, P., 1969, Tumour-specific antibodies in human malignant melanoma and their relationship to the extent of the disease, *Br. Med. J.* 3:547.

Lewis, M. G., Loughridge, L. W., and Phillips, T. M., 1971, Immunological studies on a patient with the nephrotic syndrome associated with malignancy of non-renal origin, *Lancet* 2:134.

Lewis, M. G., Hartmann, D., and Jerry, L. M., 1976, Antibodies and anti-antibodies in human malignancy: An expression of deranged immune regulation, *Ann. N. Y. Acad. Sci.* 276:316.

Lewis, M. G., Phillips, T. M., and Rowden, G., 1979, Host–tumour interactions as examples of enhancement and tolerance, in: *Immunological Tolerance and Enhancement* (F. P. Stuart and F. W. Fitch, eds.), pp. 149–184, MTP Press, Lancaster, England.

Margaretten, W., and McKay, D. G., 1971, The requirement of platelets in the active arthus reaction, *Am. J. Pathol.* 64:257.

Mastrangelo, M. J., Laucius, J. F., and Outzen, H. C., 1974, Fundamental concepts in tumor immunology: A brief review, *Semin. Oncol.* 1:291.

Minden, P., Odom, L. M., Tubergen, D. G., Hardtke, M. A., Sharpton, T. R., Rose, B., Zlotnick, A., and Carr, R. I., 1980, Immune complexes in children with leukemia: Relationship to disease characteristics and to antibody response to mycobacterium Bovis (BCG) in patients receiving BCG immunotherapy, *Cancer* 45:460.

Morton, D. L., Malmagren, R. A., Holmes, E. C., and Ketcham, A. S., 1968, Demonstration of antibodies against human malignant melanoma by immunofluorescence, *Surgery* 64:233.

Muller-Eberhard, H. J., 1976, The serum complement system, in: *Textbook of Immunopathology* (P. A. Miescher and H. J. Muller-Eberhard, eds.), pp. 45–73, Grune and Stratton, New York.

Nelson, R. A., 1953, The immune-adherence phenomenon: An immunologically specific reaction between microorgansims and erythrocytes leading to enhanced phagocytosis, *Science* 118:733.

Nisenoff, A., Hopper, J. E., and Spring, S. B., 1975, *The Antibody Molecule*, Academic Press, New York.

Old, L. J., Boyse, E. A., Geering, G., and Oettgen, H. F., 1968, Serologic approaches to the study of cancer in animals and man, *Cancer Res.* 28:1288.

Olsen, J. L., Phillips, T. M., Lewis, M. G., and Solez, K., 1979, Malignant melanoma with renal dense deposits containing tumor antigens, *Clin. Nephrol.* 12:74.

Osterland, C. K., Harboe, M., and Kunkle, H. G., 1963, Anti-gammaglobulin factors in human sera revealed by enzymatic splitting of anti-Rh antibodies, *Vox Sang.* 8:133.

Panayi, G. S., Poston, R. N., and Corrigal, V., 1977, Inhibition of antibody-mediated lymphocyte cytotoxicity by aggregated human immunoglobulin, *Ann. Rheum. Dis.* 36 (Suppl):159.

Pascal, R. R., Iannaccone, P. M., Rollwagen, F. M., Harding, T. A., and Bennett, S. J., 1976, Electron microscopy and immunofluorescence of glomerular complex deposits in cancer patients, *Cancer Res.* 36:43.

Pesce, A. J., Phillips, T. M., Ooi, B. S., Evans, A., Shank, R. A., and Lewis, M. G., 1980, Immune complexes in transitional cell carcinoma, *J. Urol.* 123:486.

Phillips, T. M., and Lewis, M. E., 1976, Immune reactions in patients with bladder and prostatic cancer, *Aust. N. Zealand J. Surg.* 48:545.

Phillips, T. M., and Lewis, M. G., 1980, Detection of circulating immune complexes by polyethylene glycol sedimentation and double countercurrent immunoelectrophoresis, in: *Serologic Analysis of Human Cancer Antigens* (S. A. Rosenberg, ed.), pp. 701–703, Academic Press, New York.

Phillips, T. M., Queen, W. D., and Lewis, M. G., 1982, The significance of circulating immune complexes in patients with malignant melanoma, in: *Melanoma Antigens and Antibodies* (R. A. Riesfeld and S. Ferrone, eds.), pp. 289–316, Plenum Press, New York.

Phillips, T. M., Queen, W. D., More, N. S., and Thompson, A. M., 1985, Induction of anti-idiotypic antibodies by naturally occurring rheumatoid factor, *Ann. N. Y. Acad. Sci.* (in press).

Piessons, W. F., 1970, Evidence for human cancer immunity: A review, *Cancer* 26:1212.

Ratnoff, O. D., and Naff, G. B., 1967, The conversion of C'1 to C'1-esterase by plasmin and trypsin, *J. Exp. Med.* 125:337.

Robbins, J., and Stetson, C. A., 1959, An effect of antigen–antibody interaction on blood coagulation, *J. Exp. Med.* 109:1.

Robins, R. A., and Baldwin, R. W., 1978, Immune complexes in cancer, *Cancer Immunol. Immunotherapy* 4:1.

Rowley, D. A., Fitch, E. W., Stuart, F. P., Kohler, H., and Cosenza, H., 1973, Specific suppression of immune responses, *Science* 181:1133.

Schroeter, A. L., Conn, D. L., and Jordon, R. E., 1976, Immunoglobulin and complement deposition in skin of rheumatoid arthritis and systemic lupus erythematosus patients, *Ann. Rheum. Dis.* 35:321.

Shiku, H., Takahashi, T., Oettgen, H. F., and Old, L. J., 1976, Cell surface antigens of human malignant melanoma. II. Serologic typing with immune adherence assays and definition of two new surface antigens, *J. Exp. Med.* 144:873.

Sinclair, N. R., and Chan, P. L., 1971, Regulation of the immune response. IV. The role of the Fc-fragment in feedback inhibition by antibody, *Adv. Exp. Med. Biol.* 12:609.

Sjögren, H. O., Hellström, I., Bansal, S. C., and Hellström, K. E., 1971, Suggestive evidence that the "blocking antibodies" of tumor-bearing individuals may be antigen–antibody complexes, *Proc. Natl. Acad. Sci. USA* 68:1372.

Snyder, H. W., Jones, F. R., Day, N. K., and Hardy, W. D., 1982, Isolation and characterization of circulating feline leukemia virus-immune complexes from plasma of persistently infected pet cats removed by ex vivo immunoadsorption, *J. Immunol.* 128:2726.

Southam, C. M., 1967, Evidence for cancer specific antigens in man, *Proc. Exp. Tumor Res.* 9:1.

Tan, E. M., and Kunkle, H. G., 1966, An immunofluorescent study of the skin lesions in systemic lupus erythematosus, *Arthritis Rheum.* 9:37.

Taylor, F. B., and Ward, P. A., 1967, Generation of chemotactic activity in rabbit serum by plasminogen–streptokinase mixtures, *J. Exp. Med.* 126:149.

Terman, D. S., 1979, Extensive necrosis of primary and metastatic canine breast adenocarcinoma after extracorporeal perfusion over *S. aureus*-Cowan I, *Clin. Res.* 27:392.

Terman, D. S., Yamamoto, T., Mattioli, M., Cook, G., Tillquist, R., Henry, J., Poser, R., and Daskal, Y., 1980, Extensive necrosis of spontaneous canine mammary adenocarcinoma after extracorporeal perfusion over *S. aureus* Cowan I, *J. Immunol.* 124:795.

Terman, D. S., Young, J. B., Shearer, W. T., Ayus, C., Lehane, D., Mattioli, C., Espada, R., Howell, J. F., Yamamoto, T., Zaleski, H. I., Miller, L., Frommer, P., Feldman, L., Henry, J., Tilquist, R., Cook, G., and Daskal, Y., 1981, Preliminary observations of the effects on breast adenocarcinoma of plasma perfused over immobilized protein A, *N. Engl. J. Med.* **305**:1195.

Theofilopoulos, A. N., and Dixon, F. J., 1980, Immune complexes in human diseases, *Am. J. Pathol.* **100**:529.

Theofilopoulos, A. N., Wilson, C. B., and Dixon, F. J., 1976, The Raji cell radioimmune assay for detecting immune complexes in human sera, *J. Clin. Invest.* **57**:169.

Thoman, M. L., Morgan, E. L., and Weigle, W. O., 1981, Fc fragment activation of lymphocytes. I. Fc fragments trigger Lyt $1^+2^+3^-$T lymphocytes to release a helper T cell-replacing activity, *J. Immunol.* **126**:632.

Twomey, J. J., Rossen, R. D., Lewis, V. M., Laughter, A. H., and Douglas, C. C., 1976, Rheumatoid factor and tumor–host interaction, *Proc. Natl. Acad. Sci. USA* **73**:2106.

Uhr, J. Q., and Phillips, J. M., 1966, In vitro sensitization of phagocytes and lymphocytes by antigen–antibody complexes, *Ann. N. Y. Acad. Sci.* **129**:792.

Vansnick, J. L., Vanroost, E., Markowetz, B., Cambiaso, C. L., and Masson, P. L., 1978, Enhancement by IgM rheumatoid factor of in vitro ingestion by macrophages and in vivo clearance of aggregated IgG or antigen–antibody complexes, *Eur. J. Immunol.* **8**:279.

Virella, G., Shuler, C. W., and Sherwood, T., 1983, Non-complement dependent adsorption of soluble immune complexes to human red cells, *Clin. Exp. Immunol.* **54**:448.

Von Pirquet, C. F., and Schick, B., 1905, *Die Serum Krankheit*, Deuticke, Leipzig.

Waaler, E., 1940, On occurrence of factors in human serum activating specific agglutination of sheep red blood corpuscles, *Acta Pathol. Microbiol. Scand.* **17**:172.

Waller, M., Curry, S., and Richard, A., 1968, Serological specificity of IgG and IgM antiglobulin antibodies in anti-Gm(a) antisera, *Exp. Immunol.* **3**:631.

Williams, R. C., Duncan, M. H., Tung, K. S. K., Stinton, E. R., Walker, L. C., and Greaves, M. F., 1983, Characterization of immune complexes in acute lymphoblastic leukemia, *Clin. Exp. Immunol.* **54**:418.

Yoshida, T. O., and Andersson, B., 1972, Evidence for a receptor recognizing antigen complexed immunoglobulin on the surface of activated mouse thymus lymphocytes, *Scand. J. Immunol.* **1**:401.

Young, J. B., Ayus, J. C., Miller, L. K., Divine, G. W., Frommer, J. P., Miller, R. R., and Terman, D. S., 1983, Cardiopulmonary toxicity in patients with breast carcinoma during plasma perfusion over immobilized protein A, *Am. J. Med.* **75**:278.

Zimmerman, S. E., Smith, F. P., Phillips, T. M., Coffey, R. J., and Schein, P. S., 1982, Gastric carcinoma and thrombotic thrombocytopenic purpura: Association with plasma immune complex concentrations, *Br. Med. J.* **284**:1432.

Zimmerman, T. S., 1974, The platelet in complement-blood coagulation interaction, *Adv. Biosci.* **2**:1.

Zubler, R. H., Lange, G., Lambert, P. H., and Miescher, P. A., 1976, Detection of immune complexes in unheated sera by modified ^{125}I-C1q binding test: Effect of heating on the bonding of C1q by immune complexes and application of the test to systemic lupus erythematosus, *J. Immunol.* **116**:232.

Chapter 4

Immune Complexes in Patients Bearing Solid Tumors

Didier Cupissol, Christian Thierry, and Bernard C. Serrou

*Department of Chemo-Immunotherapy and
Laboratory of Tumor Immunopharmacology INSERM U-236
ERA-CNRS No. 844, Centre Paul Lamarque
BP 5054, 34 033 Montpellier Cedex, France*

I. INTRODUCTION

An immune complex is an immunological association of an antigen with its antibody. The nature of this complex is determined by the characteristics of the two constituents. The immunoglobulins involved in circulating immune complexes (CIC) undergo stereochemical transformations to render them incapable of reacting with diverse elements of the immune system as well as with cells responsible for inflammatory response, e.g., platelets, histiocytes, and erythrocytes. However, as with other immune phenomena, the formation and role of CIC is subject to a control mechanism determined by the nature of the antigen itself. Numerous authors have reported that insoluble CIC levels were frequently elevated in cancer patients. The prognostic value of these variations has been discussed (Amlot *et al.*, 1976, 1978; Benveniste *et al.*, 1972; Brandis *et al.*, 1978; Camussi *et al.*, 1977; Carpentier *et al.*, 1977; Cochrane, 1968; Gauci *et al.*, 1978b,c; Jose and Seshadri, 1974; Silberberg-Sinakin *et al.*, 1977).

The goal of our study was to try to establish the physiological and pathological roles of CIC in the cancer patient.

II. DETECTION OF CIC

The method used included both a qualitative and a quantitative evaluation of CIC. CIC were precipitated in 2.5% polyethylene glycol in the presence of

Table I. CIC in the Sera of Cancer Patients

	N	CIC (IU/ml)		
		IgG	IgM	IgA
Controls	28	1.25 ± 0.4	10.6 ± 3.8	1.03 ± 0.35
Osteosarcomas	17	1.72 ± 1.15	19.4 ± 9	2.98 ± 1.19
		(P < 0.06)	(P < 0.0005)	(P < 0.0005)
Malignant melanomas	100	1.90 ± 0.92	12.5 ± 11.7	1.74 ± 0.61
		(P < 0.05)	(P < 0.0005)	(P < 0.0005)
Liver metastases	42	3.06 ± 1.43	27.9 ± 21	3.4 ± 2.4
		(P < 0.0005)		
Primary hepatomas	7	6.11 ± 3.13	49.72 ± 30	10.5 ± 6.7
		(P < 0.0005)	(P < 0.0007)	(P < 0.0005)
Carcinoid tumors	2	2.65 ± 1.06	9.53 ± 6.33	3.7 ± 8.18
Adrenal adenocarcinoma	1	1.06	10.3	2.37

10 mM ethylenediaminetetraacetic acid and 70 μg/ml purified human C1q. IgG, IgM, and IgA concentrations were determined by an immunonephelometric method and the results expressed as IU/ml Ig-CIC in serum. The technique has been the subject of several previous publications (Amlot *et al.*, 1978; Carpentier *et al.*, 1977; Gauci *et al.*, 1978a–c).

III. CIC IN THE SERA OF CANCER PATIENTS

CIC levels were significantly higher in cancer patients compared to a control group of 28 healthy adults. The results for 169 patients are presented in Table I. The study included patients with osteosarcomas, malignant melanomas, primary hepatomas or liver metastases (usually of gastrointestinal origin), carcinoid tumors, and one case of adrenal adenocarcinoma. All three types of CIC (IgG, IgM, IgA) were elevated for each tumor type. This increase was significant ($P < 0.001$) for all groups except osteosarcoma and malignant melanoma. The variability of our results is probably due to the heterogeneity of the tumors tested as a function of both histological criteria and the treatment stage of each patient. Moreover, it appears as if immune complexes vary with age since older populations had higher CIC levels than younger adults (Table II).

A. CIC and Tumor Development

To a lesser degree, the level of CIC correlates with tumor mass. For example, cancer patients with malignant melanoma had higher CIC levels with recurrent disease compared to patients with no signs of recurrence. Moreover, patients

Table II. Increased CIC as a Function of Age

Healthy controls (years)	CIC (IU/ml)			
	N	IgG	IgM	IgA
20–40	28	1.25 ± 0.4	10.6 ± 3.8	1.08 ± 0.3
75–100	26	2.5 ± 0.7	19.8 ± 19.1	2.6 ± 0.7
P value		<0.0005	<0.001	<0.005

Table III. CIC and Tumor Mass

	CIC (IU/ml)		
	IgG	IgM	IgA
Secondary cancer of the liver	1.77	20.4	4.4
with tumor mass > 2 kg	4.40	31.3	7.3
	3.84	40.1	3.4
	2.62	25.6	5.3
	1.52	21.7	2.3
	1.61	7.3	2.5
	0.34	2.3	0.7
Malignant melanomas after	0.94	5.3	1.2
surgery	3.80	58.5	2.7
	4.10	23.2	2.6
	3.12	68.8	1.7
	1.15	3.0	0.8

with clinically recurrent disease presented even higher CIC levels, particularly IgG-CIC ($P < 0.01$) and IgM-CIC ($P < 0.02$), and to a lesser degree IgA-CIC ($P < 0.06$). Although our results are based on malignant melanoma patients, these same findings are relatively constant for all solid tumor patients. However, it should be noted that the difference between patients with recurrent disease and those in remission is minimal. Nevertheless, these differences may constitute a basis for identifying patient populations with a high risk of recurrence. At times, CIC levels rise prior to discovery of metastases; however, these findings must be viewed in light of the complex relationship between CIC levels and tumor mass. Elevated CIC may be the result of increased tumor mass but may also arise from release of soluble antigen excess and suppressed immune response (Tables III and IV).

B. Immune Complexes and Pleural Effusions

We measured CIC levels in 16 patients with pleural effusions caused by cancer. Fourteen of these patients had glandular cancer and two had lymphosar-

Table IV. Relationship between Clinical Status and CIC of Malignant Melanoma Patients

	N	CIC (IU/ml)		
		IgG	IgM	IgA
Complete remission	53	1.47 ± 0.7	8.5 ± 7	1.84 ± 0.7
Recurrence	24	2.11 ± 1.3	13.9 ± 12	2.24 ± 1.1
P value		<0.01	<0.02	<0.06

comas. The mean value for IgG-CIC was 0.28 ± 0.24; that for IgM-CIC, 2.48 ± 1.54; and that for IgA-CIC, 1.27 ± 0.7. Immune complexes were also found in pleural effusions from tuberculosis patients. In fact, based on the results of a small test series, immune complexes were significantly higher for tubercular pleuritis. We found that pleural immune complexes varied in the same manner as CIC for both cancer and tuberculosis patients.

C. CIC and Autologous Rosettes

A subpopulation of T lymphocytes can be identified by its capacity to form rosettes with autologous erythrocytes in the presence of autologous serum: autologous rosette-forming cells (ARFC). This procedure has been particularly developed in our laboratory, and the optimal conditions necessary for its realization have been the object of intensive investigations.

We found that autologous rosettes contain a T lymphocyte subpopulation devoid of Fc receptor for IgG. This subpopulation is frequently diminished in patients with recurring cancer. It is pointed out that CIC were not shown to affect the formation of autologous rosettes (Table V).

D. CIC and ADCC

The antibody-dependent cell-mediated cytotoxicity (ADCC) activity of mononucleated cells was tested using lymphoma 1210 cells in the presence of

Table V. Autologous Rosettes and CIC

Autologous rosettes	CIC (IU/ml)		
	IgG	IgM	IgA
Elevated (30%)	4.18 ± 1.87	47.9 ± 15	2.35 ± 0.3
Low (4%)	6.69 ± 6.38	49.8 ± 22	3.02 ± 2.95
P value	<0.04	<0.4	<0.05

Table VI. Coefficient of Correlation

	CIC (IU/ml)		
	IgG-CIC	IgM-CIC	IgA-CIC
Antibody-dependent cell-mediated cytotoxicity	−0.09	−0.07	−0.08
Autologous rosette-forming cells	−0.15	−0.15	−0.02

xenogeneic rabbit antiserum. Results are expressed as the number of cells required to produce 50% lysis. Some authors have used inhibition of ADCC activity to measure CIC. In our patient group, the distribution of ADCC activity was heterogeneous compared to the control group. Few patients had low ADCC activity when IgG-CIC was high (26%). We found no significant statistical correlation between ADCC and CIC (Table VI).

E. CIC and Delayed Hypersensitivity

We measured delayed hypersensitivity using the Merieux multitest method, which tests sensitivity to seven antigens and one control substance. The antigens are tetanus, diphtheria, streptococcus, tuberculin, candida, trycophyton, and proteus; the control was glycerin. All reactions were read at 48 hr. Erythema and an induration greater than 2 mm were considered as positive reactions. Testing took place 3-4 weeks after chemotherapy. This method is highly reproducible using only a small amount of inoculated antigen. We tested a hypothesis proposing a correlation between delayed hypersensitivity and CIC levels. Delayed hypersensitivity is expressed as a score (in mm) representing the sum of the average diameters of all seven antigen reactions. Since 80% of patients received bacillus Calmette-Guérin during therapy, we analyzed the tuberculin delayed hypersensitivity tests separately. The IgG-CIC levels seem to correlate with tuberculin hypersensitivity since CIC levels followed the positivity or negativity of the tuberculin results. The nontuberculin delayed hypersensitivity responses followed the same pattern as the tuberculin ones, but their changes were less pronounced (Fig. 1).

F. CIC and Plasmapheresis

CIC decreased in 82% of 43 plasmapheresed cancer patients. This decrease reached 50% in 32% of patients. This procedure was most effective for IgG-CIC, which have a lower molecular weight than IgM-CIC or IgA-CIC. In our study, plasmapheresis did not affect prognosis or therapeutic effectiveness (Fig. 2).

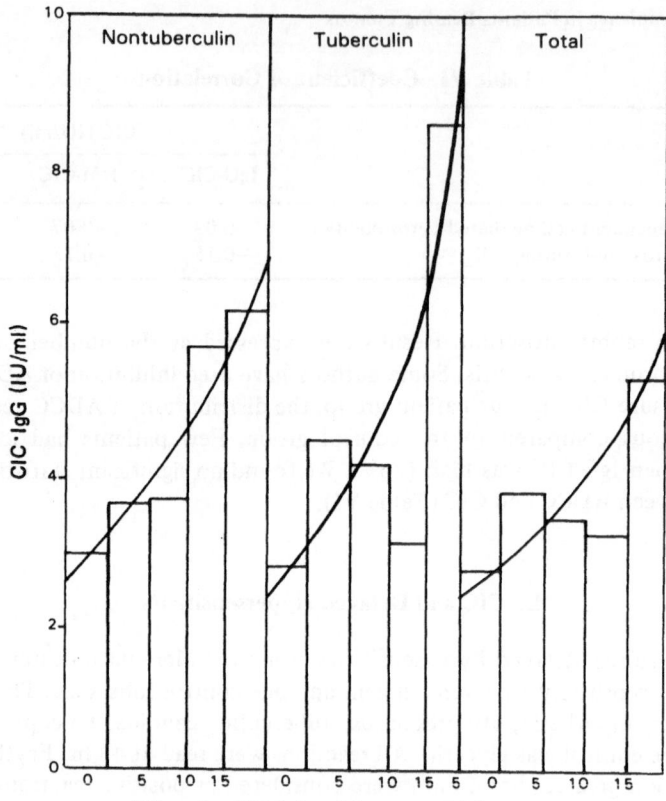

Figure 1. CIC delayed hypersensitivity.

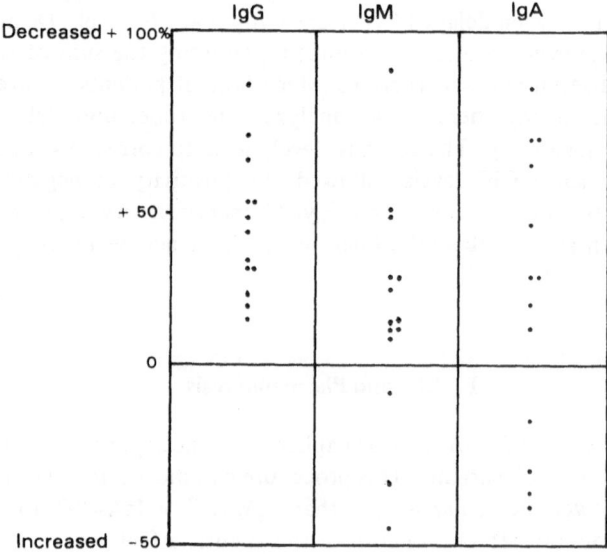

Figure 2. Percent CIC decrease following plasmapheresis.

IV. OVERVIEW AND CONCLUSION

It appears that immune complexes reflect host–tumor changes and may serve as indicators of tumor mass. For a large number of patients, pretreatment CIC levels offer a good prognostic indication. Sequential measurements show that CIC levels may foreshadow future recurrent disease prior to clinical symptomatology.

In the majority of cases increased CIC was concomitant with accelerated tumor growth. These results apparently contradict studies citing decreased CIC during evolving disease (Carr and Underwood, 1974; Heier *et al.*, 1977; Heimer and Klein, 1976). In fact, our results do not differ from those in the literature if one considers these previous results as reflecting an immunodeficient status, which may be explained by

1. Significant tumor growth inducing an antigen excess that affects tumor antigen–antibody complex stability, leading to dissociation (Jose and Seshadri, 1974).
2. Production by the tumor itself of glucocorticoid- or prostaglandinlike substances capable of dampening the immune response.
3. Induction of an activation of suppressor cells by tumor-associated antigens.

The results concerning CIC present an additional interest since they complement our studies on autologous rosettes. Moreover, the number of patients is still insufficient to determine whether there exists an interrelationship between delayed hypersensitivity CIC levels and therapeutic response.

Plasma exchange can be viewed as either a clearing process or a regulatory mechanism permitting the different elements of the immune response to respond under more optimal conditions.

At present, it is not possible to ascertain whether the elimination of immune complexes by plasmapheresis leads to induction of a better immune response and consequently an ameliorated therapeutic effect.

V. REFERENCES

Amlot, P. L., Slaney, J. M., and Williams, B. D., 1976, Circulating immune complexes and symptoms in Hodgkin's disease, *Lancet* 1:449.

Amlot, P. L., Pussel, B. Slaney, M. J., and Williams, B. D., 1978, Correlation between immune complexes and prognostic factors in Hodgkin's disease, *Clin. Exp. Immunol.* 31: 166.

Benveniste, J., Henson, P. M., and Cochrane, C. G., 1972, Leukocyte-dependent histamine release from rabbit platelets: The role of IgE, basophils and a platelet activating factor, *J. Exp. Med.* 136:1356.

Brandeis, W. E., Helson, L., Wang, Y., Good, R. A., and Day, N. K., 1978, Circulating immune complexes in sera of children with neuroblastoma: Correlation with stage of disease, *J. Clin. Invest.* 62:1201.

Camussi, G., Mencia-Huerta, J. M., and Benveniste, J., 1977, Release of platelet activating factor and histamine. I. Effect of immune complexes, complement and neutrophils on human and rabbit mastocytes and basophils, *Immunology* **33**:523.

Carpentier, N. A., Lange, G. T., Fiere, D. M., Fournie, G. J., Lambert, P. H., and Miescher, P. A., 1977, Clinical relevance of circulating immune complexes in human leukemia: Association in acute leukemia of the presence of immune complexes with unfavourable prognosis, *J. Clin. Invest.* **60**:874.

Carr, I., and Underwood, J. C. E., 1974, The ultrastructure of the local cellular reaction to neoplasia, *Int. Rev. Cytol.* **37**:329.

Cochrane, C. G., 1968, Immunologic tissue injury mediated by neutrophilic leukocytes, *Adv. Immunol.* **9**:97.

Gauci, L., Reme, T., Ursule, E., and Serrou, B., 1978*a*, Caracterisation immuno-néphélométrique des complexes immuns chez les cancéreux, *Biol. Prosp. IV Colloq. Pont. à Mousson* **236**:678.

Gauci, L., Ursule, E., and Serrou, B., 1978*b*, Circulating immune complexes in malignant melanoma, in: *Cutaneous Immunopathology* (J. Thivolet and D. Schmitt, eds.), p. 357, INSERM, Paris.

Gauci, L., Ursule, E., Pujol, H., and Serrou, B., 1978*c*, Clinical implications of elevated levels of circulating immune complexes in patients with malignant melanoma, in: *Protides of the Biological Fluids* (H. Peeters, ed.), Vol. 26, p. 349, Pergamon Press, Oxford.

Heier, H. E., Carpentier, N., Lange, G., Lambert, P. H., and Godal, T., 1977, Circulating immune complexes in patients with malignant lymphomas and solid tumors, *Int. J. Cancer* **20**:887.

Heimer, R., and Klein, G., 1976, Circulating immune complexes in sera of patients with Burkitt's lymphoma and nasopharyngeal carcinoma, *Int. J. Cancer* **18**:310.

Jose, D. G., and Seshadri, R., 1974, Circulating immune complexes in human neuroblastoma: Direct assay and role in blocking specific cellular immunity, *Int. J. Cancer* **13**:824.

Silberberg-Sinakin, I., Fedorka, M. E., Baer, R. L., Rosenthal, S. A., Berezowsky, V., and Thorbecke, G. J., 1977, Langerhans cells: Target cells in immune complex reactions, *Cell. Immunol.* **32**:400.

Chapter 5

Immunosuppressor Control as a Modality of Cancer Treatment: Effect of Plasma Adsorption with Staphylococcus aureus Protein A

Prasanta K. Ray

Department of Immunobiology
Industrial Toxicology Research Center
Lucknow 226001, India

I. INTRODUCTION

The concept of immunologic manipulation in the treatment of cancer is nothing new. Although it dates back to the late nineteenth and early twentieth centuries (Coley, 1891, 1893), little attention was paid to it for a long time. However, interest was revived with the discovery of tumor-associated antigens (TAA) on spontaneously occurring animal and human tumors (Old and Boyse, 1964; Old and Stockert, 1977; Möller, 1964; Hewitt *et al.*, 1976; Witz, 1977; Garrett *et al.*, 1977; Herberman, 1977; Prehn, 1976; Hewitt, 1978; Baker *et al.*, 1978; Billing *et al.*, 1978). These antigens are not usually found on normal cells, at least at detectable levels, and they are therefore considered to be tumor-associated. Among the various types of antigens detected so far on the cell membrane of tumor cells, besides tumor-specific antigens, are embryonic antigen, organ-specific antigen, and histocompatibility antigen (Gupta and Morton, 1983; F. Martin and Martin, 1970; Purves and Geddes, 1972; Sengupta and Ray, 1979; Ray and Seshadri, 1980, 1981). Against those antigens, both humoral and cell-mediated immune responses have been demonstrated *in vivo* and *in vitro*, implicating the "foreignness" of these antigens. An interesting review by Gupta and Morton (1983) discussed the characteristics of tumor antigens associated with animal and human tumors; the dynamic aspect of the immune response to tumor antigens; and their role in immune surveillance, rejection, and enhancement of tumor growth.

For some time it was believed that, in spite of being antigenic in nature, tumors could grow by a "sneaking through" mechanism. However, this concept seemed untenable in view of the fact that the host immune system can mount an attack against both autochthonous and syngeneic tumors (I. Hellström *et al.*, 1973; Herberman, 1974; Bansal and Sjögren, 1974; Raychaudhuri *et al.*, 1980; Ray, 1982, 1983). The question was then how a tumor could grow in the face of such opposing antitumor reactivity in the host. The ability of a tumor to grow in an otherwise immunologically competent host may be due to its ability to induce several immunosuppressor mechanisms to counteract the attack of the host against tumor growth (Gershon *et al.*, 1974; Bonnard and Herbermann, 1975; Cantor and Boyce, 1977; Klein, 1977; Kamo and Freidman, 1977; Benjamin *et al.*, 1978; Naor, 1979; Ray, 1982, 1983). We will discuss this particular phenomenon in detail in this chapter.

When one attempts to explain critically the phenomenon of tumor growth in a host, the usual picture that comes to mind is that, in order to survive and thrive, the tumor must counteract the normal cells reacting upon it on the one hand, and the immunocompetent factors (humoral and cellular) with the ability to destroy it on the other. It is between these two opposing forces that tumor cells must multiply and establish themselves, and then grow, develop, and clinically manifest their harmful effects. It has now become evident that both the normal cells and the immunocompetent factors, under suitable circumstances, are able to destroy a limited number of tumor cells. But tumor cells otherwise dominate those host factors and normally outsmart them. The major question is: How does the tumor counteract those opposing host factors?

If one looks at the profile of tumor cell growth and compares it with that of normal cell growth, it appears that the rapid turnover of tumor cells helps by increasing the total mass of the tumor at a given time, compared to that of normal cells. This is an important advantage of tumor cells, a genetically linked trait which enables them to overwhelm the surrounding pool of normal cells. It is also known that most tumor cells undergo mitosis at a rate faster than that observed in both normal and immunocompetent cells. Thus tumor cells,when allowed to grow without any interruption, can very quickly outnumber not only the surrounding opposing normal cells but also the immunocompetent cells. Yet even with that kind of advantage, tumor cells may not sit idle, because of the increasing threat of extinction by the host. In order to counteract that threat, tumor cells may induce immunosuppressive mechanisms, humoral and cellular, to depress the host's immunity. Another mechanism of tumor–host interaction may involve a direct attack on the immunocompetent cells by lymphotoxins or macrophage-migration-inhibiting factors (or similar types of molecules as yet unknown), which may be released by the tumor cells or induced by the normal cells. The tumor may also deplete the host nutritionally. Nutritional deprivation

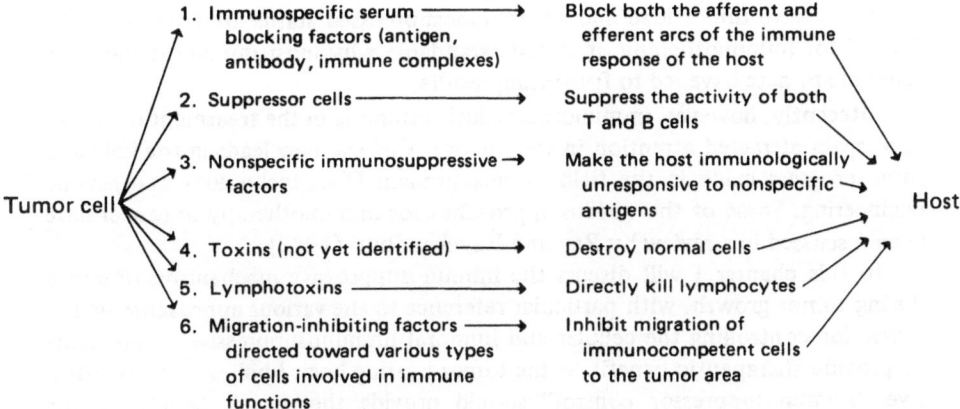

Figure 1. Tumor–host interactions facilitating continued growth of the tumor.

may in turn be responsible for immunologic suppression. As a result of such an all-around attack on the host, the tumor may attempt to create a favorable environment for uninterrupted growth, resulting in the killing of the host (Fig. 1).

Immunologic manipulation in the treatment of cancer aims at breaking the immunosuppressive environment of the host created by the tumor, so that host factors can once again become functional against the tumor. Although they have been practiced for some time now, the various immunotherapeutic measures have not been quite successful so far (Ray and Raychaudhuri, 1983). Among the several reasons for this is that the protocols utilized for cancer immunotherapy did not give adequate attention to the various factors discussed previously. Although attempts at immunotherapy to date have only brought frustration or, at best, some partial successes, those successes, however small, have been interesting enough to stimulate continued research in this area.

Although it is generally appreciated that cure rates in conventional cancer therapy have not been too high, immunotherapy is still not widely recommended. Immunotherapy is not given due consideration even though in some forms of cancer it has shown some success clinically. Another problem immunotherapists often experience is that they have to deal with the failures of conventional treatment modalities. Even though it is emphasized again and again that immunotherapy has its limitations in that it can only destroy a small mass of tumor cells, immunotherapeutic procedures are not used when the tumor mass is really small. Instead, conventional therapies are administered at this time. It has been recommended repeatedly by experts that immunotherapy would find its most appropriate application either as a treatment for early forms of cancer or as an adjunct treatment for minimal residual disease, yet this advice has, for all practical purposes, not been heeded thus far. Patients referred for immunotherapy usually have far advanced disease and a poor immunological profile.

Since excessive tumor load and an immunosuppressed status are both contraindicated for immunotherapy, it is understandable why most immunotherapeutic attempts to date have led to frustrating results.

Recently, however, immunotherapeutic attempts in the treatment of cancer have again attracted attention in view of some of the new leads in the field and some progress made in the field of recombinant DNA technology and genetic engineering. Some of the various approaches for immunotherapy of cancer have been discussed in a review by Ray and Raychaudhuri (1983).

In this chapter I will discuss the immunosuppressive mechanisms observed during tumor growth, with particular reference to the various approaches undertaken for controlling the cellular and humoral immunosuppressive components to provide therapeutic benefit to the tumor-bearing host. I believe that an effective "immunosuppressor control" should provide therapeutic benefit to the tumor-bearing host (Ray, 1982, 1983; Ray and Raychaudhuri, 1983) provided it is administered in appropriate circumstances.

Immunotherapeutic attempts have primarily centered around two goals: (1) augmentation of host immunity with the hope that this might lead to an effecttive immune attack against the tumor, and (2) counteraction of the immunosuppressor mechanisms to abrogate or decrease the "block" of the immunocompetent factors, so that the immunocompetent factors become functionally active to fight cancer (Ray, 1982, 1983). However, both the immunopotentiating factors that are utilized for augmenting the immune response of the host and attempts at specific and nonspecific immunotherapy have had mixed successes (Ray and Raychaudhuri, 1983). Most of the attempts showed either some partial response or no response at all. Some reports even showed facilitation of tumor growth (G. Moore et al., 1957; Attlic and Weiss, 1966; Andrews et al., 1967; McCredie et al., 1969; Fass, 1970; A. E. Moore and Gerner, 1970; Cohen et al., 1971; Yonemoto and Terasaki, 1972; Cohen, 1973; Dore et al., 1973; Mathe et al., 1973; Froese et al., 1974; Sparks and Breeding, 1974; Currie and McElwain, 1975; Wright et al., 1976; Albo et al., 1978; Spence et al., 1978; Ray et al., 1980b). Immunotherapy, especially with active specific agents, has been shown to have disastrous results if not properly regulated. Passive transfer of cells or serum has the potential to introduce both cellular and humoral immunosuppressor components to the host system, with obvious deleterious effects. Because of the possibility of introduction of both cellular and humoral immunosuppressor components, many uncontrolled immunotherapeutic attempts have so far shown only partial success. Thus, the hypothesis of an effective "immunosuppressor control" (Ray, 1982, 1983; Ray and Raychaudhuri, 1983) providing a valuable tool to control tumor growth under appropriate circumstances seems to provide a logical approach in cancer immunotherapy.

II. CELLULAR AND HUMORAL IMMUNOSUPPRESSIVE MECHANISMS IN THE TUMOR-HOST RELATIONSHIP

Several reports have indicated that antigenic tumors can grow *in vivo* in spite of the fact that the host may contain sensitized lymphocytes that have the ability to show antitumor cytotoxicity *in vitro*. These lymphocytes cannot deliver their cytotoxic effect against the tumor cells *in vivo* because of the presence of immunosuppressive factors (Ray, 1982, 1983; I. Hellström and Hellström, 1969; Sjögren *et al.*, 1971; Alexander, 1974; Kirchner *et al.*, 1974; Greene *et al.*, 1977; Raychaudhuri *et al.*, 1980; Ray and Raychaudhuri, 1983). Such factors can be broadly categorized into two types: humoral and cellular.

Cell-mediated immunosuppression causing facilitation of tumor growth has been described as being mediated by a specific class of cells called suppressor cells (Prehn, 1976; Treves *et al.*, 1974; Umiel and Trainin, 1974; Small, 1977; Yamagishi *et al.*, 1983). The nature of suppressor cells varies in different systems. Cells with immunosuppressive activity have been reported as being associated with T lymphocytes (Fujimoto *et al.*, 1976; Takei *et al.*, 1976; Hodes *et al.*, 1977; Pope *et al.*, 1976; Padrathsingh *et al.*, 1979; Yamagishi *et al.*, 1983), B lymphocytes (Turk *et al.*, 1972; Gorczynski, 1974; Kilburn *et al.*, 1974), and even macrophages (Kirchner *et al.*, 1974; Baird *et al.*, 1977a,b; Padrathsingh *et al.*, 1979; Yamagishi *et al.*, 1983).

Humoral factors having immunosuppressive ability are both specific and nonspecific. Tumor antigen is one of the specific humoral factors that has the ability to facilitate tumor growth (Alexander, 1974). Antitumor antibody has also been described as a specific humoral blocking agent (I. Hellström and Hellström, 1969; Pierce, 1971; K. E. Hellström *et al.*, 1977), and tumor-associated antigen-antibody complexes have been implicated as potentially effective immunosuppressive molecules in tumor hosts (Sjögren *et al.*, 1971; Baldwin *et al.*, 1972).

Several nonspecific humoral factors have also been reported to have the ability to facilitate tumor growth. These are soluble substances produced by tumor cells (Ron and Witz, 1972; Bansal *et al.*, 1972; K. E. Hellström and Hellström, 1979) or by lymphocytes (Hollander *et al.*, 1978; Isakov *et al.*, 1978, 1979; Israel *et al.*, 1977; Yamagishi *et al.*, 1983), and they will be discussed in greater detail in the following sections.

A. Immunosuppressive and Tumor-Growth-Enhancing Cells in Tumor-Bearing Hosts

Yamagishi *et al.* (1983) have described specific tumor-growth-facilitating cells in the spleens of mice pretreated with either crude 3 *M* KCl extracts or pIEF-fractionated, acidic antigen. In addition, they have also described nonspecific tumor-growth-facilitating cells in tumor-bearing mice. Adoptive transfer of a mixture of spleen cells from mice bearing methylcholanthrene-induced fibrosarcomas and the tumor cells facilitated the growth of fibrosarcomas. During the early stages of tumorigenesis, spleen cells from tumor-bearing mice indiscriminately facilitated the growth of a number of methylcholanthrene fibrosarcomas, both specific and nonspecific. Thus, Yamagishi *et al.* have concluded that the tumor-growth-facilitating cells are generated during the early stage of tumor growth, and that they are nonspecific. Nine to 15 days after tumor inoculation, tumor-bearing spleen cells inhibited the growth of specific types of tumor cells, but were not active against other types of tumor cells, suggesting the emergence of a specific cell-mediated immune response. Finally, in the late stage of tumor growth, the spleen cells neutralized the specific tumor cell growth, but facilitated the nonspecific fibrosarcoma growth, suggesting the presence of both specific tumor-neutralizing cells and nonspecific tumor-facilitating cells (Yamagishi *et al.*, 1983). They have also observed that the nonspecific tumor-facilitating cells that are present during the early stage of tumorigenesis are resistant to 700-R irradiation. They suggested that the facilitation of tumor growth was effected by preformed substances in cells that need not undergo DNA replication to promote tumor growth. Depletion of phagocytic adherent cells prior to the adoptive transfer test abrogated the tumor-facilitating activity. Thus, they concluded that the nonspecific tumor-facilitating activity was due to a radioresistant, phagocytic, adherent cell population, presumably macrophages. The tumor-bearing spleen cell population that specifically neutralized the neoplastic growth was radiosensitive and was inactivated by treatment with anti-Thy 1.2 serum and complement. Thus, the neutralizing activity of the spleen cells from the tumor-bearing host was probably mediated by a tumor-specific radiosensitive lymphocyte subpopulation. During the late stage of tumor growth, both of the cell populations were active. Irradiation of the spleen cells of the tumor-bearing host abrogated the specific tumor-neutralizing effect but did not alter the nonspecific tumor-facilitating activity.

We (Raychaudhuri *et al.*, 1980; Saha and Ray, 1982) have studied both cell-mediated and humoral effector and blocking immune reactions in C3H/Hej mice following inoculation with methylcholanthrene-induced fibrosarcomas. As shown by adoptive transfer experiments (Fig. 2), the tumor-specific cell-mediated immunity was operative as long as tumor diameter was between 0.5 cm and 1.0 cm. With the increase in tumor size, the splenocytes showed tumor growth enhancement (Table I). *In vitro* cytotoxicity assay using ^{51}Cr-labeled tumor cells showed that the cytotoxic ability of peripheral blood mononuclear cells was enhanced in the presence of plasma obtained 36 hr following tumor inoculation. From day 2 onward, plasma from animals preinoculated with the tumor cells showed a different property—blocking activity toward the cytotoxic peripheral blood mono-

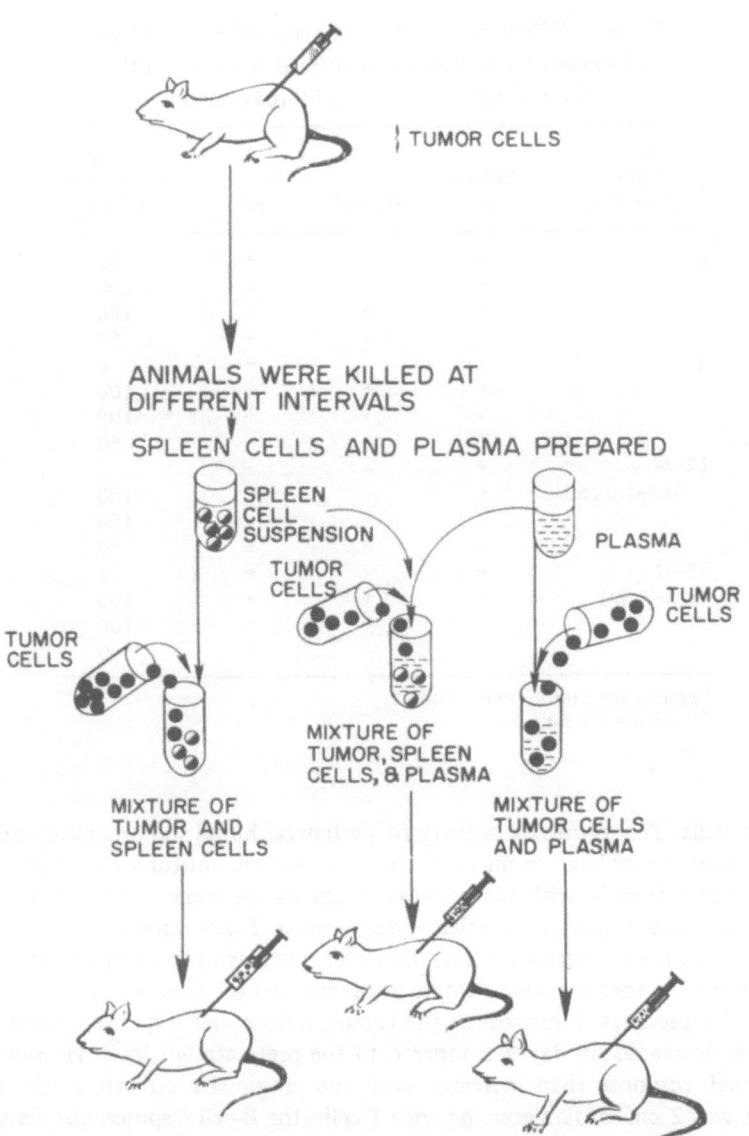

Figure 2. Scheme of adoptive transfer of spleen cells and plasma from mice inoculated with MC2 fibrosarcomas. In experiments in which mitomycin C-treated cells or KCl extracts of tumor cells were used for immunization purposes, the animals were killed on day 2 and then their cells and plasma were transferred following the above protocol.

Table I. Effect of Adoptive Transfer of Spleen Cells
and Plasma from Tumor-Inoculated Animals on the
Rate of Growth of MC2 Fibrosarcomas

Days (tumor diameter)	Spleen cell[a]	Plasma[b]	Tumor cell	Tumor incidence on day 14 (%)
2	+	−	+	50
	+	+	+	100
	−	+	+	100
	−	−	+	50
8	+	−	+	0
	+	+	+	100
	−	+	+	100
	−	−	+	50
12–24 (0.5–1.0 cm)	+	−	+	0
	+	+	+	100
	−	+	+	100
	−	−	+	0
25–35 (2–3 cm)	+	−	+	75
	+	+	+	100
	−	+	+	100
	−	−	+	0

[a]Spleen cell : tumor cell = 100 : 1.
[b]Plasma = 0.5 ml.

nuclear cells. The cytotoxic activity of peripheral blood mononuclear cells was lost in large-tumor-bearing mice. However, cytotoxic antitumor antibody activity increased directly with the increase in size of the tumor (Fig. 3). By day 2, the blastogenic response of splenocytes against T-cell mitogen was increased compared to the pretreatment level. However, the blastogenic response decreased about the time that palpable tumors appeared, and the decrease was maintained during the progressive growth of the tumor. Spleen cell response against B-cell mitogen decreased on day 2 compared to the pretreatment level. However, the spleen cell response then increased with the progressive growth of the tumor until it was 2 cm in diameter. As with T cells, the B-cell response also decreased thereafter. Interestingly, continuous stimulation of both T- and B-cell mitogen response was observed in the presence of plasma, except when the tumor size was too large (more than 2 cm) (Fig. 4).

Thus, we have observed that both blocking and effector immune reactivity changes in the tumor host during the progressive growth of fibrosarcomas in mice. These observations suggest that plasma blocking factors appear very early during tumor growth, long before the palpable tumors can be detected. The splenocytes show tumoricidal activity at this time. However, when the tumor

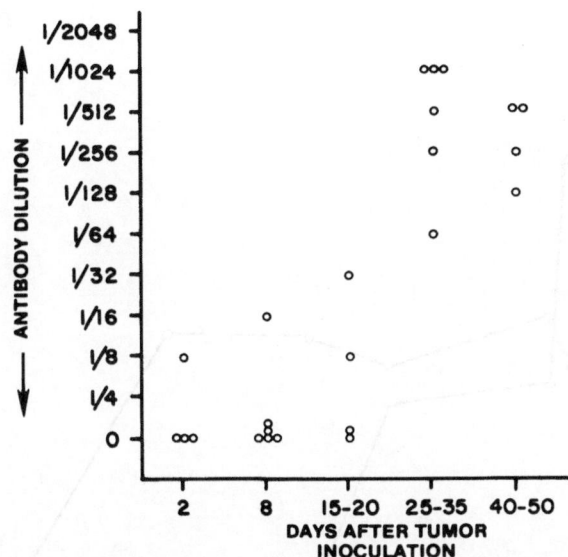

Figure 3. Rising titer of serum antitumor antibody in mice during the progressive growth of MC2 fibrosarcomas. Results show the maximal dilution at which cytotoxicity was observed in ^{51}Cr-release assays in presence of rabbit compliment.

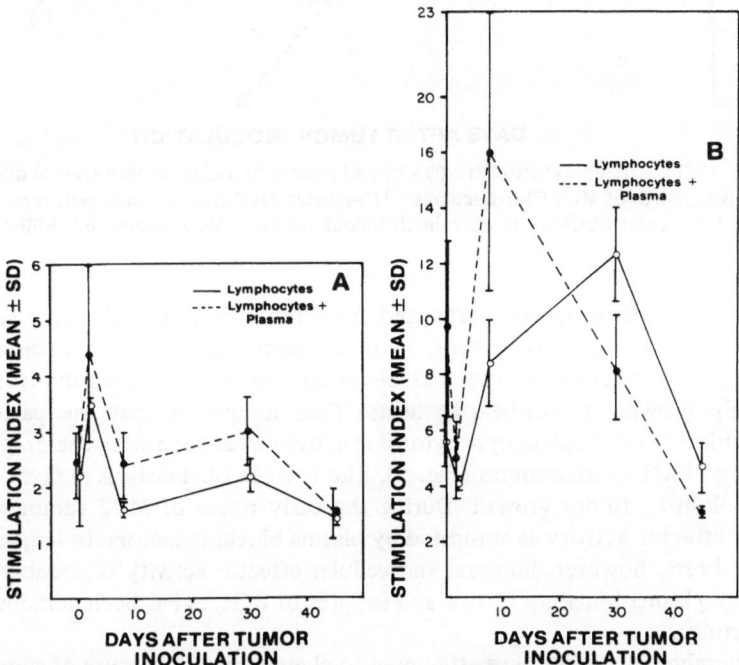

Figure 4. T-cell (A) and B-cell (B) mitogenic response in the presence or absence of plasma during the progressive growth of MC2 fibrosarcomas. Plasma collected on different days following tumor inoculation.

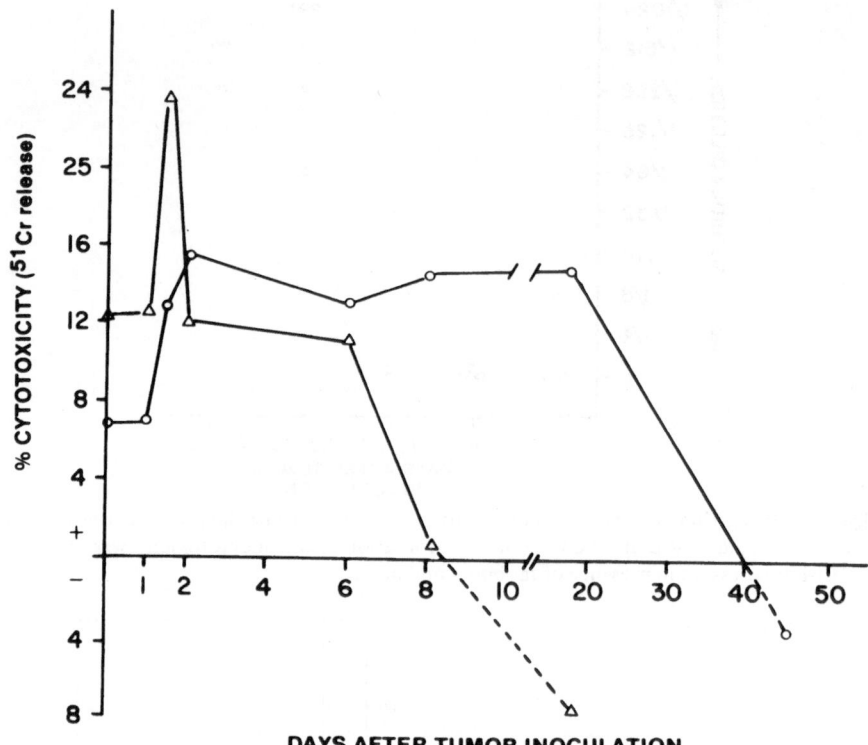

Figure 5. Cell-mediated cytotoxicity (○—○) and plasma blocking activity (△—△) during the progressive growth of MC2 fibrosarcomas. ^{51}Cr-labeled MC2 fibrosarcoma cells were reacted upon by leukocytes obtained from animals inoculated with MC2 tumor cells killed on different days.

becomes big, this property is changed from tumoricidal to enhancing activity. Plasma continues to show tumor growth enhancement. However, increasing titer of antitumor antibody activity was demonstrated *in vitro* in plasma from progressively growing tumor-bearing hosts. Thus it appears that the pattern of plasma blocking and splenocyte cytotoxic activity changes during the progressive growth of MC2 fibrosarcomas (Fig. 5). The balance obviously is in favor of factors facilitating tumor growth. During the early phase of MC2 tumor growth cellular effector activity is abrogated by plasma blocking factors. In large-tumor-bearing hosts, however, humoral and cellular effector activity is possibly eliminated by plasma blocking factors and suppressor cells, as has been demonstrated in our study.

A number of studies have attempted to characterize the nature of suppressor cells in tumor-bearing hosts.

Kirchner *et al.* (1974) suggested that the cell types that can counteract T-lymphocyte activity belong to the monocyte–macrophage series.

Poupon *et al.* (1976) investigated a nonspecific, adherent, non-T-cell splenic population from C3H mice bearing methylcholanthrene-induced fibrosarcomas. These cells had the ability to suppress *in vitro* lymphoid cell proliferation following mitogenic stimulation.

Oehler *et al.* (1977) described a population of adherent, phagocytic spleen cells that suppressed the mixed lymphocyte culture reaction and were resistant to treatment with antithymocyte serum and complement and also with radiation.

Hodes *et al.* (1977) reported that a radiosensitive T-cell population could suppress the immune response against an antigen. Small (1977) indicated that the nonspecific suppressor cells that can facilitate tumor growth may be immature cells of the T type.

Pope *et al.* (1976) reported that the suppressor cells from DBA/2J mice bearing methylcholanthrene-induced neoplasms were depleted from the spleen by passage through nylon wool columns, by treatment with carbonyl iron, or by adherence to plastic petri dishes, but not by exposure to anti-Thy 1.2 serum. However, many investigators have reported nonspecific suppressor cells to be of the B type (Padrathsingh *et al.*, 1979; Turk *et al.*, 1972; Zembala *et al.*, 1977).

Apart from experimental animal models, the nonspecific suppressor cells have also been identified in cancer patients (Naor, 1979). Patients with a variety of solid tissue tumors often have impaired cellular immunity. Zembala *et al.* (1977) reported that circulating suppressor monocytes can inhibit T-cell function in a nonspecific manner. Boder (1978) studied the role of suppressor cells in the pathogenesis of immunodeficiency, and he showed that lymphocytes from myeloma patients inhibited the *in vitro* production of polyclonal immunoglobulins. In addition, peripheral blood mononuclear cells from more than 50% of the myeloma patients suppressed polyclonal immunoglobulin production when cocultured with normal lymphocytes. The suppressor cells showed properties typical of a monocyte–macrophage type of cell.

B. Soluble Immunosuppressive Factors in the Sera of Tumor-Bearing Hosts

Some soluble mediators produced by lymphocytes have been reported to have the ability to regulate the immune response in tumor-bearing hosts. The presence of a specific suppressor T-cell factor in lymphoid cell extracts from rats and mice was demonstrated following immunization with hapten-carrier antigens (Tada *et al.*, 1975). The suppressor molecule appeared to be a small-molecular-weight (35,000–50,000) protein or polypeptide. The soluble T-cell factor showed the ability to suppress the secondary IgG response of sensitized spleen cells (Tanaguchi *et al.*, 1976). This T-cell factor was bound to the plasma membrane of cultured cells and could be released only after physical disruption of the membrane. It had the ability to modulate the IgG immune response, and it could be completely adsorbed with alloantisera specific for products of the I region of the H-2 complex. Antiimmunoglobulin antisera had no such effect. Detailed studies had indicated that it was an I-region product, probably coded by genes of the I-J subregion.

Thomas et al. (1975) reported a nonspecific soluble suppressor T-cell factor. A soluble suppressor T-cell factor was also described by Greene et al. (1977). This factor was immunologically specific, had a molecular weight of <70,000, and was susceptible to the action of pronase, implicating it as of the polypeptide type.

Waksman and Tada (1977) indicated that mice immunized with a relatively high dose of a protein immunogen release a specific suppressor T-cell factor. This factor was elaborated by the thymocytes, suppressed the development of specific antibody-forming cells in vitro, and inhibited cell-mediated immunity to the homologous tumor antigen in vivo. A nonspecific immunosuppressive factor was demonstrated to be elicited by cells either stimulated in vitro with a mitogen or sensitized in vivo by a large dose of an antigen. This factor inhibited DNA synthesis by proliferating cells. The thymocyte that produced the antigen-specific factor bore the Lyt $1^- 2^+ 3^+$ phenotype. It had the determinants of the I region of the H-2 complex. It acted only on T cells with the same I-region genes, but expressing Lyt 1^+, 2^+, and 3^+.

Sera from tumor-bearing animals have been reported to have the ability to block lymphocyte cytotoxicity against cultured tumor cells (I. Hellström and Hellström, 1969; I. Hellström et al., 1970). The serum blocking factor was reported to be a 7 S immunoglobulin, suggesting a tumor-associated antibody. It was also reported (Baldwin et al., 1972) that tumor-specific antigen–antibody complexes can block lymphocyte-mediated cytotoxicity against rat hepatoma cells. Studies on the mechanism of enhancement of allograft survival following treatment of the graft recipients with alloantiserum suggested that antitumor antibodies can protect the neoplastic cells from destruction by cytotoxic lymphocytes in vivo. Pierce (1971) observed that sera from mice bearing Moloney-virus-induced sarcoma cells facilitated tumor growth in vivo.

We have observed that mice inoculated with LD_{100} doses of methylcholanthrene induced fibrosarcoma contain plasma factor(s) that can suppress the cytotoxicity of peripheral blood mononuclear cells against autochthonous tumor cells within only 48 hr of tumor cell inoculation (Tables I and II; Fig. 5). Virtually complete suppression of mononuclear cell cytotoxicity was observed with plasma from animals with both palpable tumors and large tumors (Fig. 5). Interestingly, plasma from medium-size-tumor-bearing animals stimulated the in vitro mitogenic response of T cells, but the plasma of large-tumor bearing animals did not lead to stimulation (Fig. 4A). However, the mitogenic response of

Table II. *In Vitro* Cytotoxicity and/or Plasma Blocking Assay Using Spleen Cells, Peripheral Blood Leukocytes (PBL), and Plasma from Animals Preinjected with Tumor Cells Using a ^{51}Cr-Release Procedure[a]

Time	Spleen cells	PBL	Tumor cell	Plasma	Cytotoxicity (%)
4 hr	+	−	+	−	0
	+	−	+	+	0
	−	+	+	−	4
	−	+	+	+	8
12 hr	+	−	+	−	0
	+	−	+	+	3
24 hr	−	+	+	−	0
	−	+	+	+	1
	+	−	+	−	0
	+	−	+	+	0
	−	+	+	−	1
	−	+	+	+	15
36 hr	+	−	+	−	2
	+	−	+	+	2
	−	+	+	−	1
	−	+	+	+	12
48 hr	+	−	+	−	7
	+	−	+	+	0
	−	+	+	−	2
	−	+	+	+	6
6 days	+	−	+	−	4
	+	−	+	+	0
	−	+	+	−	12
	−	+	+	+	3
8 days	+	−	+	−	4
	+	−	+	+	0
	−	+	+	−	20
	−	+	+	+	0
12 days (0.5 cm)	+	−	+	−	0
	+	−	+	+	0
	−	+	+	−	17
	−	+	+	+	0
20-35 days (1-3 cm)	+	−	+	−	0
	+	−	+	+	0
	−	+	+	−	0
	−	+	+	+	0

[a]*Cellular cytotoxicity:* PBL or spleen cells: Tumor cells (100 : 1) incubated for 18 hr in a 5% CO_2 humidified atmosphere. Released chromium was measured to determine cytotoxicity (Ray *et al.*, 1982*a*,*b*). *Blocking assay:* Labeled tumor cells coated with plasma + PBL or spleen cells (100 : 1), other details same.

B cells was inhibited by plasma from both medium- and large-tumor-bearing animals (Fig. 4B). Ron and Witz (1972) showed that the surface eluate of chemically induced mouse sarcoma could facilitate the growth of this tumor. The eluate contained tumor-bound immunoglobulin (Witz, 1977), which was also observed in a polyoma-virus-induced sarcoma model (Bansal *et al.*, 1972). The active participation *in vivo* of tumor-specific antigen, antibody, antigen–antibody complexes, and suppressor cells in tumor growth regulation has been discussed in three reviews by Ray (1982, 1983) and Ray and Raychaudhuri (1983).

Several authors (Hollander *et al.*, 1978; Isakov *et al.*, 1978, 1979) have reported that supernatants of spleen cell cultures from tumor-bearing mice can facilitate tumor growth. This factor affects the antigenic triggering of antibody-producing B lymphocytes.

I. Hellström and Hellström (1969) described both specific and nonspecific tumor growth facilitation by cell-free tumor fluid (TF), which was obtained from culture medium of methylcholanthrene-induced sarcomas. TF could specifically inhibit cell-mediated cytotoxicity of tumor cells *in vitro*. Adoptive transfer of TF with the tumor cells had shown limited tumor growth *in vivo*. In addition, the *in vivo* facilitation of tumor growth was demonstrated when sarcoma cells and TF were inoculated together. Tumor-specific facilitation was also demonstrated when TF was given intraperitoneally, suggesting that TF had the ability to generate systemic effects. These authors have suggested that TF has both specific tumor-facilitating antigen and facilitating factors carrying no antigenic determinants.

In our study (Ray and Saha, 1985a), we have observed that both humoral and cellular tumor growth enhancement (TGE) factors are generated as early as 2 days after the injection of both mitomycin C-treated tumor cells (MTTC) and a 3 M KCl extract of tumor tissues (TAg). Adoptive transfer of plasma or splenic mononuclear cells from both MTTC and TAg-treated mice provided some interesting data (Table III, Fig. 6). Plasma of mice treated with lower doses of MTTC (2×10^6 or 7.5×10^6 cells) and TAg (1.0 mg or 3 mg) showed TGE. Splenic mononuclear cells of these animals did not show much TGE. However, when these cells were obtained from animals inoculated with large doses of MTTC (15×10^6 cells) or TAg (7.5 mg) TGE was prominent in adoptive transfer studies (Table III; Fig. 6). This property of the immunogen (MTTC, TAg) may be due to the TAA, since sera and splenic mononuclear cells from animals immunized with mixed normal tissue extract or from absolutely normal animals did not show TGE. These data can be correlated with our data obtained from animals inoculated with LD_{100} doses of viable methylcholanthrene-induced fibrosarcomas (Tables I and II; Figs. 2–5). The data obtained with small dose of immunogen (MTTC, TAg) are similar to what was observed in small-tumor-bearing animals, and the data obtained with large doses of immunogen are similar to what was observed in large-tumor-bearing animals (Tables I–III; Figs. 2–6).

Based on our data, I hypothesize that TAA may be released by tumor cells

Table III. Humoral and Cellular Blocking Factors in Mice
Inoculated with Various Doses of Both Viable Tumor
Cells and Tumor Cell Antigen or Immobilized Tumor
Antigen (Mitomycin C-Treated Tumor Cell)

Antigen type	Dose	Plasma blocking factor[a]	Cellular blocking factor[a]
1. Viable	2×10^6	+	−
tumor cell	15×10^6	+	+
2. Immobilized	2×10^6	+	−
tumor cell	7.5×10^6	+	+
(mitomycin C-treated)	15×10^6	+	++
3. Extracted tumor	1.0 mg	+	−
antigen	3.0 mg	+	±
(KCl extract)	7.0 mg	+	++

[a]Demonstrated by adoptive transfer test.

in increasing concentrations as the tumor grows larger. Small concentrations of TAA in the sera of small-tumor-bearing animals may be responsible for plasma blocking activity, while large concentrations of TAA in the sera of large-tumor-bearing animals may induce the production of suppressor cells. This may result in complete anergy in a large-tumor-bearing host, allowing the tumor to grow uninterruptedly. It is quite likely that TAA is the initiator of both suppressor cells and plasma blocking activity, although this latter effect may be due to antibody and antigen–antibody complexes as well, depending on the particular stage of the neoplastic growth (Fig. 7).

The immune responses of tumor-bearing hosts may be regulated by nonspecific humoral factors. In the sera of tumor-bearing patients several factors capable of inhibiting normal lymphocyte response to mitogenic stimuli were described by Brooks et al. (1972). They have also described an antibodylike substance with the ability to suppress lymphocyte activation in patients with intracranial tumors.

Yamazaki et al. (1973) reported three immunosuppressive factors in Ehrlich ascites fluid, with molecular weights of >100,000, <10,000, and <1000.

Nimberg et al. (1975) have fractionated cancer patients' sera by diethyl aminoethyl cellulose chromatography. The fraction containing albumin and gamma globulins showed the strongest immunosuppressive activity.

We (Ray and Saha, 1982) have analyzed the plasma of mice with methylcholanthrene-induced fibrosarcomas on Sephadex G-200 columns and separated it into five fractions with molecular weights of >440,000, >232,000, >158,000, >67,000, and <67,000. The concentration of fraction No. 1 (>440,000) did not change appreciably up to a tumor diameter of 2 cm diameter. After this, the

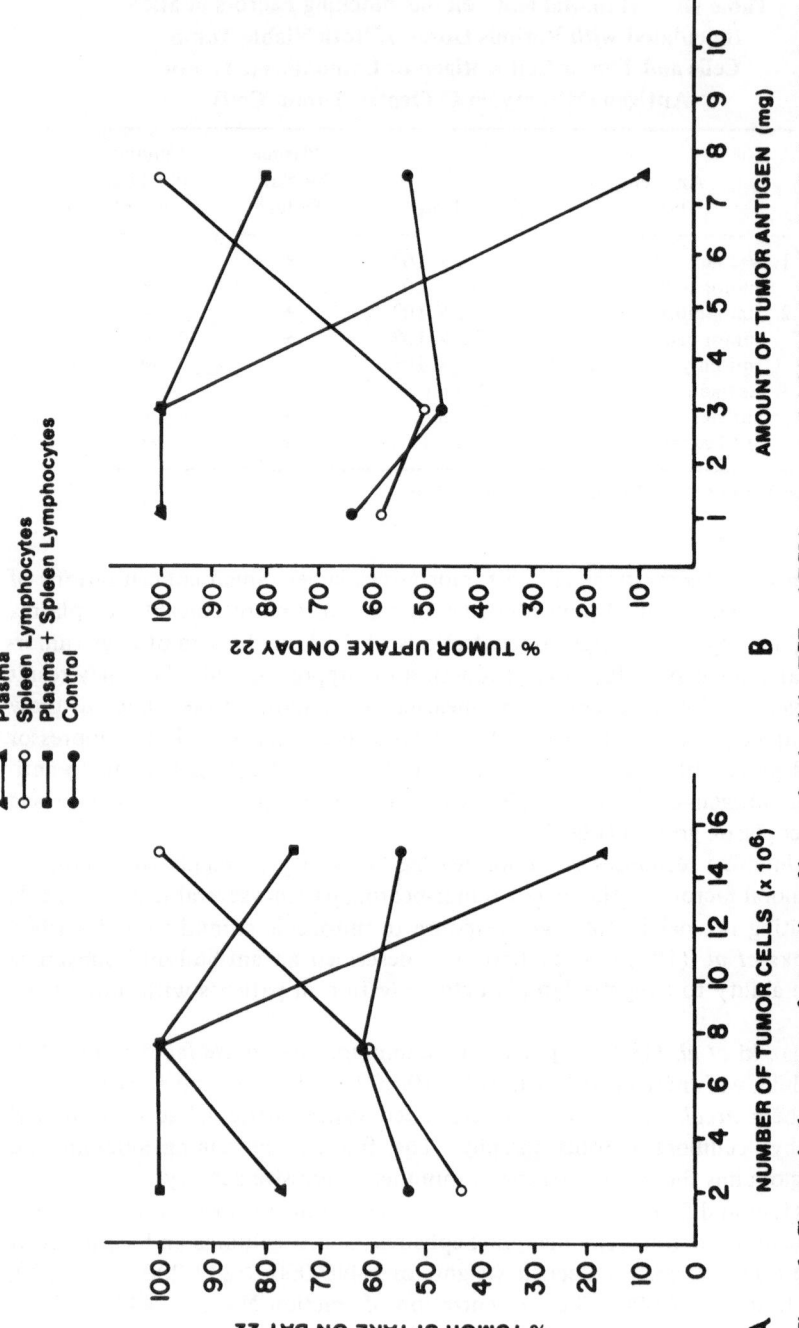

Figure 6. Changes in the pattern of generation of humoral and cellular TGE and TGI (tumor growth inhibition) factors in mice immunized with various doses of MTTC (A) and TAg (B) as measured in adoptive transfer studies. Note that plasma from large doses of MTTC- and TAg-immunized animals inhibited tumor growth. In contrast, splenic lymphocytes from animals immunized with large doses of MTTC and TAg showed tumor growth enhancement. Plasma from animals immunized with low doses of MTTC and TAg showed enhancement of tumor growth.

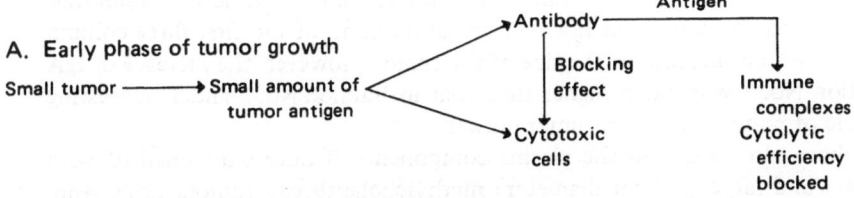

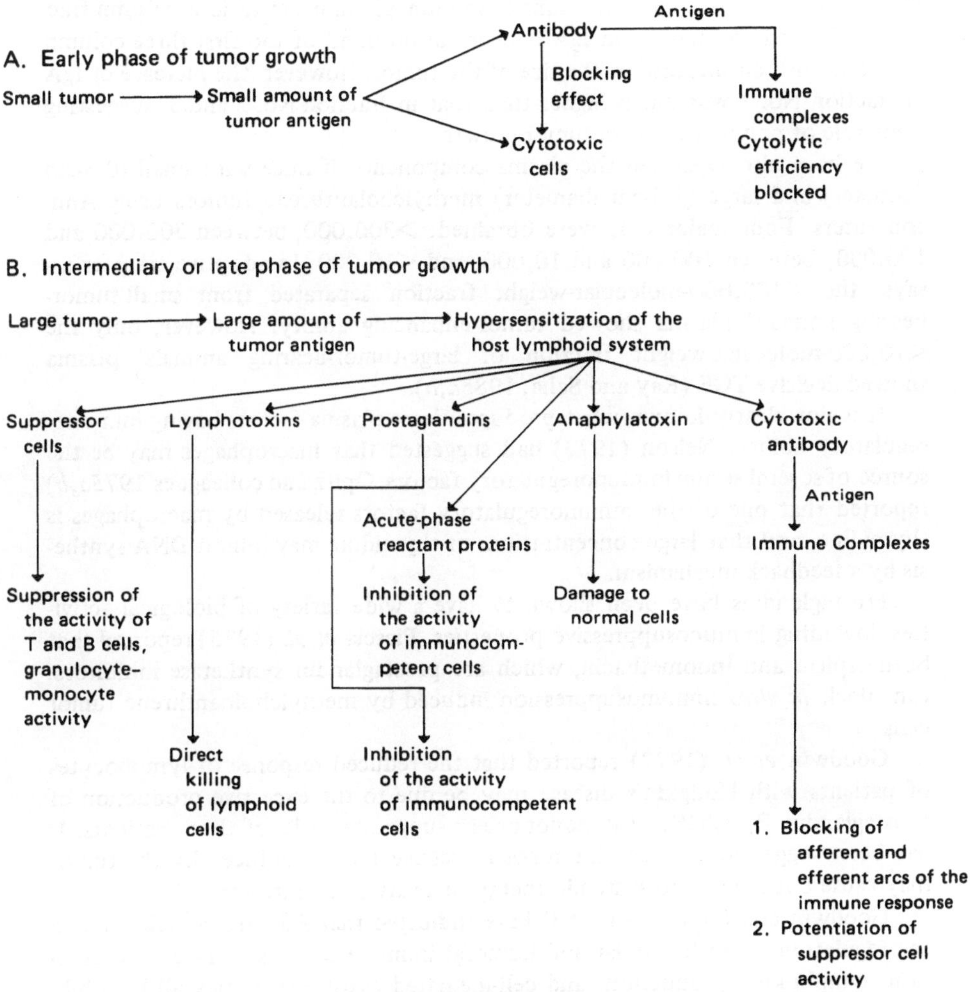

A. Early phase of tumor growth

Small tumor ⟶ Small amount of tumor antigen

Antibody ⟶ Antigen

Blocking effect

Cytotoxic cells

Immune complexes

Cytolytic efficiency blocked

B. Intermediary or late phase of tumor growth

Large tumor ⟶ Large amount of tumor antigen ⟶ Hypersensitization of the host lymphoid system

Suppressor cells — Lymphotoxins — Prostaglandins — Anaphylatoxin — Cytotoxic antibody

Acute-phase reactant proteins

Antigen

Immune Complexes

Suppression of the activity of T and B cells, granulocyte-monocyte activity

Inhibition of the activity of immunocompetent cells

Damage to normal cells

Direct killing of lymphoid cells

Inhibition of the activity of immunocompetent cells

1. Blocking of afferent and efferent arcs of the immune response
2. Potentiation of suppressor cell activity

Figure 7. Immunomodulation circuit in a tumor-bearing host.

concentration of this fraction increased progressively. The concentration of fraction No. 2 (>232,000) increased gradually up to a tumor diameter of 2 cm. The concentration of fraction No. 3 (>158,000) was lower than that of fraction No. 2 for small tumors. However, after the tumor size reached 2 cm, its concentration started increasing, and surpassed that of fraction No. 2. The concentration of fraction No. 4 (>67,000) was very large when the tumor size was 0.5 cm. It gradually decreased and remained unaltered after the tumor size increased beyond 2 cm. Fraction No. 5 (<67,000) did not show any appreciable change.

Quantification of the concentrations of immunoglobulins in various column fractions indicated an increase in IgA concentration in all of the first three column fractions with an increase in the size of the tumor. However, the increase of IgA in fraction No. 1 was much higher than that in fraction No. 2 and 3, suggesting some role of polymeric IgA in tumor growth.

We have also separated the plasma components of mice with small (0.5-cm diameter) and large (3.5-cm diameter) methylcholanthrene tumors using Amicon filters. Four major cuts were obtained: >300,000, between 300,000 and 100,000, between 100,000 and 10,000, and <10,000. In adoptive transfer assays, the <100,000-molecular-weight fraction separated from small-tumor-bearing animals' plasma showed tumor-enhancing ability. However, only the <10,000-molecular-weight fraction of large-tumor-bearing animals' plasma showed decisive TGE (Ray and Saha, 1985a,b).

It is not clearly known what produces those plasma factors having immunoregulatory ability. Nelson (1973) had suggested that macrophages may be the source of several serum immunoregulatory factors. Opitz and colleagues 1975a,b) reported that one of the immunoregulatory factors released by macrophages is thymidine, and that large concentrations of thymidine may inhibit DNA synthesis by a feedback mechanism.

Prostaglandins have been shown to have a wide variety of biological activities, including immunosuppressive properties. Plescia et al. (1975) reported that both aspirin and indomethacin, which are prostaglandin synthetase inhibitors, can block in vitro immunosuppression induced by methylcholoanthrene tumor cells.

Goodwin et al. (1977) reported that the reduced response of lymphocytes of patients with Hodgkin's disease may be due to the excessive production of prostaglandin E_2 (PGE_2) by mononuclear suppressor cells of these patients. It has been suggested that the immunosuppressive factors induced by the tumor may cause both local and systemic anergy to a variety of antigens.

Goodwin and Cauppens (1983) have indicated that PGE has a major role in the regulation of both cellular and humoral immune responses. T-cell proliferation, lymphokine production, and cell-mediated cytotoxicity may all be inhibited by PGE via a feedback-inhibition mechanism. PGE may also inhibit the activity of both macrophages and natural killer cells. In some instances, however, PGE may be responsible for cellular activation rather than inhibition.

In the control of humoral immunity, PGE production may normally be necessary for the generation of some type of T suppressor cells, whereas both increased production of PGE and/or increased sensitivity to PGE may result in the suppression of cellular immunity, and drugs that inhibit PGE production act as stimulators of cellular immunity both in vitro and in vivo.

Results from a number of laboratories have shown that in tumor-bearing hosts there is an increased activity of the prostaglandin-producing suppressor cells. Increased production of PGE by both naturally occurring and experimentally induced cancers has now been reported by a number of groups (Kline and Raisz, 1970; Bennett *et al.*, 1977; Roland *et al.*, 1980; Tashjain *et al.*, 1972). Pelus and Backman (1979) have demonstrated that macrophages from tumor-bearing mice produce significantly more PGE than cells from normal littermates. The existence of indomethacine-sensitive adherent suppressor cells has been demonstrated by Glaser (1980) in tumor-bearing mice. Spleen cells of tumor-bearing mice have been shown to inhibit *in vitro* generation of cytotoxic reactivity by spleen cells from tumor-free mice, sensitized *in vitro* with SV-40-induced tumor cells. The suppressor cells were of the macrophage type, and indomethacin eliminated the suppressive activity of these cells. Various types of cancer patients have been shown to possess prostaglandin-producing suppressor cells. It has been observed that, apart from activation of the prostaglandin-producing suppressor cells, the tumor cells themselves can also produce immunodepressing PGE.

Werner *et al.* (1973) have reported that freshly harvested tumor cells release a low-molecular-weight peptide that can inhibit both protein and DNA synthesis of normal lymphocytes. Soluble factors released from human colonic carcinomas have been found to be able to suppress stimulated lymphocytes nonspecifically.

According to Renacle-Bonnett *et al.* (1978) tumor cells produce various factors that can suppress the activation, migration, and phagocytic properties of macrophages (Anderson *et al.*, 1972; Rodey *et al.*, 1974; Stevens *et al.*, 1978).

Perry *et al.* (1978) described inhibition of tumor growth in mice pretreated with anti-I-J alloantiserum that can bind suppressor cells.

Drebin *et al.* (1983) have examined the effect of intravenous administration of monoclonal anti-I-J antibodies on tumor growth in syngeneic and semisyngeneic hosts. These antibodies, at nanogram dosages, inhibited tumor growth in mice bearing the appropriate I-J-encoded gene product on their lymphoid cells. These findings suggested that inhibition of suppressor cell function may be the mechanism by which anti-I-J antibodies inhibit tumor growth.

A number of laboratories (Fujimoto *et al.*, 1976; Naor, 1979; Berendt and North, 1980; Mills *et al.*, 1981) have suggested that an activation of the suppressor T cell is a potential mechanism by which growing tumors escape immune destruction. Our data (Tables I–III, Figs. 2–6) also provide support for such a hypothesis. We (Ray and Raychaudhuri, 1981) have shown that injection of an immunostimulatory dose of cyclophosphamide 48 hr before inoculation with an LD_{100} dose of transplantable mouse fibrosarcoma cells may cause a delay in or complete inhibition of this tumor growth. We proposed that this was due to the depletion of the suppressor cell clones by cyclophosphamide so that the host could not be immunologically suppressed by the tumor.

III. SOLUBLE IMMUNE COMPLEXES AS PREDOMINATING IMMUNOSUPPRESSOR MOLECULES IN TUMOR-BEARING HOSTS

Several studies have suggested that circulating immune complexes (CIC) may favor tumor growth since an association between the concentration of CIC and poor prognosis is frequently observed in malignancy. Carpentier and Miescher (1983) have recently reviewed the role of immune complexes in malignancy. CIC have been described in the deposits of immunoglobulin and complement in the renal glomeruli of patients with cancer (Lee *et al.*, 1963; Kiley *et al.*, 1969; Helin *et al.*, 1980; Pascal *et al.*, 1976). The presence of immune complexes in the sera of individuals with growing neoplasms, with the ability to inhibit *in vitro* lymphocyte reactivity to tumor cells, has also been described by a number of laboratories (Sjören *et al.*, 1971; Currie and Basham, 1972; Baldwin *et al.*, 1974; Jose and Sashadri, 1974; Montovanni and Sorafico, 1975).

Theofilopoulos *et al.* (1976) demonstrated CIC in 16-52% of patients with solid tumors. Of 251 patients they studied, 109 had CIC and all but 5 had clinically evident disease. In myeloma patients, higher levels of CIC were detected in patients with large tumors.

Samayoa *et al.* (1977) have estimated the level of CIC in the sera of a group of 146 cancer patients. They found significantly higher concentrations of CIC in 29% of patients with metastatic cancer. However, Teshima *et al.* (1977) and Rossen *et al.* (1977) detected CIC in 50-83% of inpatients with various types of cancer. Teshima *et al.* (1977) have observed that the presence of CIC in 67-77% of sera was associated with lower total hemolytic complement activity or reduced levels of C3 and C1q. It is possible that the level of CIC may vary with the tumor mass. In ovarian cancer patients CIC were observed only in patients with recurrent disease (Poulton *et al.*, 1978). However, in postoperative cancer patients CIC were more frequent in individuals with residual tumor than in those who were considered to be cured (Rossen *et al.*, 1977; Theofilopoulos *et al.*, 1976, 1977).

Brandeis *et al.* (1978) showed a close correlation between the amount of CIC and the tumor mass in children with neuroblastoma. The concentrations of CIC increased with the extent of the disease. The level of CIC was significantly higher in stage IV disease than in other stages and the amount of CIC decreased as treatment progressed. Reporting their results from a four-year study in 86 children with Hodgkin's disease, Brandeis *et al.* (1980) demonstrated a change in the level of CIC in patients following treatment. Before the treatment, 81% of children had elevated levels of CIC. During the treatment, 33% of patients were still positive with elevated levels of CIC during the year following the treatment, while in 37% of patients CIC levels remained above the normal value. At relapse, 63% of patients showed elevated levels of CIC, which was higher than had been observed previously.

Summarizing their six-year study, Carpentier and Miescher (1983) have described their experiences with a large number of patients with leukemia, malignant lymphoma, or solid tumors. Forty-one percent of their patients with acute leukemia and 22% of patients with chronic leukemia showed CIC. In acute myeloid leukemia and acute lymphatic leukemia as well as in blastic crisis of chronic myelocytic leukemia, CIC were detected in patients with blastic stage. In general, patients with disseminated tumor showed greater percentages of CIC. In a series of 136 women with breast carcinoma, comparative analyses of the CIC levels showed the prevalence of CIC in the disseminated tumor group.

From all the studies thus far described, it is apparent that CIC level is closely related to the extent of the disease in cancer. Very little information is available concerning either the specificity of the complexes or the nature of the antigen and antibody of which they are composed. Unless those components are identified we may not learn what type(s) of CIC are increased or decreased in various stages of the disease. However, a few studies have been reported in the literature which have attempted to look into this question.

Constanza et al. (1973) and Couser et al. (1974) have shown that CIC in colon cancer patients contained carcinoembryonic antigen (CEA), which is widely believed to be a TAA.

IgG antibody eluted from renal immune deposits of patients with Burkitt's lymphoma showed a specificity for the viral capsid and early antigens of the Epstein–Barr virus (EBV) (Oldstone et al., 1975). Heimer and Kline (1976) also showed the presence of EBV-associated glycoprotein antigens in CIC. CIC containing antilymphocyte antibodies were demonstrated in a chronic lymphatic leukemia patient (Day et al., 1976).

Long et al. (1977) have shown that patients with Hodgkin's disease contain CIC composed of antibodies that could react with cultured cells derived from lymphoma.

In infectious mononucleosis, a disease which resembles a malignant lymphoma, some of the complex antibodies of CIC were show to be directed against viral capsid antigen (Carpentier et al., 1978). Leukemia-specific antigens were demonstrated in CIC of patients with acute myelocytic leukemia (Faltt and Ankerest, 1980), while Staab et al. (1980) have reported the occurrence of CIC involving CEA in patients with gastrointestinal tumors.

We (Ray and Saha, 1985b) have studied CIC from the plasma of animals bearing methylcholanthrene-induced fibrosarcomas (MC2). The immune complexes obtained by 3.5% polyethylene glycol precipitation were dissociated by exposure to glycine-HCl buffer (pH 2.8) and then separated by the Amicon ultrafiltration technique. The fraction with molecular weight $<100,000$ showed a single protein band following PEG. It also showed a single precipitin band on immunoelectrophoresis against rabbit anti-MC2 antiserum. Upon comparison of this band with those obtained with TAg, mixed normal tissue extract (MAg),

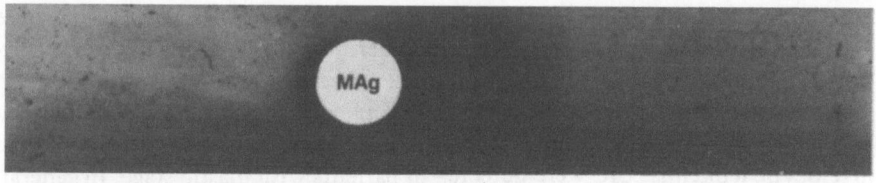

Rabbit Anti-MC2 antiserum

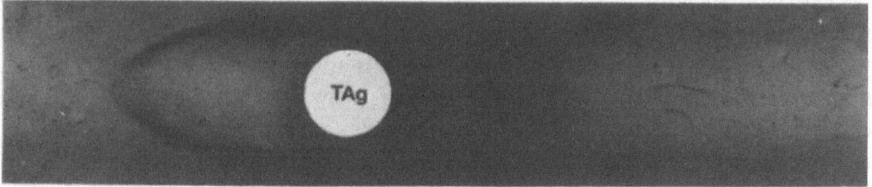

Rabbit Anti-MC2 antiserum

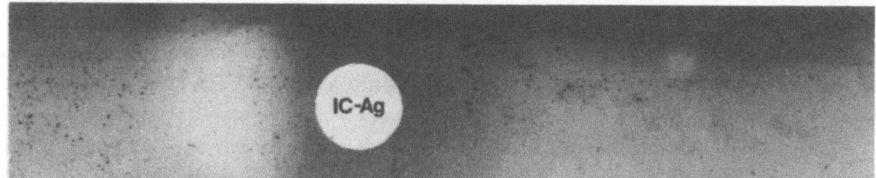

Figure 8. Immunoelectrophoresis of MAg, TAg, and Ag separated from CIC (IC-Ag). Note that IC-Ag shows a band corresponding to TAg, which is not present in MAg.

and anti-MC2 antiserum, it appeared that the antigen prepared from immune complex disassociation (MW <100,000 fraction) was also present in TAg, but absent from MAg (Fig. 8). Thus, it is possible that TAA-specific CIC may be elevated in tumor-bearing hosts, since we (Ray and Raychaudhuri, 1985) have observed that there is an increase in the plasma concentration of CIC during the progressive growth of (1) a transplantable methylcholanthrene-induced fibrosarcoma in mice, (2) dimethylbenzanthrene (DMBA)-induced mammary adenocarcinoma in rats, and (3) various human tumors, compared to normal controls (Tables IV–VI). Interesting correlations were observed in clinical studies between the presence of CIC in cancer patients and an unfavorable course of the disease.

Rossen *et al.* (1977) reported that patients with bronchiocarcinoma with high levels of CIC at the first test were more likely to have tumors that grew very rapidly or recurred. Bleme (1977) reported the presence of CIC in patients with breast cancer.

Amlot *et al.* (1978) have shown that the presence of CIC correlates not only with the extent of the disease but also with other factors that can adversely affect prognosis.

Dent *et al.* (1980) have reported that in lung cancer patients the increased se-

Table IV. Increase in the Concentration of CIC in
the Plasma of Mice Injected with an LD_{100} Dose of
a Transplantable Methylcholanthrene-Induce
Fibrosarcoma

Time after tumor cell inoculation	CIC level (PEG ppt., mg/ml)
0 hr	0.91
24 hr	1.20
48 hr	1.22
Day 6	1.45
Day 8	1.50
Days 12–16 (0.5-cm tumor)	1.75
Days 20–24 (1-cm tumor)	2.10
Days 30–40 (2- to 3-cm tumor)	2.95

Table V. Relationship between the Size of the Tumor
and the Concentration of CIC in the Plasma of Rats
Inoculated with DMBA to Produce Mammary
Adenocarcinomas

Average size of tumor	CIC level (PEG ppt., mg/ml)
0	0.90
Palpable tumor	1.75
0.5 cm	2.10
0.75 cm	2.15
1.3 cm	2.30
2.7 cm	1.9
3.1 cm	2.75
3.6 cm	2.5
Animals that did not produce any tumor following carcinogen injection	1.15

rum levels of CIC and CEA may be utilized as a prognostic factor. They showed
two- to threefold longer median survival time in patients with normal postoperative levels than in those with elevated levels. It has been reported (Hubert et al.,
1981; Carpentier et al., 1978) that leukemic patients positive for CIC at the time
of diagnosis or during a remission had a worse prognosis than those without CIC.

In patients with gastrointestinal carcinoma (Staab et al., 1980) preoperative
circulating CEA immune complexes proved to be a marker with regard to the
extent of the disease and prognosis. In addition, the occurrence of CIC during

Table VI. Concentration of CIC in the Plasma of Normal
and Cancer Patients

Diseases	No. of subjects	CIC level[a] (PEG ppt., mg/ml ± SD)
Normal	26	2.4 ± 1.2
Advanced cancer patients with various types of malignancy	30	5.58 ± 3.34

[a]$P < 0.05$.

the postoperative period appeared to be an indicator of relapse. It was also observed that survival of children with neuroblastoma (Brandeis et al., 1978) and of patients with retinoblastoma (Stein et al., 1980) or brain tumors (D. Martin et al., 1980) was shorter when high levels of CIC were present than when CIC levels were low.

It is quite apparent from the preceding discussion that at least two types of humoral immunosuppressive factors exist in a tumor-bearing host: (1) factors produced by the tumor cells and (2) factors released by the host lymphoid cells, including macrophages. The first type may be produced by the tumor cells in order to protect themselves against the host attack, and the second type may be produced by the host cells in response to a tumor-induced sensitization reaction. The latter factors are the immunoregulatory molecules normally produced by the body to provide feedback inhibition against hyperimmune reactivity. In the tumor host, these factors become self-defeating indirectly facilitating the growth of the tumor. The massive amount of TAA released by the tumor cells appears to be responsible for inducing the production of these immunosuppressive host factors.

IV. POSSIBLE MECHANISM OF GENERATION OF IMMUNOSUPPRESSIVE FACTORS IN THE TUMOR-BEARING HOST

I propose the following hypothesis regarding the generation of various types of immunosuppressive factors in a tumor host (Fig. 7): During the initial phase of tumor development, the tumor may release a small amount of antigen, which sensitizes the host and produces lymphoid cells with cytotoxic potential. However, the antigenic sensitization may lead to the production of antibodies, which may bind to the circulating antigen to form antigen–antibody complexes. The concentration of antibody produced initially may be small either because the TAA may be a weak immunogen or because their concentration may be very low, thus forming CIC, which may remain in soluble form. These CIC may be devoid of configurations needed to bind Fc receptors on macrophages, enabling them to remain in the circulation. These complexes could inhibit the activity of cytotoxic lymphoid cells, facilitating the growth of tumor cells.

With the progressive growth of tumor cells, increasing concentrations of TAA may be released. Under such circumstances, the host would be overstimulated and would begin reacting. A number of feedback inhibitors are produced: suppressor cells, prostaglandins, and several other types of soluble immunomodulators (Fig. 7). Although antitumor antibodies are found at this stage, their production may very soon be limited because of overall immunosuppressive actions on the B cells by the suppressor cells. Such antibodies may not gain access to the tumor cells because of the abundant quantity of TAA often encountered. Large immune complexes are formed, which may further stimulate the activity of suppressor cells. Other immunosuppressive soluble plasma factors may also be generated, exerting an overall immunosuppressive action and making the host partially or completely anergic—a situation that is mostly observed in advanced malignancy.

V. IMMUNOTHERAPY BY CONTROLLING THE SUPPRESSOR CELL FUNCTION

As discussed previously, there has been an impressive amount of progress in the area of suppressor cells and cancer (Prehn, 1976; Treves et al., 1974; Umiel and Trainin, 1974; Cohen and Feldman, 1976; Small, 1977; Yamagishi et al., 1983). It has also been noted that suppressor cells have been detected in both animals and humans with tumors, and that the suppressor cells may have the characteristics of T cells, B cells, or even macrophages and monocytes (Fujimoto et al., 1976; Glaser et al., 1976; Glasgow et al., 1974; Hodes et al., 1977; Turk et al., 1972; Gorczynski, 1974; Kilburn et al., 1974; Kirchner et al., 1974; Eggers and Wunderlich, 1975; Gelsner et al., 1976; Pope et al., 1976; Padrathsingh et al., 1979; Yamagishi et al., 1983).

Naor (1979) has discussed the role of suppressor cells both in the development of tumors and also for promoting their growth. It is now becoming increasingly clear that suppressor cells can block both the cellular and the humoral immunity of the host. Therefore, it is reasonable to expect that inhibition of suppressor cell activity should be of therapeutic benefit in tumor-bearing hosts.

A number of drugs or procedures have been utilized so far to kill the suppressor cells or abrogate their effects. These have included irradiation; thymectomy; splenectomy; and treatment with hydrocortisone, cyclophosphamide, antithymocyte serum, anti I-J serum, aspirin, and indomethacin. However, although these approaches have shown some promising antitumor effect, they should be utilized with caution. Complete loss of suppressor cells may lead to an autoimmune response in the host, since normally the suppressor cells provide feedback control of hyperimmune reactivity in the host. Induced hyperimmune reactivity may go out of control and cause self-destruction in the absence of this built-in control mechanism.

A number of questions remain unanswered regarding the suppressor cells, including questions regarding (1) how these cells are induced, (2) how they act, (3) whether they always act by releasing some soluble immunosuppressive factors, (4) where their specificity lies, (5) how the target cell is recognized by the suppressor cell, and (6) why the suppressor cell activity is sometimes rendered by T cells, sometimes by B cells, and sometimes by macrophases. As soon as these questions are answered, more direct and definitive control of suppressor cell activity will be possible. with consequently improved therapeutic benefit to the tumor-bearing host. I shall discuss in the following paragraphs some of the work related to the abrogation of suppressor cell activity to provide therapeutic benefit. A list of various agents used to abrogate suppressor cell activity, often providing therapeutic benefit, is given in Table VII. Some of these studies have been mentioned earlier in Section II.A.

Small (1977) observed that exposure of immature T cells to a tumor may lead to tumor enhancement, whereas interaction between mature T lymphocytes and tumor cells may be required for tumor inhibition. These thymus-derived lymphocytes were rapidly dividing cells and were susceptible to cortisone and thymic humoral factors.

Fujimoto et al. (1976) reported that the suppressive activity of thymus or splenic cells from a tumor-bearing animal was entirely abolished by treatment of those lymphocytes with anti-θ serum or antithymocyte serum (ATS). ATS treatment of normal syngeneic animals after tumor cell inoculation or splenectomy of tumor-bearing animals resulted in the suppression of tumor growth.

Blasecki and Tevethia (1976) showed that lymphoid cells from animals undergoing tumorigenesis by SV-40-transferred BALB/c cells had blocking activity, and that such activity was lost when the cells were cultured in vitro and they regained their reactivity to SV-40 tumor-specific transformation antigen.

Treves et al. (1974) reported that tumor growth could be facilitated by soluble products of T lymphocytes that were found in spleens of tumor-bearing mice and which nonspecifically suppressed the immune defense mechanisms.

Kirchner et al. (1974) demonstrated that spleen cells from MuSV-tumor-bearing mice could inhibit the proliferation of RBL-5 lymphoma cells and could also inhibit [^{3}H]-TDR incorporation.

Uchida and Hoshino (1980) daily injected a streptococcal preparation, OK-432, intradermally into patients with advanced cancer of the stomach or lung for several weeks and examined the effects of OK-432 on the mitogenic responses of cancer patients. The cells involved in the depression of the response of untreated cancer patients were characterized. The cells responsible for impaired responses were found to be nylon-wool-nonadherent and could suppress the mitogen re-

Table VII. Abrogation of Suppressor Cell Effects in Tumor-Bearing Hosts by Various Agents

Tumor type	Tumor host	Type of suppressor cell	Sensitive to:	References
3LL spontaneous tumor	C57/BL6 mice	T cell	HC BUdR X irradiation	Treves et al. (1976) Carnaud et al. (1974) Treves et al. (1974) Rotter and Trainin (1975) Small (1977)
Friend leukemia	BALB/c mice	T cell	HC	Kumar and Bennett (1977)
ALL	Man	T cell	X irradiation	Broder et al. (1978)
MCA-induced sarcoma	A/J mice	T cell	ATS treatment, not to HC	Fujimoto et al. (1976) Fujimoto et al. (1976)
DMBA-induced mammary tumor	Fisher rat	Not known	HC	Kuperman et al. (1976)
B-16 melanoma	C57/BL6 mice	Not known	X irradiation	Stelzer and Wallace (1977)
SV-40-transformed fibroblasts	BALB/c mice	Not known	HC	Blasecki and Tevethia (1975)
Murine tumor	C57/BL6 mice	Not known	Cimetidine	Gifford et al. (1981)
Cancer of stomach, lung	Man	Nylon-wool-nonadherent cell	OK-432	Uchida and Hoshino (1980)
KMT-17 tumor	WKA rats	T cell	Busulfan	Mizushima et al. (1981)
Methyl-cholanthrene-induced tumor	Mice	Not known	Indomethacin, aspirin	Fulton and Levy (1980)
Tumor-bearing mice and cancer patients	Mice and patients	T cell	Thymosin	Serrou et al. (1980)
P 815 tumor	DBA/2 mice	T cell	Radiation	Tilkin et al. (1981)
Methyl-cholanthrene-induced fibrosarcoma	C3H/Hej mice	Not known	Cyclophosphamide	Ray and Raychaudhuri (1981)
S 1509 Methyl-cholanthrene-induced fibrosarcoma	A/J mice	T cell	Monoclonal anti-I-J antibody	Drebin et al. (1983)

sponses of both autologous and allogeneic lymphocytes. These cells lost their suppressive activity during 7 days' culture *in vitro*. Following OK-432 immunotherapy, mononuclear cells from the patients showed increased responses to phytohemagglutinin and concanavalin A and the nylon-wool-nonadherent cells did not inhibit the mitogen responses. The authors suggested that the improved mitogen responses of peripheral blood lymphocytes of cancer patients treated with OK-432 probably resulted from a reduction in the number or activity of circulating nonspecific suppressor cells.

Mizushima *et al.* (1981) described an enhancement of specific transplantation resistance to a syngeneic tumor (KMT-17) in WKA rats by treatment with the antileukemia drug busulfan 5 days before and 5 days after immunization with X-irradiated KMT-17 tumor cells. They suggested that the mechanism of the enhancement by busulfan involved a selective elimination of the immunosuppressor cells from the immunized hosts.

Gifford *et al.* (1981) have shown that cimetidine, a type-2 receptor antagonist, can render protection against lethal tumor challenge in mice. Cimetidine also inhibits the metastatic spread of the tumor and prolongs the lifespan of the tumor-bearing animal. The effect was considered to be due to the action of cimetidine on suppressor cells. It has been noted that inhibitors of prostaglandin synthesis, such as indomethacin and aspirin, can cause inhibition of murine tumor growth (Fulton and Levy, 1980; Greenwich and Plescia, 1977).

Serrou and colleagues (1980) have reported that thymosin can modulate suppressor cell activity in tumor-bearing mice and cancer patients. These authors have also indicated that thymosin not only has the ability to block metastatic tumor growth, but can also significantly reduce local tumor growth. The number of primary metastases were reduced after thymosin treatment.

Tilkin *et al.* (1981) have demonstrated an inhibition of tumor growth following low-dose irradiation (150 rads). They thought that these results were due to an induction of antiidiotypic activity directed against the receptors of suppressor T lymphocytes.

Ray and Raychaudhuri (1981) observed that elimination of the precursors of suppressor cells by a low dose of cyclophosphamide can either delay or completely inhibit the growth of a lethal dose of a murine fibrosarcoma. This low dose of cyclophosphamide could stimulate host immune reactivity. Thus, the inhibition of the growth of the transplantable fibrosarcoma was thought to be due to the anti-suppressor-cell activity of cyclophosphamide.

If increased prostaglandin production either by the tumor or by the host macrophages is important in inhibiting the immune response of the host (especially in the immediate environment of the tumor) and in allowing the tumor to escape immunologic rejection, one would expect that the administration of PGE-synthesis inhibitors *in vivo* to tumor-bearing animals or cancer patients would result in either an improvement in immune function, retardation of tumor growth, or both.

Plescia *et al.* (1975) demonstrated that prostaglandin synthesis inhibitors can restore the antibody response to sheep erythrocytes in tumor-bearing mice and that they can also retard tumor growth. Several other laboratories have obtained similar results.

Brunda *et al.* (1980) have demonstrated that splenocytes from mice with Moloney-virus-induced sarcomas had severely depressed natural killer activity (NK)-cell activity. The NK-cell activity could be restored to normal by the administration of prostaglandin synthesis inhibitors, such as aspirin or indomethacin.

Hial *et al.* (1976) administered aspirin or indomethacin to tumor-bearing mice to cause substantial retardation of the growth of tumors. At higher indomethacin doses (5 mg/kg per day) the tumors were destroyed in 50% of the cases, but there were also manifestations of gastric toxicity and weight loss in the mice.

Lynch *et al.* (1978) reported that indomethacin and aspirin inhibited the growth of a methylcholanthrene-induced fibrosarcomas in mice. These drugs were not started until 7 days after tumor inoculation, when the tumor was already palpable. In approximately 20% of the indomethacin-treated mice, the tumor completely regressed and did not reappear.

Strausser and Humes (1975) have reported that indomethacin delays the growth of Moloney-virus-induced sarcomas in mice. When the drug was given at the same time as the virus, no tumors developed.

Bennett *et al.* (1979) reported that treatment with flurbiprofen (an inhibitor of prostaglandin synthesis) before the injection of mamary tumor cells inhibited tumor growth.

In a study by Pollard and Luckert (1981) indomethacin was started 14 days after carcinogen administration. It reduced significantly the appearance of intestinal tumors. Thus, prostaglandin synthesis inhibitors would possibly serve as immunomodulating agents, controlling suppressor cell activity and inhibiting tumor growth. It is possible that prostaglandins may render their immunosuppressive activity by acting elsewhere in the system. All the studies mentioned here may not provide a clear indication that inhibition of tumor growth is indeed the result of a stimulated immune system. For example, Lynch *et al.* (1978) claimed that prostaglandin synthesis inhibitors may not function through the host immune system. In support of their hypothesis, they showed that mice whose tumors had been completely eliminated with indomethacin treatment were not immune to rechallenge with the same tumor. Augmentation of the immune response in tumor-bearing mice by indomethacin did not always correlate with the antitumor effects of the drug. There still remains the possibility that PGE synthesis inhibitors work by augmentation of NK and macrophage activity. Lynch *et al.* thought that inhibition by PGE synthesis inhibitors of tumor metastases may be mediated by mechanisms unrelated to the immune system.

Disappointing results of clinical trials with nonspecific immunostimulation in cancer patients using either bacillus Calmette-Guérin (BCG) or *Corynebacterium parvum* become more understandable in light of recent results indicating that *C. parvum* and BCG, in addition to nonspecifically activating humoral and cellular immune responses, induce the generation of suppressor cells in host animals (Klimpal, 1980; Nata and Slavin, 1979; Klimpal *et al.*, 1979; Savary and Lotova, 1978), thus facilitating tumor growth.

All these data indicate that careful and well controlled intervention in suppressor cell activity may provide therapeutic benefit to the tumor-bearing host. Although a large number of laboratories have shown an effective immune response in lymphocytes of tumor-bearing hosts under *in vitro* laboratory conditions, those reactivities remained suppressed *in vivo*. It is generally believed that because of the presence of specific and nonspecific immunosuppressive components the host remains virtually anergic (Figs. 1 and 7). It is therefore conceivable that, if these immunosuppressor agents can be removed or their production controlled, the host would then be immunologically potentiated. An activated immune reactivity would then become functional against the tumor, causing inhibition of tumor growth.

VI. NATURE OF SPECIFIC PLASMA BLOCKING FACTORS IN THE TUMOR HOST

Of the various possible specific plasma blocking factors, antigen, antibody, and antigen–antibody complexes have been suspected of playing an active role. Antigen–antibody complexes have been described as having an active role in both the induction (Sulica *et al.*, 1976) and the maintenance (Voisin, 1972) of tolerance. It has also been reported that immune complexes contribute to immunologic suppression in cancer (Baldwin *et al.*, 1974). The mechanism of immune-complex-induced suppression of the host immune response is not fully understood. Among the several mechanisms proposed, it has been suggested that immune complexes can (1) bind to the Fc receptors on a target tumor cell and thus mask their antigenic sites (Kerbal and Pears, 1974), (2) react with lymphocytes, abrogating their reactivity against the tumor cells (Kerbal and Pears, 1974), or (3) act on suppressor cells, activating their suppressive effects (Raychaudhuri *et al.*, 1980; Gershon *et al.*, 1974; Oldston and Tishow, 1977). Immune complexes have also been claimed to have the ability to inhibit NK-cell activity (Oldston and Tishow, 1977; Peter *et al.*, 1975; Cowan *et al.*, 1979).

In addition to the widespread blocking activity of immune complexes, antibody has also been reported to have the ability to facilitate tumor growth. It is not certain, however, whether these same antibodies, under some circumstances, can also function as cytotoxic antibodies. It is also not known what fundamental differences confer on them the ability to facilitate tumor growth rather than destroy tumor targets. In studies involving animal tumor models, immunologic enhancement of various type of tumors was noted. These tumors included sarcomas, carcinomas, lymphomas, and leukemias (Boyse et al., 1962; Philips and Stetson, 1962). It has been reported that sarcomas and carcinomas are very easily potentiated by antibody. On the other hand, the growth of lymphomas and leukemias is usually suppressed by antibody (Borer and Kallis, 1959; E. Möller and Möller, 1962; G. Möller, 1963). However, the fundamental basis of this difference is not known.

Among the various immunoglobulin classes and subclasses, IgM, IgG, IgG2a, IgG2b, and IgA (Rubenstein et al., 1974), Fab (Chard, 1968; Chard et al., 1967), and F(ab)$_2$ (Chard et al., 1976) have been shown to have the ability to enhance tumor growth in mice.

Rubenstein et al. (1974) suggested that IgM, IgG, and IgG2 are individually capable of enhancing the growth of sarcoma I. These results are contradictory to an earlier hypothesis that tumor enhancement and suppression are mediated by different immunoglobulin subclasses. However, it was also suggested that tumor growth suppression and enhancement are dependent on the doses of the antiserum used. Usually, low or intermediate doses enhanced tumor growth, while large doses frequently suppressed tumor growth. A large number of reports are available in the literature in support of this hypothesis (Herberman, 1974; E. Möller and Möller, 1962; Deorger, 1942; Hutchin et al., 1967; Rosenberg and Perry, 1977; Bansal and Sjögren, 1971). These observations pose a very practical problem for cancer immunotherapists, since they reveal that specific antitumor antibody can cause tumor growth facilitation as well as tumor destruction. It is not certain, however, whether this is a question of the dose or of the type of antibody molecules or their classes or subclasses. Future research will yield new insights into this area.

VII. CONTROL OF SERUM BLOCKING FACTORS AS AN APPROACH TO CANCER IMMUNOTHERAPY

A. Unblocking Approach

In some in vitro models, unblocking or deblocking serum activity was first demonstrated in the sera of animals showing spontaneous regression of Moloney-virus-induced sarcoma (I. Hellström and Hellström, 1970; I. Hellström et al., 1971). Hellström and colleagues have demonstrated unblocking activity in the sera of tumor-free human cancer patients. The effect of unblocking sera in counteracting tumor growth may be due either to its ability to deactivate the serum-blocking activity or its ability to mediate antibody- and complement-dependent

cytoxicity. The latter possibility seems more probable, since increased antibody-
and complement-mediated cytotoxicity is usually seen in the sera of tumor-free
animals and human cancer patients.

Bansal and Sjögren (1973b) have shown that simultaneous use of unblocking serum and splenectomy provides therapeutic benefit in polyoma-tumor-
bearing rats. Combination therapy involving splenectomy, BCG immunization,
and unblocking sera was utilized in a rat polyoma tumor model to show partial
antitumor effect (Bansal and Sjögren, 1973a,b). Similar results have also been reported from the laboratory of K. E. Hellström (1975).

It has become evident that although unblocking sera can counteract the
blocking effect to some extent, their clinical use is questionable owing to a number of limitations:

1. Purification and identification of specific TAA for each individual tumor
   type is quite difficult. Therefore, immunization of the host with specific
   TAA does not yet appear to be a practical possibility for production of
   unblocking serum.
2. The optimal method of production of unblocking serum factor by immunization of the host with a specific TAA has not been developed. On the
   other hand, use of TAA for immunization may produce tumor-enhancing
   factors, humoral and cellular, instead of unblocking factors (Raychaudhuri
   et al., 1980; Saha and Ray, 1982).
3. A large amount of unblocking factor may be needed to unblock the serum blocking activity sufficiently to affect tumor growth. This result has
   been difficult to obtain up until now. However, if unblocking factor(s)
   is always a cytotoxic antibody, then recent advances in hybridoma technology for the production of monoclonal antibodies might offer a solution—one to be approached with cautious optimism.
4. Tumor-free individuals are not always available as a source of unblocking
   sera.

Thus it appears that the unblocking approach may provide some therapeutic
benefit only if methods are developed to (1) produce large amounts of specific
"unblocking sera," (2) isolate tumor-specific antigen free from host-related antigen, (3) abrogate serum blocking activity, and (4) elicit autogenous production
of unblocking factors while suppressing the production of blocking factors. During the recent past, a number of approaches have been utilized to meet these
needs.

B. Immune Complex Removal—Plasma Adsorption
with Protein A of *Staphylococcus aureus*

Since CIC, antigen and antibody, and a variety of other plasma components
(Figs. 1 and 7) are known to exert specific and nonspecific immunosuppressive

effects in tumor-bearing patients, therapeutic approaches have been directed toward removal or reduction of those factors interfering with the patient's immune response. The availability of blood cell separators capable of handling large volumes of blood and separating the blood cells from the plasma within a short period of time, has facilitated studies aimed at the removal of blood components or manipulation of specific blood components followed by reintroduction of the processed blood into the system. Various laboratories have reported the effects of multiple modalities of therapy for patients with disseminated cancer (Agnello, 1981; Bottino et al., 1978; Hamblin, 1979; Israel et al., 1977; Jones et al., 1980; Langvade et al., 1975; Rossen and Morgan, 1981; Suckalova et al., 1973). Plasma exchange has been shown to be clinically successful in a variety of diseases characterized by an increase in CIC (Agnello, 1981; Hamblin, 1979; McKenzie et al., 1979; Verrier-Jones et al., 1981). The successes in cancer have not been as dramatic as those reported in other diseases (McKenzie et al., 1979; Rossen and Morgan, 1981). However, using a combination of plasma exchange and cyclophosphamide, Suckalova et al. (1973) treated five patients with multiple myeloma and two patients with Waldenström's macroglobulinemia. They observed impressive remissions in their patients for 2–8 months.

Partial response to repeated plasma exchange has been reported by Israel et al. (1977) in 8 of 23 cancer patients. Hershey et al. (1976) showed partial response in 1 of 4 multiple myeloma patients following plasmapheresis. They also noticed a marked reduction in blocking of cell-mediated cytotoxicity upon addition of posttreatment plasma.

Ray et al. (1980a,d,e) observed appreciable objective improvement in a patient with IgG-type myeloma following plasmapheresis and plasma adsorption with protein A-containing Staphylococcus aureus.

Salinas et al. (1981) examined the effect of repeated plasmapheresis on the removal of specific and nonspecific factors interfering with lymphocyte activation. Modulation of mixed-lymphocyte reactivity was noted in patients showing response to plasmapheresis. Their patients showed symptomatic improvement following the initial plasmapheresis treatment, but no objective response was observed in patients with advanced disease (Salinas and Wee, 1983).

The plasmapheresis technique has its limitations as a procedure since it lacks selectivity—with the removal of whole plasma both beneficial and harmful plasma components are lost (Ray, 1981, 1983). Particularly where the effect is immunologically mediated, the removal of whole plasma eliminates the essential immunological components as well, depriving the host of benefit from the treatment.

Noonan et al. (1974) investigated the role of thoracic duct drainage in controlling the growth of tumors in mice by attempting to remove blocking factors from the lymph. While they reported some beneficial effects, a harmful effect of such an approach has also been described (Proctor et al., 1973). In human cancer patients, thoracic duct drainage has been of very little therapeutic benefit (Isbister et al., 1975). However, all these methods have their limitations in that they also remove beneficial serum factors, such as immune components, enzymes, and a large number of other biochemical, hormonal, and nutritional components (Ray, 1981, 1983).

In 1969, I. Hellström and Hellström reported that the plasma of both tumor-bearing animals and human cancer patients contained circulating specific blocking factors which could block the ability of sensitized lymphocytes to destroy tumor cells *in vitro*. The blocking factors have since been characterized as TAA, antibody, and antigen–antibody complexes. It was thought that the presence of these blocking agents in the sera of a tumor-bearing host helped the tumor to escape host immunologic attack. Any procedure to remove them or control their production may be therapeutically beneficial.

An attempt to adsorb extracorporeally the serum proteins of colon carcinoma and hypernephroma patients was made by Langvade and colleagures in 1975. They used F(ab)$_2$ fragments as ligand to adsorb plasma proteins in an extracorporeal adsorption system and reported some partial therapeutic benefit in their patients.

Steele *et al.* (1975) observed that plasma from polyoma- and carcinoma-bearing rats lost its blocking activity when adsorbed *in vitro* with protein A-containing *S. aureus* Cowan I. These authors performed their study under *in vitro* conditions and did not investigate the effect of infusion of the adsorbed serum into the tumor-bearing animal for any possible therapeutic benefits.

An extracorporeal method of adsorbing plasma IgG and immune complexes using protein A-containing *S. aureus* Cowan I as the adsorbent has been described by Bansal and colleagues (1978). This method was used first in normal dogs and later in one colon carcinoma patient (Bansal *et al.*, 1978). Tumoricidal responses were seen and tumor regression was observed in this patient. Histopathologic data indicated tumor necrosis and replacement by fibrous tissues. There was a transient reduction in the serum blocking activity and appearance of complement-dependent serum cytotoxicity. An increase in serum IgM levels, a transient increase in the Ig surface-bearing lymphocytes, and a decrease in E-rosetting lymphocytes in the first 24–48 hr postperfusion were noted, particularly during the early treatments.

Expanding on Bansal's studies, Ray *et al.* extended their investigations in three tumor models to show that, irrespective of the tumor model and the tumor type, plasma adsorption can cause tumor regression (Ray *et al.*, 1979*a*,*b*; 1980 *a*,*c*,*e*,*f*; 1981*a*–*c*; 1982*a*,*b*; 1984*a*,*b*). Ray and colleagues have described regressions of tumors in (1) a chemically induced primary mammary adenocarcinoma model; (2) a transplantable canine venereal tumor model, including several cases of spontaneously occurring dog tumors; and (3) human colon carcinoma patients and other human malignancies. A number of other laboratories subsequently investigated the use of the intact *S. aureus* plasma perfusion technique, the protein A-collodion-charcoal adsorption method, protein A-silica adsorption, or the protein A-Sepharose adsorption procedure (Terman *et al.*,

1980*a,b*, 1981; Jones *et al.*, 1980; Holohan *et al.*, 1982; Gordon *et al.*, 1983; Bensinger *et al.*, 1982; MacKintosh *et al.*, 1983). These studies have described tumor regression in various animal tumor models and also in human cancer patients. Although various types of protein A adsorbents were used by various laboratories, tumor regressions were reported consistently in a number of tumor models. Some of these studies (Terman *et al.*, 1980*a,b*, 1981; Jones *et al.*, 1980) used a combination of plasma adsorption and chemotherapy or radiation to cause tumor regression.

VIII. PLASMA ADSORPTION IN RATS BEARING A CHEMICALLY INDUCED MAMMARY ADENOCARCINOMA

For greater flexibility and well controlled experimentation, we have developed a rat primary mammary tumor model (Ray *et al.*, 1979*b*, 1980*f*, 1981*a*, 1982*b*, 1984*a,b*) to study the effect of plasma adsorption on tumor growth. This model has provided several advantages: (1) Results of plasma adsorption can be compared with those in untreated tumor-bearing hosts. (2) Large numbers of tumor-bearing animals can be included in the studies, to establish the statistical significance of the data. (3) Adsorption can be provided with various frequencies in various groups to study its effect on tumor regression. (4) Immunological studies can be done in both treated and untreated tumor-bearing hosts to evaluate changes in immunologic reactivity in plasma-adsorbed hosts compared to that in the untreated tumor-bearing controls. (5) Finally, it is less expensive a model compared to others used in this field.

We (Ray *et al.*, 1979*b*, 1981*a*, 1982*b*) have observed that weekly adsorption of plasma of rats bearing DMBA-induced mammary adenocarcinomas over *S. aureus* for a period of 6 weeks caused regression of the tumors. The treated animals showed a decrease in plasma blocking activity and an increase in complement-dependent, antibody-mediated cytotoxicity. Instead of blocking the cellular cytotoxicity, the plasma showed potentiation of cell-mediated lysis of DMBA-induced mammary tumor cells. In a separate study (Ray *et al.*, 1984*a,b*) we have studied the effect of frequency of plasma adsorption on the regression of rat mammary adenocarcinomas. Weekly, biweekly, and alternate-day adsorptions were performed. Alternate-day adsorption showed highly significant ($P <$ 0.001) and early regression of tumors compared to other protocols, in which tumor regression was delayed. Potentiated immunological reactivities were observed in the treated host, as noted in our previous studies (Ray *et al.*, 1979*b*, 1982). In addition, histological analyses of biopsied sections of tumors from treated animals showed disruption of tumor cell architecture, loss of glandular structure, shrinkage of epithelial cells, and moderate mononuclear cell infiltration. Animals from both the control and treated groups were kept for observation for a period of 6 months after termination of the experiment to follow the pattern of their tumor growth and longevity. While tumors in the control animals continued to grow, tumors in the treated animals regressed or else regressed for a while and then grew slowly. The treated animals survived longer than the controls (Ray et al., 1984a). In one study, 14 of 14 untreated animals died one month after termination of the experiment, whereas only 3 of 14 treated animals died during the same period. In the treated group, 11 of 14 animals survived several months longer than the controls, and one has remained tumor-free for an indefinite period.

Interestingly, we have also noted that autologous plasma adsorbed with non-protein A-containing S. aureus Wood 46 also caused tumor regression in this tumor model (Ray et al., 1984a), as did freshly perpared normal rat plasma adsorbed over S. aureus and then infused into DMBA-induced-tumor-bearing animals (Ray et al., 1984b). Infusion of normal rat plasma adsorbed over S. aureus into tumor-bearing rats caused an approximately 20% regression of tumor volume at a time when the untreated tumor's volume had increased by 70% over that at the beginning of the experiment. We also studied NK-cell activity using peripheral blood mononuclear cells (PBMNC) as effector and YAC_1 as target (obtained by courtesy of Dr. Ronald B. Herberman, NCI, NIH, Bethesda, Maryland). Antibody-dependent cell-mediated cytotoxicity (ADCC) against DMBA-induced mammary adenocarcinoma cells was also measured using PBMNC and rat mammary adeno-carcinoma cells either coated with or without autologous serum (Table VIII). Both NK activity and ADCC [chicken red blood cell (CRBC)–anti-CRBC system] were not changed in treated animals. However, as noted previously (Ray et al., 1982b, 1984a) there was a potentiation of the cytotoxic activity in PBMNC of treated rats compared to untreated controls (Table VIII). There was also some increase in the complement activity (CH50 units) in the treated sera.

IX. PLASMA ADSORPTION IN DOGS BEARING A TRANSPLANTABLE CANINE VENEREAL TUMOR AND VARIOUS SPONTANEOUSLY OCCURRING TUMORS

On-line adsorption of the entire plasma volume of dogs with transplantable canine venereal tumors (TVT) and spontaneous tumors led to very impressive tumor regressions (Ray et al., 1980f, 1981a, 1984b). Regressions were noted that ranged from as low as a 24% decrease in tumor volume to a 99% decrease. A few animals did not respond. This observation was true in both the TVT system and spontaneously occurring tumor-bearing dogs. Similar results have been reported by a number of laboratories (Terman et al., 1980a, b; Holohan et al., 1982; Gordon et al., 1983).

Table VIII. NK-Cell Activity, ADCC (CRBC–Anti-CRBC System), and Cytotoxicity against DMBA-Induced Mammary Tumor Cells by PBMNC of Treated and Untreated Rats

Group	Percent specific ^{51}Cr release by PBMNC from labeled YAC$_1$ cells (NK) Effector:target ratio		Percent specific ^{51}Cr release by PBMNC from antibody-coated labeled CRBC (ADCC) Effector:target ratio		Percent specific ^{51}Cr release by PBMNC from labeled DMBA-induced mammary tumor cells in presence of medium or autologous plasma[a]	Plasma dilution	
	25:1	50:1	25:1	50:1	Medium	1:8	1:32
Untreated tumor-bearing control rats	16.35 ± 7.93 (N = 4)	20.00 ± 7.43	27.13 ± 6.55 (N = 4)	31.37 ± 7.16	22.85 ± 6.30	10.39 ± 9.03 (−54.52)[b]	21.14 ± 3.65 (−7.48)
Treated tumor-bearing rats	18.99 ± 8.42 (N = 6)	19.10 ± 9.19	25.36 ± 13.38 (N = 6)	26.30 ± 16.08	30.5 ± 5.82	12.83 ± 6.23 (−57.93)	31.03 ± 3.11 (1.73)

[a]Note that PBMNC of treated rats show increased cytotoxicity compared to PBMNC of untreated controls. While 1:32 dilution of plasma of untreated rats still retains its blocking activity, the blocking effect is reversed at the same dilution of plasma of treated rats. Values represent average of four rats ± SD.

[b]Values in parentheses represent percent blocking (−)/percent augmentation (+) by autologous plasma compared to autologous cellular cytotoxicity.

X. PLASMA ADSORPTION IN HUMAN CANCER PATIENTS

We (Ray, 1979; Ray *et al.*, 1979*a,b*, 1980*a,c-f*, 1981*a-c*, 1982*a,b*, 1984*a,b*) have performed plasma adsorption in a total of 40 human cancer patients, a selected group of which are shown in Table IX. Most of the patients belonged to the colon carcinima category, although patients with other forms of cancer were also included in this study. Patients were treated for anywhere from 1 week to 12 months. During this period, they received 2-26 adsorptions. Usually two adsorptions were done in a week, and each time plasma equivalent to one half of the total blood volume was processed. The patients all showed some form of response—subjective, objective, or both. As soon as there were indications of disease proliferation or no response, they were excluded from the study. We wanted to investigate the following three aspects: (1) whether the plasma adsorption procedure can be offered safely to all types of patients, (2) whether immunostimulation can be shown in plasma-adsorbed hosts, and (3) whether any subjective and/or objective response can be documented.

During the past six years (1978-1984) of our study, we have administered more than 320 plasma adsorption procedures in 40 human cancer patients. Varying numbers of plasma adsorption procedures were administered for a varying period of time in patients having different types of prognoses (Table IX). Obviously, the response varied. In some 21 patients, we observed subjective improvements. But in only a small number of patients (9 of 40) was some partial objective response noted. Interestingly, eight of these nine patients were treated over a long period of time (7-12 months). Nineteen of 40 patients received only two to four plasma adsorptions and did not show any response. They were dropped from the study for a variety of reasons. In general, most of the responsive patients showed a decrease in CIC level, IgG, C3, Ca^{2+}, and CEA; an increase in skin sensitivity to an anergy panel (*Candida*, mumps, triphyton); an increase in the phytohemagglutinin blastogenic response of lymphocytes and CH50; and some positive histological and radiological changes reminiscent of tumor destruction.

We had the opportunity to study the cytotoxic effect of PBMNC from a colon carcinoma patient against his own cryopreserved tumor cells. Out results showed a marked increase in PBMNC cytotoxicity against autochthonous tumor cells during the postadsorption period (35%) compared to the preadsorption period (9%). Post adsorption plasma could further potentiate the PBMNC cytotoxicity (66%), but plasma from the preadsorption period could not do so (9.5% cytotoxicity).

A. Clinical Observations

During each immunoadsorption procedure, vital signs were monitored every 5 min during and after the procedure until they were stable for a total period of

Table IX. Effect of Plasma Adsorption in Human Cancer Patients

Patient profile[a]	Total no. of adsorptions (period of treatment)[b]	Response: subjective (S) or objective (O)
1. 55 F, Ca-colon, ovarian mets.	17 (12 months)	S, for 12 months
2. 61 M, Ca-colon, liver mets.	3 (1 week)	S, O; liver scan showed decreased size of the defect
3. 82 M, Ca-colon, liver mets.	11 (10 months)	S. stable for 10 months; liver scan showed nonhomogeneous tumor size
4. 58 F, Ca-rectum	10 (8 months)	S, stable for 8 months
5. 59 F, Ca-rectum, mets. nodes, bone	3 (1 week)	S, discontinued
6. 56 F, glioblastoma	11 (12 months)	S, O (scan); CAT scan showed decrease in tumor size; stable for 12 months
7. 52 F, Ca-breast, mets. bone	6 (3 months)	S
8. 56 F, Ca-colon, mets. liver, colon	8 (3 months)	S, O; histopathological data indicated fibrosis and necrosis around the tumor
9. 40 M, Ca-colon, mets. lung, liver	7 (1 month)	S
10. 54 F, Ca-colon, mets. liver	13 (6 months)	S, O; liver scan showed decrease in the liver defect, stable for 6 months
11. 58 M, Ca-colon, mets. omentum, liver	7 (7 months)	S, O; stable for 7 months; complete regression of a small tumor nodule in the tumor area and necrosis in another
12. 55 F, Ca-colon, mets. liver	24 (8 months)	S, stable for 8 months
13. 50 F, Ca-colon, mets. liver	26 (10 months)	S, O; stable for 10 months; decrease in liver defect was seen in liver scan
14. 66 F, glioma	8 (3 months)	S, stable for 3 months
15. 30 F, unknown primary, mets. bone, cervical lymphs	12 (7 months)	S, stable for 7 months
16. 41 M, Ca-colon, mets, liver	7 (3 months)	S, stable for 3 months
17. 55 F, Ca-colon, mets. liver	12 (3½ months)	S, O; histopathological data showed fibrosis and necrosis around the tumor
18. 61 M, Ca-colon	4 (1 month)	S, stable for a month
19. 47 M, Ca-stomach	5 (1 month)	S, stable for a month
20. 56 M, Ca-colon	10 (10 months)	S, stable for 10 months
21. 68 M, Ca-kidney, mets. skull, neck, back	8 (5 weeks)	S, O; actual size of many metastatic nodules decreased

[a]Nineteen other patients received only two to four adsorptions and did not show much improvement.
[b]During this therapy no other treatment was given.

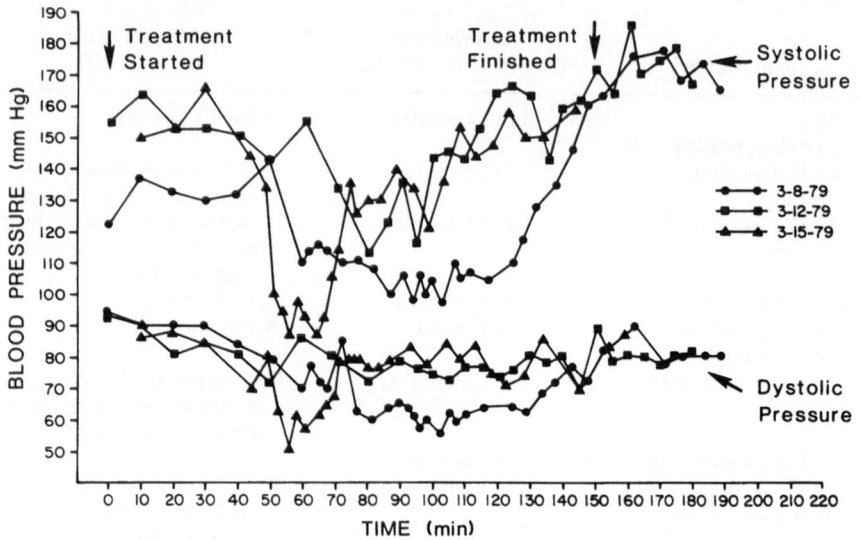

Figure 9. Changes in blood pressure during and after plasma adsorption in a colon carcinoma patient.

2 hr. The temperature over the tumor was continuously recorded and the oral or rectal temperature was taken every 30 min. The clinical changes seen during and following each procedure were similar. In general, during every procedure the patient showed symptoms of hypovolemia 20-30 min after the initiation of the procedure. This was corrected by fluid replacement (5% albumin in Ringer's lactate). This condition lasted 10-15 min. The systolic blood pressure rose gradually to about 180 mm Hg during some of the procedures. Usually it varied between 160 and 180 mm Hg (Fig. 9). After about 45 min to an hour, the patient started to shake and complained of a burning pain around the tumor area. There was an increase in the temperature on the surface of the tumor by 2-3°F. Body temperature also increased to 102-104°F (Fig. 10). There was no clinical, biochemical, or electrocardiographic evidence of cardiopulmonary dysfunction. Patient discomfort caused by the procedure was limited to the burning pain in the tumor, chills, and nausea. There was subjective improvement in the general condition of many patients, together with a significant decrease of pain in the tumor area.

B. Studies on Plasma Adsorbed over *S. aureus*

Radiolabeled *S. Aureus* (labeled with [³H]thymidine, [³H]leucine, [³H]palmitic acid, and [³H]glucose) was used *in vitro* for adsorption with normal and cancer patients' plasma. The plasma was filtered through a bacterial filter (0.2

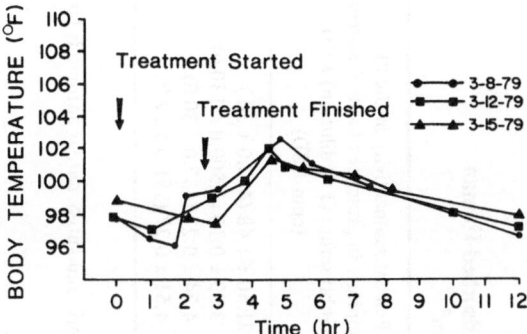

Figure 10. Increase in body temperature during and after plasma adsorption in a colon carcinoma patient.

μm) and examined for radioactivity following precipitation with rabbit anti-*S. aureus* antiserum (Table X). Radioactivity was noted in the postadsorbed plasma. During an *ex vivo* adsorption of dog plasma with radiolabeled *S. aureus* a procedure similar to that used in dogs and human patients, we also noted radioactivity in the postfilter plasma and in postadsorption plasma (collected from the body of the dog). These results indicate that bacterial components are released during the plasma adsorption procedure with *S. aureus* (Bandyopadhyay and Ray, 1985).

C. Other Studies

Terman *et al.* (1980*a,b,* 1981) studied *S. aureaus* plasma adsorption and protein A–collodion charcoal plasma adsorption effects in dogs with spontaneously occurring tumors and in human patients with mammary tumors. In some tumors both gross and microscopic tumor necrosis was observed. Healing of some large ulcerated areas of cutaneous tumor was also reported, including deposition of IgG and C3 on tumor cell membranes. There was an increase in C1q-binding complexes and a decrease in C3 levels in serum following perfusion, as well as an increase in TAA levels in plasma. These results are consistent with our findings (Ray, 1979; Ray *et al.,* 1979*a,b,* 1980*a,c-f,* 1981*a-c,* 1982*a,b,* 1984*a,b*).

Jones *et al.* (1980) used a feline leukemia virus (FeLV) model and demonstrated a reaction in circulating lymphoblasts within two weeks of plasma adsorption over *S. aureus* and radiation treatment. Three of five cats showed clinical improvement. Two of five cats remained FeLC-negative and tumor-free 7–8 months posttherapy.

Holohan *et al.* (1982) observed objective regression of spontaneous mammary adenocarcinomas in dogs following extracorporeal plasma adsorption over *S. aureus.*

Table X. Radioimmunoprecipitation of Eluted Bacterial Molecules from Postadsorbed Human Plasma by Normal Rabbit Serum and Rabbit Anti-S. *aureus* Serum[a]

Precursors used to radiolabel S. *aureus*	Total radioactivity in 0.2 mol postadsorbed plasma (cpm ± SD)	Percent radioactivity in the PEG precipitate in presence of normal rabbit serum (1:2 dilution) ± SD (cpm ± SD)	Percent radioactivity in the PEG precipitate in presence of anti-S. *aureus* rabbit serum (1:2 dilution) ± SD (cpm ± SD)
[^{3}H] leucine	100.0% (1,874.41 ± 148.48)	2.35 ± 0.15 (44.0 ± 4.0)	21.50 ± 1.48 (403.0 ± 30.)
[^{3}H] palmitic acid	100.0% (69,637.88 ± 3,454.90)	0.94 ± 0.06 (655.0 ± 68.0)	3.59 ± 0.10 (2,500.0 ± 130.0)
[^{3}H] glucose	100.0% (10,069.12 ± 691.24)	1.34 ± 0.09 (135.0 ± 13.0)	4.34 ± 0.27 (437.0 ± 30.0)
[^{3}H] thymidine	100.0% (4,390.24 ± 487.80)	2.99 ± 0.10 (131.0 ± 15.0)	4.51 ± 0.27 (198.0 ± 22.0)

[a] All values represent an average of triplicate sets.

[b] Note that total percent radioactivity in the precipitate of plasma absorbed with [^{3}H] leucine-labeled bacteria and anti-S. *aureus* antisera is far greater than that of other groups.

Gordon et al. (1983) reported tumoricidal responses in dogs with spontaneous tumors following extracorporeal plasma adsorption on both S. aureus and S. aureus Wood 46. However Terman et al. (1980a) reported that they could not find any antitumor activity following plasma perfusion over S. aureus Wood 46. Contrary to this observation, Ray et al. (1984b) have observed tumor regression in rats following plasma adsorption over S. aureus Wood 46.

Cooper and Masinello (1983) described an increase in median survival time in mice inoculated with cultured B-16 melanoma cells when they received S. aureus adsorbed serum from either tumor-bearing or normal mice. If serum was given for a period of 7 days or less after B-16 inoculation, the median survival time of the mice was greatly increased (up to 32%).

Yamamoto et al. (1983) reported that treatment of FeLV-positive cats by ex vivo plasma adsorption with S. aureus or AMF Staph protein A filters twice a week for 10 weeks was associated with a dramatic increase in serum interferon titer prior to remission of leukemia.

Pickett et al. (1983) showed an inhibition of growth of transitional cell carcinoma in mice treated with either normal mouse plasma passed over protein A–Sepharose beads or progressor animals' plasma treated with protein A–Sepharose beads.

All of these studies had at least one common observation—tumor regression irrespective of the tumor type or plasma adsorption procedure used.

D. Role of Immune Complex Removal in Plasma Adsorption Procedure

Diener and Feldman (1972) have suggested that immune complexes may be involved in the regulatory mechanism in the body and that they can act by delivery of a signal to induce tolerance. If this is true, an alteration in the concentration of immune complexes by the plasma adsorption procedure discussed previously may break that tolerance of the host for its tumor. As a result, the host immune components should be able to recognize the tumor as foreign and exert their cytotoxic effects, resulting in the killing of the tumor cells.

Gershon et al. (1974) have suggested that tumor antigen–antibody complexes can activate suppressor T cells, which then inhibit the antitumor activity of macrophages. Therefore, removal of immune complexes may be beneficial by causing activation of macrophages to make them functional against tumors.

It appears that immune complexes play a major role in both humoral and cellular blocking phenomena. Therefore, effective removal of immune complexes from the plasma may be therapeutic by potentiating the antitumor immune reactivity of tumor-bearing hosts, leading to tumor regression.

So far, we have been successful in inducing tumor regression in a number of tumor models: (1) in primary-mammary-tumor-bearing rats (Ray et al., 1979b, 1982a,b, 1984a,b; (2) in dogs with both TVT and spontaneously occurring canine lymphosarcoma, fibrosarcoma, and rectal carcinoma (Ray *et al.*, 1980*f*, 1981*b*, 1984*b*); (3) in a number of metastatic colon carcinoma patients (Ray, 1979; Ray *et al.*, 1979*a*,*b*, 1980*a*,*c-f*, 1981*a-c*, 1982*a*,*b*, 1984*a*,*b*); and (4) in a few other types of cancer patients. These observations have been confirmed by a number of other laboratories in both humans and animals (Terman *et al.*, 1980, 1981; Jones *et al.*, 1980; Gordon *et al.*, 1983; Holohan *et al.*, 1982; Messerschmidt *et al.*, 1982; Day *et al.*, 1983; Yamamoto *et al.*, 1983; Pickett *et al.*, 1983; Cooper and Masinello, 1983).

One of the major drawbacks of most of these studies has been that no such protocol was ever employed to remove most of the blocking components from whole plasma. This was either because of some technical difficulty with complete adsorption of CIC or because of inappropriate experimental design. Obviously, all the results reported so far in the literature cannot be explained as due exclusively to the direct removal of plasma blocking components. Yet whatever the mechanisms, tumor regressions were obtained in a large number of these studies. This obviously raises the possibility that physical adsorption of the plasma blocking components may not be the mechanism behind the tumor regression process, particularly in view of the following facts: (1) Both we (Ray *et al.*, 1984*a*,*b*) and others (Gordon *et al.*, 1983) have reported that plasma adsorption with non-protein A-containing *S. aureus* Cowan I can cause similar tumor regression. (2) Normal animals' plasma adsorbed over *S. aureus* and infused into a tumor-bearing host can also cause tumor regression (Ray *et al.*, 1984*a*,*b*; Cooper and Masinello, 1983). (3) In most of the studies reported little reduction in plasma IgG or CIC levels was effected. (4) Perfusion of a small volume of adsorbed plasma can also induce tumor-regressive response. We may therefore pose the following question: Is there any other mechanism(s) responsible for the reduction in the level of plasma blocking factor(s), causing immunological stimulation and tumor regression? I shall discuss such a possibility in the following section.

XI. POSSIBLE MECHANISMS OF TUMOR REGRESSION IN PLASMA-ADSORBED HOSTS—AN IMBALANCE IN THE DYNAMIC EQUILIBRIUM OF IMMUNE COMPLEXES ACTIVATING THE HOST IMMUNITY TO FIGHT CANCER

Ray *et al.* have studied the mechanisms responsible for tumor regression in the plasma-adsorbed host. These have been described in greater detail in several publications (Ray, 1982; Ray *et al.*, 1980*c*, 1981*a*,*c*, 1982*a*,*b*, 1984*a*,*b*). I believe that the rationale behind this approach is sound, and that, if by some manipulation the plasma blocking immune complexes can be removed, or their concentration reduced, then the dynamic balance of the equilibrium (Fig. 11) will

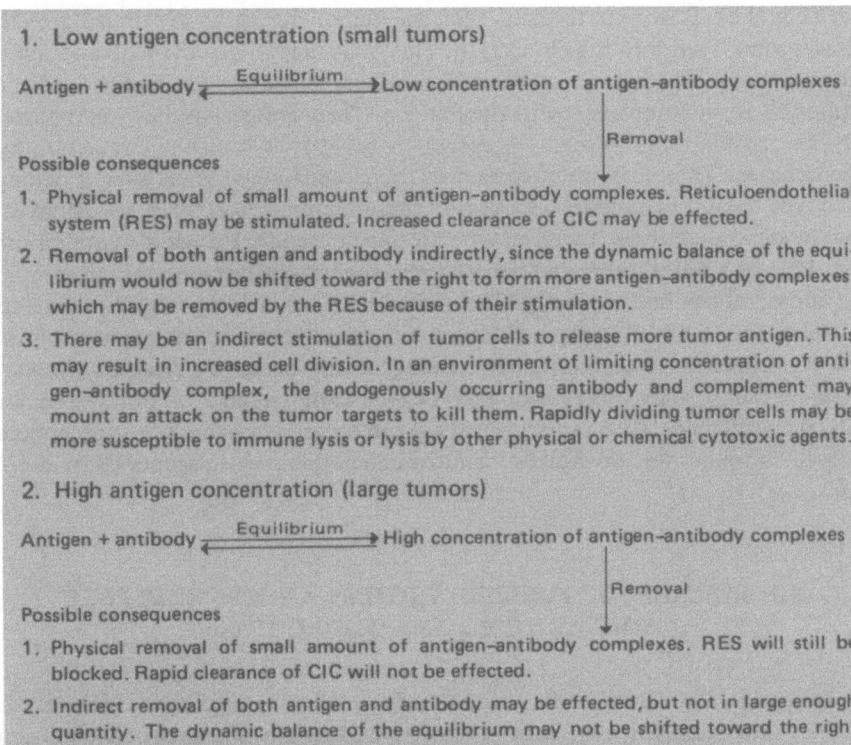

1. Low antigen concentration (small tumors)

Antigen + antibody $\xleftrightarrow{\text{Equilibrium}}$ Low concentration of antigen–antibody complexes

Removal

Possible consequences

1. Physical removal of small amount of antigen–antibody complexes. Reticuloendothelial system (RES) may be stimulated. Increased clearance of CIC may be effected.

2. Removal of both antigen and antibody indirectly, since the dynamic balance of the equilibrium would now be shifted toward the right to form more antigen–antibody complexes, which may be removed by the RES because of their stimulation.

3. There may be an indirect stimulation of tumor cells to release more tumor antigen. This may result in increased cell division. In an environment of limiting concentration of antigen–antibody complex, the endogenously occurring antibody and complement may mount an attack on the tumor targets to kill them. Rapidly dividing tumor cells may be more susceptible to immune lysis or lysis by other physical or chemical cytotoxic agents.

2. High antigen concentration (large tumors)

Antigen + antibody $\xleftrightarrow{\text{Equilibrium}}$ High concentration of antigen–antibody complexes

Removal

Possible consequences

1. Physical removal of small amount of antigen–antibody complexes. RES will still be blocked. Rapid clearance of CIC will not be effected.

2. Indirect removal of both antigen and antibody may be effected, but not in large enough quantity. The dynamic balance of the equilibrium may not be shifted toward the right because of larger concentration of antigen–antibody complexes.

3. There may not be any stimulation of tumor cell mitosis, because of the antigen excess situation. In this case, tumor cells may not be too susceptible to either immune lysis or lysis by physical and/or chemical agents.

4. Endogenously available antibody and complement may not gain access to the tumor targets to mount an attack because of antigenic excess.

5. When an environment is created for the elimination of the bulk of antigen, removal of antigen–antibody complexes may provide the same benefit as described under (1) above.

Figure 11. Possible mechanism of CIC clearance leading to endogenous immunological stimulation and tumor destruction in plasma-adsorbed hosts.

be shifted to the right. The host would then be immunologically activated to mount an attack on the tumor cells. Even a small amount of CIC removal may be able to disturb the equilibrium. In fact, it is known that the reticuloendothelial system (RES) may be blocked when there is an immune complex excess and the RES system may be made functional following a partial clearance of CIC (Frank *et al.*, 1979; Lockwood *et al.*, 1979).

I would like to propose the following hypothesis as a possible mechanism for how plasma adsorption may lead to immunological activation and tumor regression (Fig. 11). It is hypothesized that the tumor during its continued growth releases some TAA into the circulation. This TAA migrates to the RES and sensitizes the host. The host responds and produces antitumor antibodies, and the antibodies form complexes with the antigen. These antigen-antibody complexes may not develop complement receptors to be cleared from the circulation by macrophages. Therefore, they remain in the circulation to exert their blocking effect on the host immune response. If these immune complexes are removed, even in small quantities, there may be an imbalance in the dynamic equilibrium (Fig. 11). As a result, more and more complexes may be formed, consuming more and more antigen and antibody. The tumor cells may undergo rapid mitosis to replenish the depleted antigen. In such an environment of limited concentration of antigen-antibody complexes, endogenously occurring effector lymphocytes, antibody, and complement may be able to mount an attack on the tumor cells and kill them. The rapidly dividing tumor cells may be more susceptible both to immune lysis or radiation and to chemotherapeutic agents (Ray et al., 1980a,d,e).

XII. INFUSION OF PURIFIED PROTEIN A SHOWING EFFECT SIMILAR TO PLASMA ADSORPTION

Recently, Ray (1982), Ray and Bandyopadhyay (1983), and Ray et al. (1984c) have adopted a strategy to lower the immune complex concentration in the plasma of a tumor-bearing host by direct intravenous infusion of purified protein A of S. aureus. It has been observed that direct inoculation of purified protein A in rats carrying primary mammary adenocarcinomas may cause impressive regression of this tumor. Protein A infusion results in an activation of the cell-mediated cytotoxicity of the tumor, a decrease in plasma-blocking activity, and an increase in the complement-dependent antibody-mediated lysis of the tumor target (Ray and Bandyopadhyay, 1983; Ray et al., 1984c).

In a canine TVT model, we have also observed tumor regression following infusion of purified protein A (Table XI). The regressor animals showed potentiation of cell-mediated cytotoxicity and an increased antibody-complement mediated lysis of TVT cells.

We have also observed that within an hour of protein A infusion plasma CIC concentration decreased significantly, although it reverted back to the preinfusion level within 48 hr (Ray et al., 1984c). However, a quick decrease in the concentration of CIC may cause an imbalance in the dynamic equilibrium of CIC concentration and suppressed host immune reactivity. The equilibrium may now be shifted to favor the reaction of endogenously occurring host immunocompetent factors against the tumor. If this condition is maintained for a long period of time, or even intermittently, the tumor may be subjected to attack by the host immune components, causing its destruction (Fig. 11).

**Table XI. Effect of Intravenous Administration of Purified Protein A
on Regression of Canine TVT[a]**

Group	Drug used	Dog no.	Tumor volume (cm³)		Percent increase (+) or decrease (−) in tumor volume
			Before treatment	After treatment (14 days)	
Control	Saline	1	4.5	4.8	+6.66
		2	0.77	12.77	+1558.44
		3	3.18	8.43	+165.09
Experimental I	Protein A	1	5.3	Palpable	>−90.00
	(500 μg)	2	6.37	Not measurable	>−90.00
		3	0.35	Not measurable	>−90.00
Experimental II	Protein A	1	8.18	1.59	−80.56
	(1000 μg)	2	4.85	Palpable	>−90.00
		3	0.60	Not measurable	−100.00

[a] Protein A was given in 10 ml of sterile normal saline on alternate days.

During protein A infusion, Ray (1982) observed that tumors in regression turned black or blue-black in the course of treatment. Biopsy of the treated tumors showed necrosis, inflammatory cell infiltration, and replacement by fibrous tissues (Ray et al., 1984c). Furthermore, protein A in doses that had antitumor activity in rats did not show any significant toxicity toward either the hematopoietic stem cells, any major organs, or even the hepatic mixed-function oxidase system (Ray et al., 1984c). These results offer the promise that protein A, an immunomodulator, can be used to reduce the plasma level of immune complexes for the potentiation of antitumor activity in the tumor-bearing host. Detailed investigations, however, are necessary prior to its future use in experimental cancer therapy.

It is not certain, however, that the observed effect of purified protein A infusion is due to protein A alone, since protein A has been reported to be contaminated with small quantities of staphylococcal enterotoxin A (SEA) (Smith et al., 1983), which may also contribute to the observed phenomena. Further work will shed more light on this subject.

XIII. ENTEROTOXIN CONTAMINATION OF PROTEIN A AND ITS POSSIBLE EFFECTS

Smith et al. (1983) studied commercial preparations of protein A to detect the presence of SEA by SDS-PAGE analysis and observed about 5% contamination of protein A with SEA. A low-molecular-weight fraction of about 25,000 daltons, which was obtained by chromatographic separation of protein A, showed about 90% of the interferon-inducing ability of the protein A preparation. This fraction is likely to be SEA, since the molecular weight of SEA is 28,000 and the activity of this fraction was abrogated by treatment with anti-SEA. Therefore, the protein A utilized in our study and elsewhere is very likely to contain a small amount of SEA. Its contribution cannot be ruled out, since SEA in very small concentrations may exert very potent biological actions, such as T-cell mitogenic activity (Langford et al., 1978; Peavy et al., 1970), gamma-interferon induction (Smith et al., 1983), endothelial cell lesion formation (Finegold, 1967), and stimulation of other immunocytes. The enterotoxin may be reponsible for the hemodynamic changes observed in plasma-absorbed hosts, since similar changes were observed in monkeys following the infusion of enterotoxin B (Beisel, 1972; Hodoval et al., 1968).

XIV. POSSIBLE MECHANISM OF GENERATION OF VARIOUS BIOREACTIVE PRODUCTS FOLLOWING PLASMA ADSORPTION OVER S. AUREUS OR S. AUREUS WOOD 46 AND DURING DIRECT INFUSION OF PROTEIN A

Plasma adsorption over S. aureus may result in the release of a number of staphylococcal agents, including protein A and enterotoxin (Fig. 12). Released protein A would combine with serum IgG to form a series of complexes, the largest one being $(IgG)_4$ -(Protein A)$_2$, as depicted in Fig. 13. Such a molecule (19 S) is most likely to be formed when the four binding sites of the protein A molecule and the two binding sites of the IgG molecule are all saturated, particularly since IgG is available in large excess in the serum of the host. CIC will also bind with released protein A to form large complexes, such as $(CIC)_4$ - (Protein A)$_2$. These large molecular species obviously would give rise to a series of reactions:

1. Inflammatory reactions may be initiated in the microenvironment of the tumor when these complexes bind with complement-receptor-binding cells present in and around the tumor, resulting in the activation of the endothelial cells (Linder, 1981) and the release of histaminelike substances.
2. The complement activation (Langone et al., 1978) may result in the formation of chemoattractants (like C3a and C5a) that could draw polymorphonuclear leukocytes to the tumor site.
3. Granulocytes may also be activated to induce hydrolytic reactions.
4. The tumor destruction process may thus begin with the formation of edema at the tumor site, causing pain in the tumor area—an observation we have made in most of the patients we have treated. In our TVT model, we observed that immediately after the plasma adsorption procedure the tumors inflated in size and felt softer.

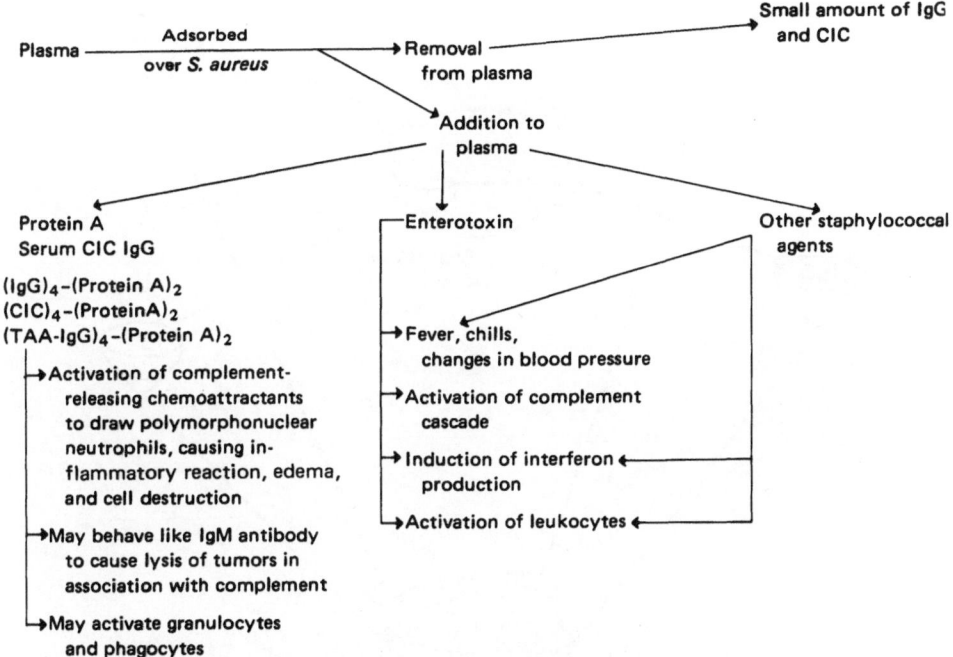

Figure 12. Removal and addition of various molecules during plasma adsorption over *S. aureus* Cowan I and their possible reactions.

5. The large complexes may behave like an IgM molecule and may be responsible for immune lysis of the tumor. Necrotic reactions have been observed by us and others in the tumor biopsies of plasma-absorbed hosts.

6. Enterotoxin entering into the system may be responsible for the induction of the fever, chills, and blood pressure changes (Biesel, 1972; Hodoval *et al.*, 1968) observed in plasma-adsorbed patients. Enterotoxin may activate lymphocytes (Langford *et al.*, 1978; Peavy *et al.*, 1970) and induce interferon (Smith *et al.*, 1983). Complement activation and direct lesion formation of tumor cells may also be effected by enterotoxins, leading to increased permeability and facilitated lysis of the tumor cells. The increased susceptibility of chemotherapeutic drugs of plasma-adsorbed patients had earlier been reported by us (Ray *et al.*, 1981*a,d-f*). This was perhaps due to the increased permeability of chemotherapeutic drugs into the tumors of these patients.

In our study, we have observed a number of staphylococcal agents being leached during the plasma absorption process with *S. aureus* (Bandyopadhyay and Ray, 1985). These molecules, apart from protein A and enterotoxin, may also serve as nonspecific immunomodulators in the plasma-adsorbed hosts, tak-

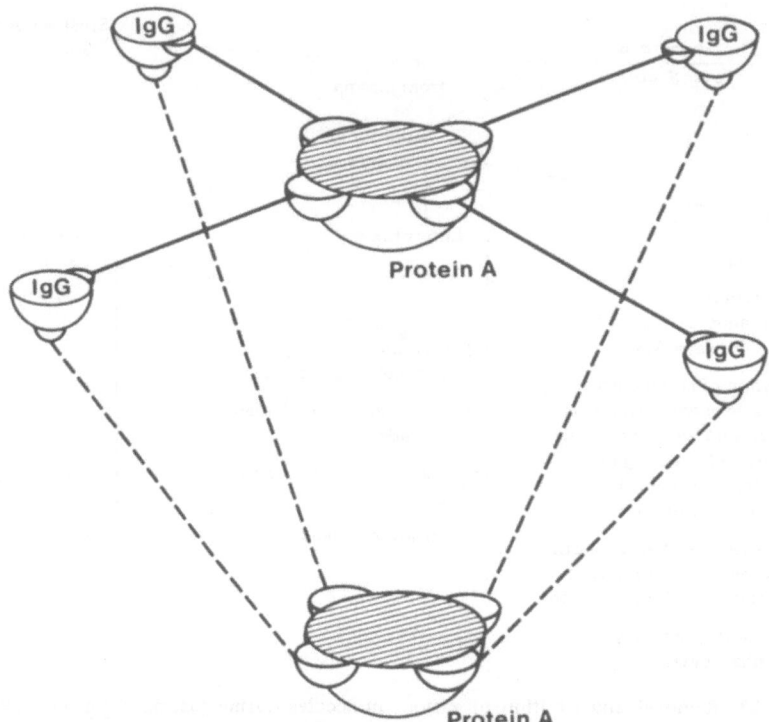

Figure 13. Hypothetical structure of IgG–protein A complex under IgG conditions of excess. Note that this $(IgG)_4$–$(Protein A)_2$ is a stable high-molecular-weight (19 S) complex. A number of relatively lower-molecular-weight complexes should also be formed because of interactions among IgG, CIC, and protein A.

ing part particularly in the activation of macrophages, which may kill the tumor cells.

Interestingly, this proposed mechanism fits in quite well to explain the mechanism of tumor regression observed in dogs (Gordon *et al.*, 1983) and rats (Ray *et al.*, 1984*b*) following plasma adsorption over *S. aureus* Wood 46, and also in rats following direct infusion of protein A (Ray, 1982; Ray and Bandyopadhyay, 1983; Ray *et al.*, 1984*c*). In the case of plasma adsorption with *S. aureus* Wood 46, enterotoxin and other staphylococcal agents may play an active role, in the manner described above, in causing tumor regression. However, in the case of direct infusion of protein A, the reaction described above for both protein A and enterotoxin (which enters as a contaminant of protein A) may result in tumor destruction.

It is significant to note, however, that the *in vivo* reactions owing to the dynamic imbalance in the equilibrium of CIC as a result of direct adsorption with *S. aureus* may also induce reactions contributing to the tumor-regressive phenomena (Fig. 12).

At this point it is not clear what role each of the components described in Fig. 12 plays in the observed tumor-regressive phenomena following plasma adsorption over *S. aureus* or *S. aureus* Wood 46, or direct infusion of protein A. Until purified molecules of protein A and enterotoxin are obtained, understanding of the exact mechanism of tumor regression may not be possible. However, in view of our results (Ray, 1982; Ray and Bandyopadhyay, 1983; Ray *et al.*, 1984*c*) demonstrating tumor regression by direct infusion of protein A in rats carrying mammary adenocarcinomas, it appears that the complex plasma perfusion procedure with *S. aureus*, *S. aureus* Wood 46, or other immobilized protein A columns may be irrelevant. Our observations showing that inoculation with a solution of protein A can provide the same tumor-regressive response strongly negate the use of the complex plasma adsorption procedures. Furthermore, our results with rat tumors should provide a model to dissect the mechanism of protein A effects in tumor destruction.

XV. SUMMARY

In tumor-bearing hosts both cellular and humoral tumor-growth-enhancing factors are present. They cause immunosuppression and facilitate the growth of tumors. Very early during tumor growth these factors are either elicited by the tumor cells or induced by the host immunocytes. Among these immunosuppressive agents, circulating immune complexes appear to play a predominant role. They also activate suppressor cell activity. Plasma adsorption of CIC and IgG by protein A of *Staphylococcus aureus* has been reported to cause tumor regression. Plasma adsorption with protein A–collodion charcoal, protein A–silica, or protein A–Sepharose also induced tumorilytic reactions. Even direct infusion of protein A induced tumor regressions in rat mammary tumors. Recent studies showing tumor regressions following *S. aureus* Wood 46 plasma adsorption or infusion of normal plasma adsorbed over *S. aureus* indicate that specific blocking factor removal by plasma adsorption may not be the mechanism for causing tumor destruction. Results indicate that *S. aureus* plasma adsorption leaches a number of staphylococcal agents. Thus, it appears that staphylococcal agents, protein A, enterotoxin, and other factors are responsible for the induction of reactions leading to tumor destruction. A unified mechanism explaining the results obtained with plasma adsorption using protein A of *S. aureus*, or *S. aureus* Wood, or direct protein A infusion, was presented.

ACKNOWLEDGMENTS

The author gratefully acknowledges financial assistance from R. J. Reynolds Industries, Inc., the W. W. Smith Charitable Trust, and the Fannie E. Rippel

Foundation for carrying out various investigations in our laboratory, some of which were described here. The author would like to thank Mrs. Monica Dent for her unfailing support in typing this manuscript. Thanks are also due to many of my co-workers, whose valuable contributions have expanded our knowledge in this area of research, and to all the referring physicians, for allowing us to study the effect of the plasma adsorption procedure in their patients. I would in addition like to record my thanks to those patients' families, whose courageous attitude made this work possible. Finally, thanks are due to Drs. Donald R. Cooper and James G. Bassett for their continued encouragement and sincere support during the course of this investigation.

XVI. REFERENCES

Agnello, V., 1981, Immune complex assays: The first 10 years, *Ann. Intern. Med.* **94**:266.

Albo, V., Krivit, W., and Hartman, J., 1978, Fresh plasma as adjuvant to the chemotherapy of acute lymphatic leukemia in children, *Proc. Am. Assoc. Cancer Res.* **9**:104.

Alexander, P., 1974, Escape from immune destruction by the host through shedding of surface antigens: Is this a characteristic shared by malignant and embryonic cells? *Cancer Res.* **34**:2077.

Amlot, P. L., Pussel, B., Slaney, J. M., and Williams, B. D., 1978, Correlation between immune complexes and prognostic factors in Hodgkin's disease, *Clin. Exp. Immunol.* **31**:166.

Anderson, R. J., McBridge, C. M., and Hersch, E. M., 1972, Lympocyte blastogenic responses to cultured allogeneic tumor cells *in vitro*, *Cancer Res.* **32**:988.

Andrews, S., Congdon, G. A., and Edwards, C. C., 1967, Preliminary trials of clinical immunotherapy, *Cancer Res.* **27**:2535.

Attlic, M. A. M., and Weiss, D. W., 1966, Immunology of spontaneous mammary carcinomas in mice. V. Acquired tumor resistance and enhancement in strain A mice infected with mammary tumor virus, *Cancer Res.* **26**:1787.

Baird, L. G., and Kaplan, A. M., 1977a, Macrophage regulation of mitogen-induced blastogenesis. I. Demonstration of inhibitor cells in the spleens and peritoneal exudate of mice, *Cell. Immunol.* **28**:22.

Baird, L. G., and Kaplan, A. M., 1977b, Macrophage regulation of mitogen-induced blastogenesis. II. Mechanism of inhibitor cell, *Cell. Immunol.* **28**:36.

Baker, M. A., Falk, J. A., and Taub, R. M., 1978, Immunotherapy of human acute leukemia: Antibody response to leukemia associated antigens, *Blood* **52**:469.

Baldwin, R. W., Price, M. R., Robins, R. A., 1972, Blocking lymphocyte-mediated cytotoxicity for rap hepatoma cells by tumor specific antigen–antibody complexes, *Nature* **238**:185.

Baldwin, R. W., Embleton, M. J., Price, M. R., and Robins, R. A., 1974, Immunity in the tumor-bearing host and its modification by serum factor, *Cancer* **34**:1452.

Bandyopadhyay, S. K., and Ray, P. K., 1985, Introduction of bacterial components in post-adsorbed plasma during adsorption with *Staphylococcus aureus*, *Cancer* (in press).

Bansal, S. C., and Sjögren, H. O., 1971, Unblocking serum activity *in vitro* in polyoma system may correlate with antitumor effects of antiserum *in vivo*, *Nature* **233**:76.

Bansal, S. C., and Sjögren, H. O., 1973a. Effects of BCG on various facets of the immune response against polyoma tumors in rats, *Int. J. Cancer* **11**:116.

Bansal, S. C., and Sjögren, 1973b, Regression of polyoma tumors, tumor metastasis by combined unblocking and BCG treatment: Correlation with induced alterations in tumor immunity status, *Int. J. Cancer* 12:179.

Bansal, S. C., and Sjögren, H. O., 1974, Antitumor immune response and its manipulation in a tumor-bearing host, *Isr. J. Med. Sci.* 10:939.

Bansal, S. C., Hargraves, R., and Sjögren, H. O., 1972, Facilitation of polyoma tumor growth in rat by blocking sera and tumor eluates, *Int. J. Cancer* 9:97.

Bansal, S. C., Bansal, B. R., Thomas, J. L., Siegel, P. D., Rhoads, J. E., Jr., Cooper, D. R., Terman, D. S., and Mark, R., 1978, *Ex vivo* removal of serum IgG in a patient with colon carcinoma, *Cancer* 42:1.

Beisel, W. R., 1972, Pathophysiology of Staphylococcal enterotoxin, Type B (SEB) toxemia after intravenous administration to monkeys, *Toxicon* 10:433.

Benjamin, E., Theilen, G. H., Torten, M., Fong, S., Crow, S., and Hennes, A. M., 1978, Specific active immunotherapy (tumor vaccines) for cancer: Tumor vaccines for immunotherapy of canine lymphosarcoma, *Ann. N.Y. Acad. Sci.* 277:305.

Bennett, A., DelTacca, M., Stamford, I. F., and Zebro, T., 1977, Prostaglandins from tumors of human large bowel, *Br. J. Cancer* 35:881.

Bennett, A., Houghton, J. K., Lepar, D. J., and Standord, I. F., 1979, Cancer growth response to treatment and survivial time in mice: Beneficial effect of the prostaglandin synthesis inhibitor Flurbiprofen, *Prostaglandins* 17:179.

Bensinger, W. I., Kinet, J. P., Hennen, G., Frankenne, F., Schaus, C., Saint-Remy, M., Hoyoux, P., and Mahien, P., 1982, Plasma perfused over immobilized protein A for breast cancer, *N. Engl. J. Med.* 306:935.

Berendt, M. J., and North, R. J., 1980, T cell-mediated suppression of anti-tumor immunity: An explanation for progressive growth of an immunogenic tumor, *J. Exp. Med.* 151:69.

Billing, R., Minowad, J., Cline, M., Clark, B., and Lee, K., 1978, Acute lymphocyte leukemia-associated cell membrane antigen, *J. Natl. Cancer Inst.* 61:423.

Blasecki, J. W., and Tevethia, S. S., 1976, *In vitro* studies on the cellular immune response of tumor-bearing mice to SV-40 transformed cells, *J. Immunol.* 114:244.

Bleme, R. W., 1977, Circulating immune complexes in patients with breast cancer, *Br. Med. J.* 2:218.

Boder, S., 1978, Suppressor cells in the humoral immunodeficiency of multiple myeloma, *Ann. Intern. Med.* 88:226.

Bonnard, E. D., and Herberman, R. B., 1975, Suppression of lymphocyte proliferative responses by murine lymphoma cells, in: *Immune Recognition* (A. Rosenthal, ed.), p. 819, Academic Press, New York.

Borer, T., and Kallis, N., 1959, The effect of isoantibodies *in vivo* on three different transplantable neoplasms in mice, *Cancer Res.* 19:824.

Bottino, J. C., Rosen, R. D., Hirsh, E. M., Foster, J. B., and McBride, C. H., 1978, Response of malignant melanoma to plasma exchange surgical debulking and *Corynebacterium parvum*, *Int. J. Artif. Organs* 1:53.

Boyse, E. A., Old, L. F., and Stockert, E., 1962, Immunologic enhancement of a leukemia, *Nature* 194:114.

Brandeis, W. E., Hellson, L., Wang, Y., Good, R. A., and Day, N. K., 1978, Circulating immune complexes in sera of children with neuroblastoma: Correlation with stage of the disease, *J. Clin Invest.* 62:1201.

Brandeis, W. E., Tan, C., Wang, Y., Good, A., and Day, N. K., 1980, Circulating immune complexes, complement and complement component levels in childhood Hodgkin's disease, *Clin. Exp. Immunol.* 39:551.

Broder, S., Poplack, D., Whang-Peng, J., Durm, M., Goldman, C., Muul, L., and Waldmann, T. A., 1978, Characterization of a suppressor-cell leukemia: Evidence for the requirement of an interaction of two T cells in the development of human suppressor effector cells, *N. Engl. J. Med.* 298:66.

Brooks, W. H., Netsky, M. G., Normansell, D. E., and Horwitz, D. A., 1972, Depressed cell-mediated immunity in patients with primary international tumors: Characterization of a humoral suppressive factor, *J. Exp. Med.* **136**:1631.

Brunda, M. J., Herberman, R. B., and Holden, H. T., 1980, Inhibition of murine natural killer activity by prostaglandins, *J. Immunol.* **124**:2682.

Cantor, H., and Boyce, E., 1977, Regulation of the immune reponse by T cell subclasses, *Contemp. Top. Microbiol.* **7**:47.

Carnaud, C., Markowicz, O., and Trainin, N., 1974, The influence of a graft-versus-host reaction on the incidence of metastases after tumor transplantation, *Cell Immunol.* **14**:87.

Carpentier, N. A., and Miescher, A., 1983, The clinical relevance of circulating immune complexes in cancer, kidney transplantation and pregnancy, in: *Immunobiology of Transplantation, Cancer and Pregnancy* (P. K. Ray, ed.), p. 375, Pergamon Press, New York.

Carpentier, N. A., Docquier, C. E., Pugin, P., Lambert, P. H., and Miescher, A., 1978, Incidence et specificité des complexes immune circulants dans la mononucleose infectieuse, *Schweiz. Med. Wochenschr.* **108**:1601.

Chard, T., 1978, Immunological enhancement by mouse isoantibodies: The importance of complement fixation, *Immunology* **14**:383.

Chard, T., French, M. E., and Batchelor, J. R., 1967, Enhancement of the C57 BL leukemia EL4 by fragments of isoantibodies, *Transplantation* **5**:1266.

Chard, T., Kallis, N., Sinclair, N. R., and Cantrell, J. L., 1976, Immunologic enhancement of a murine tumor allograft by passive alloantibody IgG and F(ab), *Eur. J. Immunol.* **6**:38.

Cohen, R. R., 1973, The recruitment of specific effector lymphocytes by antigen-reactive lymphocytes in cell-mediated autosensitization and allosensitization reactions, *Cell. Immunol.* **8**:209.

Cohen, R. R., and Feldman, M., 1976, Suppressor factor secreted by T-lymphocytes from tumor-bearing mice, *J. Natl. Cancer Inst.* **57**:409.

Cohen, R. R., Crolberson, A., and Feldman, M., 1971, Lymphoid cells sensitized *in vitro* against allogeneic or syngeneic fibroblasts produce immune effects *in vitro* and *in vivo*, *Transplant. Proc.* **3**:891.

Coley, W. B., 1891, Contribution to the knowledge of sarcoma, *Ann. Surg.* **14**:199.

Coley, W. B., 1893, Treatment of malignant tumors by repeated inoculations of erysipelas with a report of 10 cases, *Med. Res.* **43**:60.

Cooper, P. D., and Masinello, G. R., 1983, Protein A treatment of cancer: Activation of a serum component with trans-species anti-B-16 melanoma activity, *Int. J. Cancer* **32**:737.

Costanza, M. E., Pinn, V., Schwartz, R., and Nathanson, L., 1973, Cardioembryonic antigen-antibody complexes in a patient with colonic carcinoma and nephrotic syndrome, *N. Engl. J. Med.* **289**:520.

Couser, W. B., Wagenfeld, J. B., Spargo, B. H., and Lewis, E. J., 1974, Glomerular disposition of tumor antigen in membranous nephropathy associated with colonic carcinoma, *Ann. J. Med.* **57**:962.

Cowan, F. M., Klein, D. L., Armstrong, G. R., and Pearson, J. W., 1979, Neutralization of immune complex inhibition of antibody-independent cellular cytotoxicity *in vitro* by *Staphylococcus aureus* protein A, *Biomedicine* **30**:23.

Currie, G. A., and Basham, C., 1972, Serum mediated inhibition of the immunological reactions of the patient to his own tumor: A possible role for circulating antigen, *Br. J. Cancer* **26**:427.

Currie, G. A., and McElwain, T. J., 1975, Active immunotherapy as an adjunct to chemotherapy in the treatment of disseminated malignant melanoma: A pilot study, *Br. J. Cancer* **31**:143.

Day, N. K., Winfield, J. G., Gee, T., Tashima, H., and Gunkle, H. G., 1976, Evidence for immune complexes involving antilymphocyte antibodies associated with hypocomplementemia in chronic lymphocytic leukemia, *Clin. Exp. Immunol.* **26:**198.

Day, N. K., Tyler, R., Engelman, R., Harr, K., Glaser, R., Wang, C. Y., Yamamoto, J., Machida, K., Nabkas, F., Tran, X., and Good, R., 1983, Immunologic and bone marrow changes associated with remission of leukemia in cats following treatment with AMF protein A filter, *Fed. Proc.* **42:**5283.

Dent, P. B., Louis, J. A., McCullock, P. B., Dunnett, C. W., and Cerottini, J. C., 1980, Correlation of elevated C1q binding activity and carcinoembryonic antigen levels with clinical features and prognosis in bronchogenic carcinoma, *Cancer* **45:**130.

Deorger, T., 1942, The role of antibodies in immunity to transplanted leukemia in mice, *J. Pathol.* **54:**41.

Diener, M., and Feldman, C., 1972, Relationship between antigen and antibody induced suppression of immunity, *Transplant. Rev.* **8:**76.

Dore, J. G., Hadjlyannakis, M. J., and Goudert, A., 1973, Use of antigenic treated cells in immunotherapy of leukemia, *Lancet* **1:**600.

Drebin, J. A., Waltenbaugh, C., Schatten, S., Benaceraff, B., and Greene, M. I., 1983, Inhibition of tumor growth by monoclonal anti-I-J antibodies, *J. Immunol.* **130:**506.

Eggers, A. E., and Wunderlich, K. R., 1975, Suppressor cells in tumor-bearing mice capable of nonspecific blocking of immunization against transplant antigen, *J. Immunol.* **114:**1554.

Faltt, R., and Ankerest, J., 1980, Possibly specific immune complexes in the sera of patients with untreated acute myelogenous leukemia, *Int. J. Cancer* **26:**309.

Fass, L., 1970, Patients with Burkitt's lymphoma: Evaluation of the effect of remission plasma on untreated host, *J. Natl. Cancer Inst.* **44:**145.

Finegold, M. J., 1967, Interstitial pulmonary edema—An electron microscopic study of the pathology of the Staphylococcal exterotoxemia in rhesus monekys, *Lab. Invest.* **16:**912.

Frank, S. J., Specter, S., Nowotny, A., and Friedman, H., 1979, Effect of immune sera upon enhanced *in vitro* antibody responses, in: *Macrophages and Lymphocytes: Nature, Functions, and Interaction* (M. R. Escobar and H. Friedman, eds.), Advances in Experimental Medicine and Biology, Volume 121A, p. 261, Plenum Press, New York.

Froese, G., Berczi, I., and Sehon, A. H., 1974, Neuraminidase induced enhancement of tumor growth in mice, *J. Natl. Cancer Inst.* **52:**1905.

Fujimoto, S., Greene, M. I., and Sehon, A. H., 1976, The nature of immunosuppressor cells in tumor-bearing hosts, *J. Immunol.* **116:**800.

Fulton, A. M., and Levy, J. G., 1980, Inhibition of murine tumor growth and prostaglandin synthesis by indomethacin, *Int. J. Cancer* **26:**669.

Garrett, T. J., Takahashi, T., Clarkson, B. D., and Old, L. J., 1977, Detection of antibody to autologous human leukemia cells by immune adherence assays, *Proc. Natl. Acad. Sci. USA* **74:**4587.

Gelsner, M., Kirchner, H., Holden, H. T., and Herberman, R. B., 1976, Inhibition of cellmediated cytotoxicity against tumor associated antigens by suppressor cells from tumorbearing mice, *J. Natl. Cancer Inst.* **56:**865.

Gershon, R. K., Birnbaum-Mokyr, M., and Mitchell, M. S., 1974, Activation of suppressor T cells by tumor cells and specific antibody, *Nature* **250:**594.

Gifford, R. R., Boss, B. V., and Ferguson, R. M., 1981, Cimetidine protection against lethal tumor challenge in mice, *Surgery* **90:**344.

Glaser, M., 1980, Indomethacin sensitive suppressor cells regulate the cell mediated cytotoxic response to SV 40 induced tumor associated antigens in mice, *Eur. J. Immunol.* **10:**489.

Glaser, M., Kirchner, H., Holden, J., and Herberman, R. B., 1976, Cytotoxicity against tumor-associated antigens by suppressor cells from tumor-bearing mice, *J. Natl. Cancer Inst.* 56:865.

Glasgow. A. H.. Nimberg, R. B., Menzoian, J. O., Inna Saporoshetz, B. A., Cooperband, S. R., Schmid, K., and Mannick, J. A., 1974, Association of anergy with an immunosuppressive peptide fraction in the serum of patients with cancer, *N. Engl. J. Med.* 291:1263.

Goodwin, J. S., and Cauppens, J., 1983, Regulation of the immune response by prostaglandins, *J. Clin. Immunol.* 3:295.

Goodwin, J. S., Messner, R. P., Bankhurst, A. D., Peake, G., Sasiki, J. H., and Williams, R. C., Jr., 1977, Prostaglandin in suppressor cells in Hodgkin's disease, *N. Engl. J. Med.* 297:963.

Gorczynski, R., 1974, Immunity to murine sarcoma virus-induced tumors. II. Suppression of T cell-mediated immunity by cells from progressor animals, *J. Immunol.* 112:1826.

Gordon, B. R., Matus, R. E., Saal, S. D., MacEwen, G. E., Hurvitz, A. I., Stenzel, K. H., and Rubin, A. L., 1983, Protein A-independent tumoricidal responses in dogs after extracorporeal perfusion of plasma over *Staphylococcus aureus*, *J. Natl. Cancer Inst.* 70:1127.

Greene, M. I., Fuzimoto, S., and Shahan, H., 1977, Regulation of the immune response to tumor antigens. III. Characterization of immunosuppressor factor produced by tumor-bearing hosts, *J. Immunol.* 119:757.

Greenwich, K. D., and Plescia, O. J., 1977, Tumor mediated immunosuppression: Prevention by inhibitors of prostaglandin synthesis, *Prostaglandins* 14:1175.

Gupta, R. K., and Morton, D. L., 1983, Tumor antigens, in: *Immunobiology of Transplantation, Cancer and Pregnancy* (P. K. Ray, ed.), p. 113, Pergamon Press, New York.

Hamblin, T. J., 1979, Plasmapheresis and plasma exchange, *Res. Rev.* 1:1.

Heimer, R., and Kline, G., 1976, Circulating immune complexes in sera of patients with Burkitt's lymphoma and nasopharyngeal carcinoma, *Int. J. Cancer* 19:310.

Helin, H., Pasternack, A., Hakala, T., Penttinen, K., and Wager, O., 1980, Glomerular electron-dense deposits and circulating immune complexes in patients with malignant tumours, *Clin. Nephrol.* 14:23.

Hellström, I., and Hellström, K. E., 1969, Studies on cellular immunity and its serum mediated inhibition in Moloney virus induced mouse sarcoma, *Int. J. Cancer* 4:587.

Hellström, I., and Hellström, K. E., 1970, Colony inhibition studies on blocking and non-blocking serum effects on cellular immunity to Moloney sarcomas, *Int. J. Cancer* 4:195.

Hellström, I., Hellström, K. E., and Sjögren, H. O., 1970, Serum mediated inhibition of cellular immunity to methylcholanthrene induced murine sarcoma, *Cell. Immunol.* 1:18.

Hellström, I., Hellström, K. E. Sjögren, H. O., and Warner, G. A., 1971, Serum factors in tumor-free patients cancelling the blocking of cell mediated tumor immunity, *Int. J. Cancer* 7:1.

Hellström, I., Hellström, K. E., Warner, G. A., and Sjögren, H., 1973, Sequential studies on cell mediated immunity and blocking serum activity in 10 patients with malignant myeloma, *Int. J. Cancer* 11:280.

Hellström, K. E., 1975, The role of blocking serum factors in immunity to embryonic tumor antigens, in: *Critical Factors in Cancer Immunology* (J. Schultz and R. C. Leif, eds.), p. 211, Academic Press, New York.

Hellström, K. E., and Hellström, I., 1979, Enhancement of tumor outgrowth by tumor associated blocking factor, *Int. J. Cancer* 23:366.

Hellström, K. E., Hellström, I., and Nepom, P., 1977, Specific blocking factors—Are they important? *Biochem. Biophys. Acta* 473:121.

Herberman, R. B., 1974, Cell mediated immunity to tumor cells, *Adv. Cancer Res.* 19:207.

Herberman, R. B., 1977, Mechanism of tumor immunity, in: *Immunotherapy of Cancer* (I. Green, S. Cohen, and R. T. McClosky, eds.), p. 175, Wiley, New York.

Hershey, T., Edward, A., Adam, E., Isbister, W. H., Murray, A., and Biggs, J., 1976, Antibody dependent cell mediated cytotoxicity against myeloma cells induced by plasmapheresis, *Lancet* 1:825.

Hewitt, H. B., 1978, The choice of animal tumors for experimental studies of cancer therapy, *Adv. Cancer Res.* 27:149.

Hewitt, H. B., Blake, E. R., and Walder, A. S., 1976, A critique of the evidence for active host defence against cancer based on personal studies of 27 murine tumors of spontaneous origin, *Br. J. Cancer* 33:241.

Hial, B., Horokova, A., Shaff, R. E., and Beven, M. A., 1976, Alteration of tumor growth by aspirin and indomethacin: Studies with 2 transplantable tumors in mice, *Can. J. Pharmacol.* 37:367.

Hodes, R. J., Nadler, L. M., and Hathcock, S., 1977, Regulatory mechanisms in cell mediated immune response. III. Antigen specific and nonspecific suppressor activities generated during MLC, *J. Immunol.* 119:961.

Hodoval, L. F., Morris, E. L., Crawley, G. J., and Beisel, W. R., 1968, Pathogenesis of lethal shock after intravenous Staphylococcal enterotoxin B in monkeys, *Appl. Microbiol.* 19:187.

Hollander, N., Isakov, N., Segal, S., and Feldman, M., 1978, Immunoregulatory factor associated with spleen cells from tumor-bearing animals. II. Characterization of the cell population involved in its production and release, *Int. J. Cancer* 22:471.

Holohan, T. V., Phillips, T. M., Bowles, C., and Deisseroth, A., 1982, Regression of canine mammary carcinoma after immunoadsorption therapy, *Cancer Res.* 42:3663.

Hubert, R. A., Aggio, M. C., Lozzio, B. B., and Wust, C. J., 1981, Relation of circulating immune complexes and disease status in patients with leukemia, *Clin. Exp. Immunol.* 43:46.

Hutchin, P., Amos, D. B., and Prioleau, W. H., Jr., 1967, Interaction of humoral antibody and immune lymphocytes, *Transplantation* 4:68.

Isakov, N., Segal, S., Hollander, N., and Feldman, M., 1978, Immunoregulatory factor associated with spleen cells from tumor-bearing animals. I. Effect on tumor growth and antibody production, *Int. J. Cancer* 22:465.

Isakov, N., Hollander, N., Segal, S., and Feldman, M., 1979, Immunoregulatory factor associated with spleen cells from tumor-bearing animals. III. Characterization of the factor's target cell, *Int. J. Cancer* 23:410.

Isbister. W. H., Noona, F. P., Halliday, W. J., and Clunie, G., 1975, Human thoracic duct cannulation: Manipulation of tumor-specific blocking factors in a patient with malignant melanoma, *Cancer* 35:145.

Israel, L., Edelstein, R., Mannoni, P., Rodot, E., and Greenspan, E. M., 1977, Plasmapheresis in patients with disseminated cancer: Clinical results and correlations with changes in serum protein. The concept of nonspecific blocking factors, *Cancer* 40:3146.

Jones, F. R., Yoshida, L. H., Ladiges, W. C., and Kennedy, M. A., 1980, Treatment of feline leukemia and reversal of FeLV by *ex vivo* removal of IgG: A preliminary report, *Cancer* 46:675.

Jose, D. G., and Sashadri, R., 1974, Circulating immune complexes in human urogastroma: Direct assay and role in blocking specific cellular immunity, *Int. J. Cancer* 13:824.

Kamo, I., and Freidman, H., 1977, Immunosuppression and the role of suppressive factors in cancer, *Adv. Cancer Res.* 25:271.

Kerbal, R. S., and Pears, A. J. S., 1974, The possible biological significance of Fc receptors on mammalian lymphocytes and tumor cells, *Cell* 3:105.

Kilburn, D. G., Smith, J. B., and Gorczynsky, R. M., 1974, Nonspecific suppression of T lymphocyte responses in mice carrying progressively-growing tumors, *Eur. J. Immunol.* 4:784.

Kiley, J. M., Wagoner, R. G., and Holley, K. E., 1969, Renal complications of lymphoma, *Ann. Intern. Med.* 71:1159.

Kirchner, H., Chused, T. M., and Herberman, R. B., 1974, Evidence of suppressor cell activity in spleens of mice bearing primary tumors induced by Moloney sarcoma virus, *J. Exp. Med.* 139:1473.

Klein, E., 1977, Tumor immunology escape mechanism, *Ann. Inst. Pasteur* 122:593.

Klimpal, G. R., 1980, A soluble factor for BCG induced suppressor cells inhibits *in vitro* PFC responses but not cytotoxic response, *Cell. Immunol.* 47:218.

Klimpal, G. R., Idada, M., and Henney, C. S., 1979, Inhibition of *in vitro* cytotoxic responses by BCG induced macrophage-like suppressor cells. II. Suppression occurs at the level of a "helper" T cell, *J. Immunol.* 123:350.

Kline, B. C., and Raisz, L. G., 1970, Prostaglandins: Stimulation of bone resorption in tissue culture, *Endocrinology* 86:1436.

Kumar, V., and Bennett, M., 1977, H-2 compatibility requirements for T-suppressor cell functions induced by Friend leukaemia virus, *Nature* 265:345.

Kuperman, O., Fortner, G. W., and Lucas, Z. J., 1975, Immune response to a syngeneic mammary adenocarcinoma. III. Development of memory and suppressor functions modulating cellular cytotoxicity, *J. Immunol.* 115:1282.

Langford, M. P., Stanton, G. J., and Johnson, H. M., 1978, Biological effects of Staphylococcal enterotoxin A on human peripheral lymphocytes, *Infect. Immun.* 22:62.

Langone, J. J., Boyle, M. D. P., and Borsos, T., 1978, Studies on the intersection between protein A and immunoglobulin G. II. Composition and activity of complexes formed between protein A and IgG, *J. Immunol.* 121:333.

Langvade, E., Hyden, H., Wolf, H., and Kroeigard, N., 1975, Extracorporeal immunoadsorption of circulating specific serum factors in cancer patients, *Br. J. Cancer* 32:680.

Lee, J. C., Yamachui, H., and Hopper, S., Jr., 1963, The association of cancer and the nephrotic syndrome, *Ann Int. Med.* 64:41.

Linder, E., 1981, Binding of C1q and complement activation by vascular endothelium, *J. Immunol.* 126:648.

Lockwood, C. M., Worlledge, S., Nicholas, A., Cotton, C., and Peters, D. K., 1979, Reversal of impaired splenic function in patients with nephritis or vasculitis (or both) by plasma exchange, *N. Engl. J. Med.* 300:524.

Long, K. C., Hall, C. L., Brown, C. A., Stamatos, C., Weitzman, S. A., and Carey, E. K., 1977, Binding of soluble immune complexes in serum of patients with Hodgkin's disease to tissue cultures derived from the tumor, *N. Engl. J. Med.* 297:295.

Lynch, N. R., Casatel, M., Estonim, M., and Solmen, J. C., 1978, Mechanism of inhibition of tumor growth by aspirin and indomethacin, *Br. J. Cancer* 38:305.

McCredie, J. A., Brown, E. R., and Cole, W. H., 1959, Immunological treatment of tumors, *Proc. Soc. Exp. Biol. Med.* 100:31.

McKenzie, P. E., Taylor, A. E., Woodruff, A. J., Seymour, A. E., Chang, Y. L., and Clarkson, A. L., 1979, Plasmapheresis in glomerular nephritis, *Clin. Nephrol.* 12:97.

MacKintosh, F. R., Bennett, K., Schiff, S., Shield, J., and Hall, S. W., 1983, Treatment of advanced malignancy with plasma perfused over Staphylococcal protein A, *West. J. Med.* 139:36.

Martin, D., Achard, A., Todd, D. E., Tribole, T., Lewis, J. A., and Zander, E., 1980, Immune complexes associated with brain tumors: Correlation with prognosis, *Surg. Neurol.* 13:161.

Martin, F., and Martin, S. M., 1970, Demonstration of antigens related to colonic cancer in human digestive system, *Int. J. Cancer* 6:362.

Mathe, G., Hale-Pannenko, O., and Bourut, C., 1973, Active immunotherapy in spontaneous leukemia of AKR mice, *Exp. Hematol.* 1:110.

Messerschmidt, G., Bowles, C., Alsaker, R., McCormick, K., and Deiseroth, A., 1982, Toxic, immunologic and pathologic changes in dogs with spontaneous neoplasia treated with i.v. infusions of purified staph protein A (spA), *Fed. Proc.* **41**:325.

Mills, C. C., North, R. J., and Dye, E. S., 1981, Mechanism of antitumor action of *Corynebacterium parvum*. II. Potentiated cytolytic T cell response and its tumor-induced suppression, *J. Exp. Med.* **154**:621.

Mizushima, Y., Sendo, F., Takeichi, N., Hosohawa, M., and Kobayashi, H., 1981, Enhancement of anti-tumor transplantation resistance in rats by appropriately timed administration of Busulfan, *Cancer Res.* **41**:2917.

Möller, E., and Möller, G., 1962, Quantitative studies of the sensitivity of normal and neoplastic mouse cells to the cytotoxic action of isoantibodies, *J. Exp. Med.* **115**:527.

Möller, G., 1963, Studies on the mechanism of immunological enhancement of tumor homografts. II. Effect of isoantibodies on various tumor cells. *J. Natl. Cancer Inst.* **30**:1177.

Möller, G., 1964, Effect on tumor growth in syngeneic recipients of antibodies against tumor specific antigens in methylcholanthrene induced mouse sarcomas, *Nature* **204**:846.

Montovanni, A., and Sorafico, F., 1975, On the nature of blocking factors and their lymphoid target cells in an alogeneic tumor system, *Eur. J. Cancer* **11**:451.

Moore, A. E., and Gerner, R. E., 1970, Cancer immunity hypothesis and clinical trial of lymphocyte therapy for malignant diseases, *Ann. Surg.* **172**:733.

Moore, G., Scandberg, A., and Amos, D. B., 1957, Experimental and clinical adventures with large doses of gamma and other globulins as anticancer agents, *Surgery* **41**:972.

Noar, D., 1979, Suppressor cells: Parameters and promoters of malignancy, *Adv. Cancer Res.* **29**:45.

Nata, R., and Slavin, S. B., 1979, Endurance in the induction of suppressor cells, *Infect. Immun.* **23**:360.

Nelson, D. S., 1973, Production of stimulated macrophages of factors depressing lymphocyte transformation, *Nature* **246**:306.

Nimberg, R. B., Glasgow, J. H., Menzoian, J. O., Constantine, M. B., Cooperband, S. R., Mannick, J. A., and Schmid, K., 1975, Isolation of a γ immunosupressive type fraction from the serum of cancer patients, *Cancer Res.* **35**:1489.

Noonan, P. F., Gasdrin, M. A. H., Clunie, G. J., Isbister, W. H., and Halliday, W. J., 1974, Control of tumor growth in mice by thoracic duct drainage: Relationship to blocking factor in lymph, *Int. J. Cancer* **13**:640.

Oehler, J. R., Herberman, R. B., Campbell, D. A. J., and Jeu, J. Y., 1977, Inhibition of rat mixed lymphocyte cultures by suppressor macrophages, *Cell. Immunol.* **29**:238.

Old, L. J., and Boyse, E. A., 1964, Immunology of experimental tumors, *Annu. Rev. Med.* **15**:167.

Old, L. J., and Stockert, E., 1977, Immunogenetics of cell surface antigens of mouse leukemia, *Annu. Rev. Genet.* **11**:1.

Oldston, M. B., and Tishow, A., 1977, Active thymus derived lymphocytes in human cord blood, *Nature* **269**:333.

Oldston, M. B., Theofilopoulus, A. N., Kline, G., and Guvin, T., 1975, Immune complexes associated with neoplasia: Presence of Epstein-Barr virus antigen–antibody complexes in Burkitt's lymphoma, *Intervirology* **4**:292.

Opitz, H. G., Niethammer, D., Jackson, R. D., Lemke, H., Huget, R., and Glad, H. G., 1975*a*, Biochemical characterization of a factor released by macrophages, *Cell. Immunol.* **18**:70.

Optiz, H. G., Niethammer, D., Lemke, H., Glad, H. D., and Huget, R., 1975*b*, Inhibition of tritiated thymidine incorporation of lymphocytes by a soluble factor from macrophages, *Cell. Immunol.* **16**:379.

Padrathsingh, M. L., Dean, J. H., and Jarrell, T. R., 1979, Evidence for and characterization of suppressor cells in Balb/C mice bearing ADJ/TC 5 plasmacytoma, *J. Natl. Cancer Inst.* 61:1235.

Pascal, R. R., Ianaconne, P. N., Rollwagen, F. M., Harding, T. A., and Bennett, S. J., 1976, Electron microscopy and immunofluorescence of glomerular immune complex deposits in cancer patients, *Cancer Res.* 36:43.

Peavy, D. L., Adler, W. H., and Smith, R. T., 1970, The mitogenic effects of endotoxin and Staphylococcal enterotoxin B on mouse spleen cells and human peripheral lymphocytes, *J. Immunol.* 105:1453.

Pelus, C., and Backman, R., 1979, Increased prostaglandin synthesis by macrophages from tumor-bearing mice, *J. Immunol.* 123:1979.

Perry, L. L., Benacerraf, B., and Greene, M. L., 1978, Regulation of the immune response to tumor antigens. IV. Tumor antigen specific suppressor factors: Their IJ determinants and induced suppressor T cells *in vivo*, *J. Immunol.* 121:2144.

Peter, J. J., Pavie-Fischer, D., Fridman, W. H., Aubert, C., Cesarini, J. P., Roubin, R., and Kourilsky, F., 1975, Cell mediated cytotoxicity *in vitro* of human lymphocytes against a tissue culture animal cell line (IG R3), *J. Immunol.* 115:539.

Philips, M., and Stetson, C., 1962, Basic transfer of immunity to sarcoma I with serum, *Proc. Soc. Exp. Biol. Med.* 111:265.

Pickett, S. H., Reichert, D. F., Lucio, R. M., and Lamm, D. L., 1983, *Staphylococcus* protein A immunotherapy of transitional cell carcinoma, *Fed. Proc.* 42:3197.

Pierce, G. E., 1971, Enhanced growth of primary Moloney virus induced sarcoma in mice, *Int. J. Cancer* 8:22.

Plescia, O. J., Smith, A. H., and Greenwich, K., 1975, Suppression of immune system by tumor cells and role of prostaglandins, *Proc. Natl. Acad. Sci.* 72:1848.

Pollard, M., and Luckert, H., 1981, Effect of indomethacin on intestinal tumors induced in rats by the acetate derivative of dimethyl nitrosamine, *Science* 214:558.

Pope, B. L., Witney, R. B., Levy, J. G., and Kilburn, D. G., 1976, Suppressor cells in the spleens of tumor-bearing mice: Enrichment by centrifugation on hypaque–Ficoll and characterization of the suppressor population, *J. Immunol.* 116:1342.

Poulton, T. A., Crowther, M. E., Hay, F. C., and Nineheim, M. J., 1978, Immune complexes in ovarian cancer, *Lancet* 2:72.

Poupon, M. F., Kolb, J. P., and Lespinats, G., 1976, Evidence of suppressor cells in C3H/HEJ T cell deprived and nude mice bearing a 3-methylcholanthrene induced fibrosarcoma, *J. Natl. Cancer Inst.* 57:1241.

Prehn, R. T., 1976, Tumor progression and homeostasis, *Adv. Cancer Res.* 23:203.

Proctor, J. W., Rudenstam, C. M., and Alexander, P., 1973, A factor preventing development of lung metastases in rats with sarcoma, *Nature* 242:29.

Purves, L., and Geddes, E., 1972, Proceedings, symposium on mycotoxin in human health, *Lancet* 1:47.

Ray, P. K., 1981, L'adsorption *ex vivo* d'immunoglobulines pathologiques ou de complexes immuns: Est-elle à preferer a l'échange de plasma? *Med. Hyg.* 39:1737.

Ray, P. K., 1982, Suppressor control as a modality of cancer treatment: perspectives and prospects in the immunotherapy of malignant disease, *Plasma Ther. Transfusion Technol.* 3:101.

Ray, P. K., 1983, Extracoproreal adsorption of pathologic gammaglobulins and immune complexes in various diseases including cancer, *Plasma Ther. Transfusion Technol.* 4:289.

Ray, P. K., and Bandyopadhyay, S., 1983, Inhibition of rat mammary tumor growth by purified protein A–A potential anti-tumor agent, *Immunol. Commun.* 12:453.

Ray, P. K., and Raychaudhuri, S., 1981, Low-dose cyclophosphamide inhibition of tumor growth by augmenting the immume response of the host, *J. Natl. Cancer Inst.* 67:1341.

Ray, P. K., and Raychaudhuri, S., 1983, Immunotherapy of cancer—Present status and future trends in: *Immunobiology of Transplantation, Cancer and Pregnancy* (P. K. Ray, ed.), p. 210, Pergamon Press, New York.

Ray, P. K., and Raychaudhuri, S., 1985, Increasing concentration of polyethylene glycol precipitable immune complexes during progressive tumor growth, *Eur. J. Cancer* (in press).

Ray, P. K., and Saha, S., 1982, Changes in elution profile of plasma proteins from mice with progressive methycholanthrene fibrosarcoma on Sephadex G-200 column, *Proc. Am. Assoc. Cancer Res.* 73:978.

Ray, P. K., and Saha, S., 1985a, Tumor antigen induced generation of humoral and cellular suppressor factors, *Ind. J. Exp. Biol.* (in press).

Ray, P. K., and Saha, S., 1985b, Isolation of tumor specific antigen from plasma of mice carrying methycholanthrene-induced fibrosarcomas, *J. Immunol. Methods* (in press).

Ray, P. K., and Seshadri, M., 1980, Effect of immunization of mice with syngeneic embryos on their ability to inhibit the growth of a challenging fibrosarcoma, *Ind. J. Exp. Biol.* 18:1027.

Ray, P. K., and Seshadri, M., 1981, Influence of parity status of female mice on growth of a transplantable chemically-induced fibrosarcoma, *Ind. J. Exp. Biol.* 19:404.

Ray, P. K., Idiculla, A., Rhoads, J. E., Jr., Mark, R., Besa, E., Thomas, H., Bassett, J. G., and Cooper, D. R., 1979a, Extracorporeal immunoadsorption of pathologic plasma immunoglobulin G and its complexes: A novel approach for the selective removal from the plasma, in: *First Annual Plasmapheresis Symposium: Current Topics and Future Trends*, p. 203, American Red Cross, Mid-America Region, Chicago.

Ray, P. K., Cooper, D. R., Bassett, J. G., and Mark, R., 1979b, Antitumor effect of *Staphylococcus aureus* organisms, *Fed. Proc.* 38:4558.

Ray, P. K., Idiculla, A., Besa, E., Bassett, J. G., and Cooper, D. R., 1980a, Immunoadsorption of IgG molecules of the plasma of multiple myeloma and autoimmune hemolytic anemia patients, *Plasma Ther. Transfusion Technol.* 1:11.

Ray, P. K., De, B. K., and Guha, S., 1980b, Facilitation and/or inhibition of growth of sarcoma 190 ascites tumor by BCG: Effect of BCG on tumor cell membrane, *Ind. J. Exp. Biol.* 18:123.

Ray, P. K., Idiculla, A., Rhoads, J. E., Jr., Bassett, J. G., and Cooper, D. R., 1980c, Immunoadsorption of blocking immune complexes using protein A column—A novel approach for immunotherapy of cancer, *Fourth Int. Cong. Immunol.* 10:5.

Ray, P. K., Besa, E., Idiculla, A., Rhoads, J. E., Jr., Bassett, J. G., and Cooper, D. R., 1980d, Extracorporeal immunoadsorption of myeloma IgG and autoimmune antibodies: A clinically feasible modality of treatment, *Clin. Exp. Immunol.* 42:308.

Ray, P. K., Besa, E., Idiculla, A., Rhoads, J. E., Jr., Bassett, J. G., and Cooper, D. R., 1980e, Efficient removal of immunoglobulin G from the plasma of a multiple myeloma patient—Description of a new method for treatment of hyperviscosity syndrome, *Cancer* 45:263.

Ray, P. K., Idiculla, A., Rhoads, J. E., Jr., Bassett, J. G., and Cooper, D. R., 1980f, Extracorporeal immunoadsorption using protein A-containing *Staphylococcus aureus* column: A method for the quick removal of abnormal IgG and/or its complexes from the plasma, in: *Plasma Exchange Therapy, International Symposium* (H. Borberg and P. Reuther, eds.), p. 150, Karger, Basel.

Ray, P. K., McLaughlin, D., Mohammed, J., Idiculla, A., Rhoads, J. E., Jr., Mark, R., Bassett, J. G., and Cooper, D. R., 1981a, *Ex vivo* immunoadsorption of IgG or its complexes—A new modality of cancer treatment, in: *Immune Complexes and Plasma Exchanges in*

Cancer Patients (B. Serrou and C. Rosenfeld, eds.), p. 197, Elsevier/North-Holland, Amsterdam.

Ray, P. K., Idiculla, A., Clark, A., Clarke, L., Rhoads, J. E., Jr., Bassett, J. G., and Cooper, D. R., 1981*b*, Immunoadsorption of plasma IgG and or its complexes from colon carcinoma patients—An adjunct therapy for cancer, in: *Third International Conference on Adjuvant Therapy*, University of Arizona, Tucson, Arizona, p. 29.

Ray, P. K., Raychaudhuri, S., McLaughlin, D., Idiculla, A., Rhoads, J. E., Jr., and Bassett, J. G., 1981*c*, Ability of nonviable *Staphylococcus aureus* Cowan I to bind ionized calcium in *in vitro* and *ex vivo* perfusion systems, *Cancer Res.* 41:5010.

Ray, P. K., Idiculla, A., Mark, R., Rhoads, J. E., Jr., Thomas H., Bassett, J. G., and Cooper, D. R., 1982*a*, Extracorporeal immunoadsorption of plasma from a metastatic colon carcinoma patient by protein A—containing nonviable *Staphylococcus aureus*, *Cancer* 49:1800.

Ray, P. K., Raychaudhuri, S., and Allen, P., 1982*b*, Mechanism of regression of mammary adenocarcinomas in rats following plasma absorption over protein A—containing *Staphylococcus aureus*, *Cancer Res.* 42:4970.

Ray, P. K., Mohammed, J., Allen, P., Raychaudhuri, S., Dohadwala, M., Bandyopadhyay, S., and Mark, R., 1984*a*, Effect of frequency of plasma adsorption over protein A—containing *Staphylococcus aureus* on regression of rat mammary adenocarcinomas: Modification of antitumor immune response and tumor histopathology, *J. Biol. Resp. Modif.* 3:39.

Ray, P. K., McLaughlin, D., Allen, P., Bandyopadhyay, S., Idiculla, A., Clarke, L., Mark, R., Rhoads, J. E., Jr., Bassett, J. G., and Cooper, D. R., 1984*b*, Plasma adsorption of tumor-bearing hosts with protein A containing nonviable *Staphylococcus aureus* Cowan I—therapeutic implications and possible mechanisms, *J. Biol. Resp. Modif.* 3:293.

Ray, P. K., Bandyopadhyay, S., Dohadwala, M., Canchanapan, P., and Mobini, J., 1984*c*, Antitumor activity with non-toxic doses of protein A, *Cancer Immunol. Immunother.* 18:29.

Raychaudhuri, S., Ray, P. K., Bassett, J. G., and Cooper, D. R., 1980, High dose antigen induced suppressor generation in normal and tumor-bearing hosts, *Fed. Proc.* 39:696.

Renacle-Bonnett, M. M., Pommier, G. J., Rance, R. J., and Depieds, R. C., 1978, Nonspecific suppressor and cytostatic activities mediated by human colonic carcinoma tissue on cultured extract, *J. Immunol.* 121:44.

Rodey, G. E., Spreader, J. C., and Bortin, M. M., 1974, Inhibition of normal allogeneic responder cells in mouse mixed leukocyte culture by long passage AKR leukemic lymphoblasts, *Cancer Res.* 34:1289.

Roland, P. H., Martin, P. M., Jacquemier, J., Rolland, A. M., and Toga, M., 1980, Prostaglandin in human breast cancer: Evidence suggesting that an elevated prostaglandin production is a marker of high metastatic potential for neoplastic cells, *J. Natl. Cancer Inst.* 64:1061.

Ron, M., and Witz, I. P., 1972, Tumor associated immunoglobulins: Enhancement of syngeneic tumors by IgG2-containing eluates, *Int. J. Cancer* 9:242.

Rossen, R. D., and Morgan, A. C., 1981, Blockage of the humoral immune response: Immune complexes in cancer, in: *The Handbook of Cancer Immunology*, Vol. 9 (H. Walters, ed.), p. 209, Garland STM Press, New York.

Rossen, R. D., Reisberg, M., Hersh, E. M., and Gutterman, J. V., 1977, The C1q binding test for soluble immune complexes: Clinical correlation obtained in patients with cancer, *J. Natl. Cancer Inst.* 58:1205.

Rosenberg, S. A., and Perry, W. B., 1977, Passive immunotherapy of cancer in animals and man, *Adv. Cancer Res.* 25:323.

Rotter, V., and Trainin, N., 1975, Inhibition of tumor growth in syngeneic chimeric mice mediated by a depletion of suppressor T cells, *Transplantation* 20:68.

Rubenstein, P., Decary, R., and Strum, E. W., 1974, Quantitative studies on tumor enhancement in mice. I. Enhancement of SaI induced IgM, IgG$_1$ and IgG$_2$, *J. Exp. Med.* 140:591.

Saha, S., and Ray, P. K., 1982, Regulatory role of tumor antigen in the generation of humoral and cellular tumor growth enhancing factors in mice, *Fed. Am. Soc. Exp. Biol.* 41:411.

Salinas, F. A., Silver, H. K. B., Grossman, L., and Thomas, J. W., 1981, Plasmapheresis: A new approach in the management of advanced malignant melanoma, in: *Immune Complexes and Plasma Exchanges in Cancer Patients* (B. Serrou and C. Rosenfeld, eds.), p. 253, Elsevier/North-Holland, Amsterdam.

Salinas, F. A., and Wee, K. H., 1983, Immune complexes and human neoplasia. I., *Biomed. Pharmacother.* 36:119.

Samayoa, E. H., McDuffie, F. C., Nelson, A. M., Go, V. L. Luthar, H. S., and Brumfield, H. N., 1977, Immunoglobulin complexes in sera of patients with malignancy, *Int. J. Cancer* 19:12.

Savary, C. A., and Lotova, 1978, Suppression of natural killer cell cytotoxicity by splenocytes from *Corynebacterium parvum* injected bone marrow tolerant and infant mice, *J. Immunol.* 120:239.

Sengupta, J., and Ray, P. K., 1979, Sharing of antigens between sarcoma 180 tumors and mouse embryos, *Fed. Am. Soc. Exp. Biol.* 38:5857.

Serrou, B., Cupisol, D., and Caraux, J., 1980, Ability of thymosin to decrease *in vivo* and *in vitro* suppressor cell activity in tumor-bearing mice and cancer patients, *Recent Results Cancer Res.* 75:110.

Sjögren, H. O., Hellström, I., Bansal, S. C., and Hellström, K. E., 1971, Suggestive evidence that blocking antibodies of tumor-bearing hosts may be antigen–antibody complexes, *Proc. Natl. Acad. Sci. USA* 68:1372.

Small, M., 1977, Characterization of the immature cells involved in T cell mediated enhancement of syngeneic tumor, *J. Immunol.* 118:1517.

Smith, E. M., Johnson, H. M., and Blaylock, J. E., 1983, *Staphylococcus aureus* protein A induces the production of interferon-γ in human lymphocytes and interferon-α in mouse spleen cells, *J. Immunol.* 130:773.

Sparks, F. C., and Breeding, J. H., 1974, Tumor regression and enhancement resulting from immunotherapy with Bacillus Calmette–Guèrin and neuraminidase, *Cancer Res.* 34:3262.

Spence, R. J., Simon, R. M., and Baker, A. R., 1978, Failure of immunotherapy with neuraminidase treated tumor cell vaccine in mice bearing established 3-methylcholanthrene induced sarcomas, *J. Natl. Cancer Inst.* 60:451.

Staab, H. J., Anderer, F. A., Stump, F. E., and Fischer, R., 1980, Are circulating immune complexes a prognostic marker in patients with carcinoma of the gastrointestinal tract? *Br. J. Cancer* 42:26.

Steele, G., Ankerest, J., and Sjogren, H. O., 1974, Alteration of *in vitro* antitumor activity of tumor bearers' sera by adsorption with *Staphylococcus aureus* Cowan I, *Int. J. Cancer* 14:83.

Stein, P. C., Christiansen, N., and Char, D. H., 1980, Characterization of retinoblastoma immune complexes, *Invest. Ophthalmol. Verseral. Sci.* 19:302.

Stelzer, G. T., and Wallace, J. H., 1977, Suppressor cells in mice bearing the B-16 melanoma, *Proc. Am. Assoc. Cancer Res.* 18:68.

Stevens, R. H., Brooks, G. P., Osborn, J. W., Hoffman, K. L., and Lawson, A. J., 1978, Lymphocyte cytotoxicity in X irradiation induced rat small bowel adenocarcinoma III: Blocking by 3 M KCl extract, *J. Immunol.* 12:335.

Strausser, H. R., and Humes, J. L., 1975, Prostaglandin synthesis inhibition: Effect on bone changes and sarcoma tumor induction in mice, *Int. J. Cancer* 15:724.

Suckalova, A., Gazzola, S., Hrubisko, M., and Slakova, J., 1973, Clinical utilization of plasmapheresis and cyclophosphamide in the treatment of malignant lymphoproliferated processes, *Neoplasma* 20:335.

Sulica, A., Kaly, M., Gherman, M., Ghetie, V., and Sjoquist, J., 1976, Arming of lymphoid cells by IgG antibodies treated with protein A from *Staphylococcus aureus*, *Scand. J. Immunol.* 5:1191.

Tada, T., Taniguchi, M., and Takemori, T., 1975, Properties of primed suppressor T cells and their products, *Transplant. Rev.* 26:106.

Takei, F., Levy, J. G., and Kilburn, B. G., 1976, *In vitro* induction of cytotoxicity against syngeneic mastocytoma and its suppression by spleen and thymus cells from tumor-bearing mice, *J. Immunol.* 116:288.

Tanaguchi, M., Hayaka, W. A., and Tada, T., 1976, Properties of antigen-specific suppressor T cell factor in the regulation of antibody response of the mouse. II. *In vitro* activity and evidence for the I region gene product, *J. Immunol.* 116:542.

Tashjain, A. H., Voekel, E. F., Levine, L., and Goldhaber, P., 1972, Evidence that the bone resorption stimulator factor produced by mouse fibrosarcoma cells is prostaglandin, *J. Exp. Med.* 136:1329.

Terman, D. S., Yamamoto, T., Tillquist, R. L., Cook, G., Silvers, A., and Shearer, W. T., 1980a, Tumoricidal response induced by cytosine arabinoside after plasma perfusion over protein A, *Science* 209:1257.

Terman, D. S., Yamamoto, T. Mattioli, M., Cook, G., Tillquist, R., Henry, J., Poser, R., and Daskal, Y., 1980b, Extensive necrosis of spontaneous canine mammary adenocarcinoma after extracorporeal perfusion over *Staphylococcus aureus* Cowan I. I. Description of acute tumoricidal response, morphologic, histologic, immunohistochemical, immunologic and serologic findings, *J. Immunol.* 124:795.

Terman, D. S., Young, J. B., Shearer, W. T., Ayus, C., Mattioli, C., Lehane, D., Espada, R., Howell, J. F., Yamamoto, T., Zeleski, H. I., Henry, J. F., Feldman, L., Miller, L., Frommer, P., Tillquist, R., Cook, G., and Daskal, Y., 1981, Preliminary observations of the effects on breast carcinoma of plasma perfused over immobilized protein A, *N. Engl. J. Med.* 305:1195.

Teshima, H., Wanebo, H., Pinsky, C., and Day, N. K., 1977, Circulating immune complexes detected by ^{125}I-C1q deviation test in sera of cancer patients, *J. Clin. Invest.* 59:1134.

Theofilopoulos, A. N., Wilson, C. B., and Dixon, F. J., 1976, The Raji cell radioimmunoassay for detecting immune complexes in human sera, *J. Clin. Invest.* 57:169.

Theofilopoulos, A. N., Andrews, B. S., Urist, M. M., Morton, D. L., and Dixon, F. J., 1977, The nature of immune complexes in human cancer sera, *J. Immunol.* 119:657.

Thomas, D. W., Rover, W. K., and Talmage, D. W., 1975, Regulation of the immune responses: Production of a soluble suppressor by immune cells, *J. Immunol.* 114:1616.

Tilkin, A. F., Schaff-Lafontaine, N., Vanker, A. C., Boccadoro, M., and Urbain, J., 1981, Reduced tumor growth after low-dose irradiation or immunization against blastic suppressor T cells, *Proc. Natl. Acad. Sci. USA* 78:1809.

Treves, A. J., Carnaud, C., and Trainin, N., 1974, Enhancing T lymphocytes from tumor-bearing mice suppressed host resistance to a syngeneic tumor, *Eur. J. Immunol.* 4:722.

Treves, A. J., Cohen, I. R., and Feldman, M., 1976, Suppressor factor secreted by T-lymphocytes from tumor-bearing mice, *J. Natl. Cancer Inst.* 57:409.

Turk, J. L., Parker, D., and Poulter, L. W., 1972, Functional aspects of the selective depletion of lymphoid tissue by cyclophosphamide, *Immunology* 23:493.

Uchida, A. and Hoshino T., 1980, Reduction of suppressor-cells in cancer patients treated with OK-432 immunotherapy, *Int. J. Cancer* 26:401.

Umiel, T., and Trainin, N., 1974, Immunological enhancement of tumor growth by syngeneic thmus-derived lymphocytes, *Transplantation* 18:244.

Verrier-Jones, J., Klough, J. D., Klinburg, G. R., and Davis, P., 1981, The role of therapeutic plasmapheresis in the pneumatic diseases, *J. Lab. Clin. Med.* 97:589.

Voisin, G. A., 1972, Immunity and tolerance: A unified concept, *Cell Immunol.* 2:670.

Waksman, B. H., and Tada, T., 1977, Specific and nonspecific suppressor T-cell factors derived from thymic lymphocytes, *Cell Immunol.* 30:189.

Werner, D., Maier, G., and Lommel, R., 1973, A factor reducing protein synthesis from Ehrlich ascites cells, *Eur. J. Cancer* 9:819.

Witz, I. P., 1977, Tumor-bound immunoglobulins' *in situ* expression of humoral immunity, *Adv. Cancer Res.* 25:95.

Wright, P. W., Hellström, K. E., and Hellström, I., 1976, Serotherapy of malignant melanoma, *Med. Clin.N. Am.* 60:607.

Yamagishi, H., Nitta, K., and Umezawa, H., 1973, Immunosuppression induced with cell-free fluid of Ehrlich carcinoma ascites and its fractions, *Gann* 64:83.

Yamagishi, H., Pellis, N. R., and Kahan, B. D., 1983, Specific and nonspecific immunologic tumor growth facilitation, in: *Immunobiology of Transplantation, Cancer and Pregnancy* (P. K. Ray, ed.), p. 179, Pergamon Press, New York.

Yamamoto, J. K., Good, R. A., Johnson, H. M., Engleman, R., Tyler, R., Machida, K., Tran, X., and Day, N. K., 1983, Augmentation of serum interferon titre prior to remission of leukemia in cats treated with *ex vivo* immunoadsorption, *Fed. Proc.* 42:838.

Yonemoto, R. H., and Terasaki, P. I., 1972, Cancer immunotherapy with HLA compatible thoracic duct lymphocyte transplantation, *Cancer* 30:1438.

Zembla, M., Mytar, B., and Popiela, T., 1977, Depressed *in vitro* peripheral blood lymphocyte response to mitogens in cancer patients, *Int. J. Cancer* 19:605.

Chapter 6

Blocking (Suppressor) Factors, Immune Complexes, and Extracorporeal Immunoadsorption in Tumor Immunity

Karl Erik Hellström and Ingegerd Hellström

Oncogen
Seattle, Washington 98121

and Departments of Pathology, and
Microbiology and Immunology
University of Washington
Seattle, Washington 98195

and Harry W. Snyder, Jr., Joe P. Balint, and Frank R. Jones

Immune Response Program
Pacific Northwest Research Foundation
Seattle, Washington 98104

and Imré Corporation
Seattle, Washington 98109

I. INTRODUCTION

Some animal neoplasms, particularly many of those induced by chemical carcinogens, have tumor-specific transplantation antigens. These are detected by their ability to induce the rejection of tumors grafted onto properly immunized syngeneic hosts (Prehn and Main, 1957; Old and Boyse, 1964; Sjögren, 1965; K. E. Hellström and Brown, 1979), and the tumors expressing the antigens are commonly referred to as *immunogenic*. It is being debated whether "spontaneous" tumors, like most human tumors, have antigens that can be immunogenic in the native host (Klein and Klein, 1977; Hewitt *et al.*, 1976; Hellström *et al.*, 1983).

Animals in which immunogenic tumors are growing often reject a second transplant of cells from the same tumor while their original tumors continue to grow. This phenomenon is often referred to as *concomitant immunity* (Gershon *et al.*, 1967). It is at least partially due to an antigen-specific mechanism, since lymphocytes from a tumor-bearing animal are commonly cytotoxic to cells from the same neoplasm *in vitro* (I. Hellström *et al.*, 1968), and since the outgrowth

213

of transplanted tumor cells can be prevented by adding lymphocytes from an animal bearing the original tumor (Mikulska *et al.*, 1966). Better understanding of the mechanisms underlying concomitant tumor immunity may be helpful toward development of therapy for immunogenic tumors and may contribute to our understanding of why many "spontaneous" tumors are not immunogenic.

The fact that a tumor can grow in an animal that displays concomitant tumor immunity implies that there must be some mechanisms that prevent the antitumor response from being effective *in vivo*, and that these mechanisms are more effective at a local than at a systemic level. Several potential mechanisms of this type have been identified and are not mutually exclusive (see, for example, Old and Boyse, 1964; K. E. Hellström and Brown, 1979). Among these, specific blocking factors (SBF) have attracted much interest (I. Hellström *et al.*, 1969; K. E. Hellström *et al.*, 1977). They were identified by their ability to suppress ("block") cell-mediated immune responses to tumor antigens in an antigen-specific way, thereby inhibiting tumor destruction.

Initial studies on SBF led to the detection of immune complexes (IC) in the sera of animals and human patients with cancer, and subsequent work showed that IC, as well as tumor antigens *per se*, can activate a suppressor cell response that down-regulates the host's reactivity to tumor-associated antigens. Circulating T-cell-derived suppressor factors are among the mediators of this down-regulation. These findings, and particularly those on circulating IC (CIC), provided an impetus for attempts to remove various circulating factors by extracorporeal immunoadsorption.

In this chapter, we shall discuss specific blocking (suppressor) factors and IC with particular reference to the use of extracorporeal immunoadsorption for their possible removal from tumor hosts. We have recently reviewed the nature and role of both SBF (I. Hellström *et al.*, 1983; Nelson *et al.*, 1985) and suppressor cells (Nepom *et al.*, 1983) in tumor immunity and refer the reader to these reviews for a more detailed discussion of these topics. In this chapter we shall not discuss the evidence that nonspecific suppressor factors of various types may be also important in inhibiting tumor immunity and that extracorporeal removal of the nonspecific factors may be beneficial to the tumor-bearing host; however, we continue to have an interest in such factors as well.

II. SPECIFIC BLOCKING FACTORS

Most studies of SBF have used colony inhibition (I. Hellström, 1967) and microcytotoxicity (I. Hellström and Hellström, 1971) techniques. Both of these assays involve long exposure of effector and target cells to each other (4–6 days for the colony inhibition assay and about 40 hr for the microcytotoxicity assay). Therefore, they probably measure a combination of lymphocyte activation and such effects of the activated lymphocytes on the target cells as killing, inhibition of growth, and loss of adherence.

The experiments that led to the discovery of SBF were inspired by the demonstration of "enhancing antibodies" in certain hyperimmune sera (Kaliss, 1958: K. E. Hellström and Möller, 1965), which could prevent both the induction of cell-mediated immune responses and the effectiveness of these responses once activated. It was therefore investigated whether sera from tumor-bearing animals could inhibit ("block") the reactivity of specifically immune lymphocytes to the appropriate tumor cells (I. Hellström et al., 1969, 1970; I. Hellström and Hellström, 1969; Heppner, 1969). Such inhibition was, indeed, detected and found to be specific for the antigens of each tumor. Subsequent work extended these findings to a variety of animal and human neoplasms (for review, see K. E. Hellström and Hellström, 1974; Baldwin and Robins, 1977; K. E. Hellström and Brown, 1979), and the serum factors responsible for the inhibitory effects were called SBF (K. E. Hellström et al., 1977). In a study of transplated methylcholanthrene (MCA)-induced sarcomas it was found that the concentration of SBF was much higher within a growing sarcoma than systemically (K. E. Hellström and Hellström, 1979). This suggested that a high local concentration of SBF provides at least part of the explanation for why a tumor can grow in an animal displaying concomitant immunity.

When the blocking phenomenon was discovered, it seemed likely that it was due to a "blocking" or "masking" of target cell antigens by antibodies (Möller, 1965) and represented a case of "efferent" immunological enhancement (K. E. Hellström and Hellström, 1970). However, this interpretation was abandoned when it was found that the blocking serum effect disappeared within 3–4 days of tumor removal (I. Hellström et al., 1970) and that antibodies from tumor-immunized animals not only lacked inhibitory activity but could cancel ("unblock") the inhibitory activity of sera from animals bearing the same tumor (I. Hellström and Hellström, 1970).

A new hypothesis had to be introduced to take into account the evidence that the blocking factors cannot be circulating antibodies but can nevertheless be removed by absorption with the specific tumor cells (I. Hellström and Hellström, 1971). The hypothesis stated that antigen–antibody complexes were the most important components of SBF, and experiments were designed to test this possibility (Sjögren et al., 1971). Sera from mice with growing Moloney sarcoma virus (MSV)-induced sarcomas were absorbed onto MSV-induced syngeneic sarcoma cells, eluted from these cells at low pH, and subjected to ultrafiltration to isolate material with molecular weights of 10,000–100,000 ("E10") or higher than 100,000 ("E100"). After filtration, the E10 and E100 fractions were tested for biological activity, using the microcytotoxicity assay. When tested alone, neither fraction could prevent specifically immune lymphocytes from reacting against MSV-induced sarcoma cells. However, pretreatment of either the lymphocytes or the target cells with a combination of the E10 and E100 fractions blocked reactivity. Furthermore, reactivity was blocked when E10 was added to the lymphocytes and allowed to remain in contact with the cells during the assay. Sjögren *et al.* (1971) tentatively concluded that the E10 fraction contained tumor antigen, that the E100 fraction contained antitumor antibodies, and that the combination of the two contained antigen–antibody complexes. They postulated that SBF act by inhibiting effector lymphocytes (effector cell blockade) and not be "masking" tumor antigens (as "blocking antibodies" are presumed to do). In view of the fact that a 48- to 72-hr assay was used, however, one must be aware that the SBF need not necessarily interact with the effector cells. It is equally possible that they recruit T suppressor cells or directly (or indirectly via suppressor cells) prevent the formation of lymphocyte-dependent antibodies involved in target cell killing. The main point of the paper of Sjögren *et al.* (1971) was, nevertheless, that IC could be detected in tumor-bearing mice, that they were found to act on lymphocytes rather than on target cells, and that their blocking effect had immunological specificity.

Baldwin *et al.* (1972, 1973) subsequently analyzed the blocking of cell-mediated antitumor immunity by sera, cell-free tumor homogenates, and mixtures of the two (presumably containing antigen–antibody complexes). Inhibition of reactivity was detected following incubation of lymphocytes with tumor homogenates and tumor-bearer sera. Suppressed killing was also observed upon incubation of the target cells with tumor-bearer sera or mixtures of antitumor antibodies with tumor homogenates (believed to represent IC), while tumor homogenates ("antigens") were not inhibitory under these conditions. Blocking at the target cell level or inhibition of the reactivity of preincubated and washed lymphocytes was detected during different phases of tumor growth (Baldwin and Robins, 1977).

III. IMMUNE COMPLEXES IN CANCER

As reviewed in the preceding section, CIC have been implicated as SBF. There are many reports that tumor-bearing animals and human cancer patients have higher levels of IC than do healthy individuals, that these levels decrease after tumor removal, and that they may be of prognostic significance (see, e.g., Gutterman, 1977; Theofilopoulos *et al.*, 1977; Theofilopoulos and Dixon, 1980; Hofken *et al.*, 1978; Brandeis *et al.*, 1978; Amlot *et al.*, 1978; Carpentier *et al.*, 1982; Gupta *et al.*, 1983; Snyder *et al.*, 1984).

In most cases it is unknown whether CIC do indeed contain antibodies to tumor-associated antigens, even if work on certain animal tumors (Oldstone *et al.*, 1975; Jennette and Feldman, 1977; Tucker *et al.*, 1978; Balint, 1982; Snyder *et al.*, 1984) and on patients with Burkitt's lymphoma (Oldstone *et al.*, 1975; Heimer and Klein, 1976) and melanoma (Gupta *et al.*, 1983) suggests this by showing that CIC with tumor antigen as a component do occur.

When SBF in the form of tumor antigen or IC are present in tumor-bearer serum, it should be possible to isolate them by immunoadsorption, using an antibody with proper specificity. Based on this assumption, Tamerius *et al.* (1976) and Nepom *et al.* (1977) attempted to isolate SBF from the sera of BALB/c mice carrying transplanted MCA-induced sarcomas. Immunoadsorbent columns were used that had been prepared using "unblocking" sera (I. Hellström and Hellström, 1970) from mice that had been repeatedly immunized with tumor. When tumor-bearer serum was passed through such a column, its SBF activity, as measured by microcytotoxicity testing, was removed and could be recovered by elution of the column at low pH (Tamerius *et al.*, 1976). The SBF purified on the basis of immunoaffinity had the same specificity as SBF in the corresponding tumor-bearer serum (Nepom *et al.*, 1976). Only sera from mice immunized against the MCA-induced sarcoma borne by the respective tumor-bearers could be used to make an effective immunoadsorbent (Nepom *et al.*, 1976, 1977).

Nepom *et al.* (1976, 1977) found that the SBF purified by immunoadsorption were glycoproteins with a molecular weight of approximately 56,000. Isolates that had SBF activity contained this protein consistently, while isolates lacking SBF activity did not (Nepom, 1977; K. E. Hellström *et al.*, 1977). The 56,000-molecular-weight SBF could be specifically removed by adsorption with cultivated cells from the respective tumor (Nepom *et al.*, 1977), a finding consistent with previous observations on whole tumor-bearer sera (I. Hellström and Hellström, 1969). In view of the 56,000 molecular weight of the factor isolated, it could not be an antibody, and the fact that SBF activity was removed by adsorption with tumor cells indicated that it was not an antigen either. Thus, these data differed from what was originally expected and indicated that a new type of "blocking" molecule had to be contemplated. In view of what had been reported about the role of T cells in immune regulation (Gershon, 1974; Asherson and Zembala, 1976), and the findings of Nelson *et al.* to be described shortly, Nepom *et al.* postulated (1977) that the 56,000-molecular-weight SBF were T-cell-derived, antigen-specific suppressor molecules, and speculated that the "unblocking" antibodies used for their isolation bound to an idiotype-specific determinant on the SBF (K. E. Hellström *et al.*, 1977).

The evidence of Nelson *et al.* just referred to, indicating that there are SBF in the form of immunosuppressive molecules different from antibodies (or antigens), came from studies on SBF production by cultured T cells from tumor-bearing mice. Nelson *et al.* (1975*a*–*c*) showed that spleen cells from BALB/c mice bearing either a progressively growing MSV-induced sarcoma or a transplanted MCA-induced sarcoma could produce factors that blocked the *in vitro* cytotoxic effect of specifically tumor-immune T cells, as assessed by a 30- to 40-hr microcytotoxicity assay. These factors, which had a molecular weight of less than 100,000 (Nelson, 1975), could bind specifically to tumor cells carrying the appropriate antigens (Nelson *et al.*, 1975*c*). Removal of Thy-1-positive cells from the cultures stopped the production of SBF, and this production was restored if Thy 1$^+$ cells from spleens of tumor-bearing or normal syngeneic mice were added back to the cultures (Nelson *et al.*, 1975*b*). Removal of adherent cells or of immunoglobulin-carrying cells did not interfere with SBF synthesis.

We conclude that there is evidence for circulating SBF of at least three types, namely tumor antigen, IC, and antigen-specific factors that are probably suppressor-T-cell derived. In the following section we shall discuss the relationship of the first two factors to suppressor T cells.

IV. RELATIONSHIP BETWEEN SBF AND SUPPRESSOR CELLS

Tumor antigen can inhibit tumor immunity *in vivo* (Vaage, 1972; Paranjpe *et al.*, 1976). This may be due to a direct effect of antigen on helper or effector cells or it may result from a more indirect mechanism, for example, from the induction of suppressor cells. Convincing evidence that tumor antigen can have a direct inhibitory effect comes from the demonstration of "cold target cell inhibition" *in vitro* (Cerrotini and Brunner, 1974), an inhibition that is due to competition by antigen for available effector cells. However, this competitive inhibition occurs when the antigen is provided in the form of intact cells, and it is questionable whether circulating (soluble) antigen can give competitive inhibition (Berke, 1980).

K. E. Hellström and Hellström (1978) investigated whether the inhibition of tumor immunity by antigen *in vivo* was due to a direct antigen effect on the effector cells, or whether it, for example, resulted from an activated suppressor cell response. The studies were performed with MCA-induced BALB/c sarcomas, transplanted into syngeneic hosts, and heavily irradiated tumor cells were employed as the source of antigen; the irradiated cells were similar to those routinely used to induce tumor-specific transplantation immunity (Klein *et al.*, 1960; Sjögren, 1965). As expected, small numbers of sarcoma cells were rejected by mice that had been immunized with irradiated cells from the original sarcoma. This effect was abolished, however, when the tumor cells used for challenge were mixed with an excess of heavily irradiated cells from the sarcoma; cells from an antigenically different MCA-induced sarcoma were used as a negative control. The findings confirmed that tumor antigen can, under certain circumstances, inhibit an immune response to itself *in vivo*.

Since most suppressor-cell-mediated reactions include a radiosensitive component (reviewed in Katz, 1977), while transplantation immunity to tumor antigens is not diminished following whole-body irradiation (Klein *et al.*, 1960), the next step was to study whether inhibition of tumor rejection by excess antigen was possible in immune mice that had received whole-body irradiation (400–450 rads). The data showed unequivocally that rejection was not inhibited by antigen in the irradiated mice, suggesting that the *in vivo* effect of antigen was not based on competitive inhibition. If, however, the irradiated, immune mice were given Thy 1[+] cells (for example, from normal spleens), added antigen could inhibit tumor rejection. It was concluded that tumor antigens can inhibit the development of a rejection response, but only in the presence of radiosensitive T cells, which probably are suppressor cells (K. E. Hellström and Hellström, 1978).

Other studies have strengthened this view and demonstrated that inactivation of radiosensitive cells by whole-body irradiation can cause inhibition of tumor growth in mice (F. R. Jones, 1978; K. E. Hellström et al., 1978; Enker and Jacobitz, 1980; Tilkin et al., 1981), unless the mice are reconstituted with normal T cells. As an alternative to irradiating the mice, they can be injected with cyclophosphamide (North, 1982).

The findings that we have discussed agree with the evidence from other types of studies that suppressor cells play an important role in regulating tumor immunity (Hayami et al., 1972; Gershon, 1974; Umiel and Trainin, 1974; Kall et al., 1975; Rotter and Trainin, 1975; Kripke et al., 1977; Greene et al., 1977; Fujimoto and Tada, 1978; Daynes and Spellman, 1977; Naor, 1979; Greene, 1980; Fisher and Kripke, 1982; Nepom et al., 1983). At least two types of T cells are involved in this regulation, namely antigen-specific, Lyt 1[+] (Rao et al., 1980; Mulé et al., 1982), radioresistant (I. Hellström et al., 1979) suppressor activator cells and radiosensitive, naive, suppressor acceptor cells (I. Hellström et al., 1979; Rao et al., 1980; Mulé et al., 1982). IC appear to be more effective than free antigen in inducing the suppressor activator cells (Rao et al., 1980).

The suppressor activator cells are highly antigen-specific. They require contact with the specific antigen for suppression to occur. After this contact, however, the immune response to third-party antigens may be suppressed as well (K. E. Hellström and Hellström, 1981a,b; Mulé et al., 1982). This implies that if a tumor cell expresses an antigen that preferentially induces suppression, immunity to other antigens on the tumor cell surface may sometimes also be inhibited. This "secondary" suppression may contribute to the lack of immunogenicity of many tumors when tested for tumor-specific transplantation immunity (Hewitt et al., 1976).

V. ANALYSIS OF SUPPRESSOR FACTORS PRODUCED USING HYBRIDOMA TECHNOLOGY

The finding that Thy 1[+] cells from the spleens of tumor-bearing mice produce SBF in vitro provided a starting point for work that has led to the development of T-cell hybridoma clones that form tumor-specific suppressor factors (Nelson et al., 1980, 1985; Cory et al., 1981). An analysis of the activities of these factors has led to better insight into the nature and role of suppressor factors in tumor immunity.

T-cell hybridomas were derived by fusing thymocytes from BALB/c mice carrying a transplanted, syngeneic sarcoma, MCA-1490, with BW5147 thymoma cells (Nelson et al., 1980, 1985). Like most other MCA-induced sarcomas, this tumor expresses individually unique tumor-specific transplantation antigens. Most work has been done on one clone, I82K54, which forms a suppressor factor called K54SF. This factor suppresses the ability of Thy 1⁺ lymphocytes from BALB/c mice immunized to MCA-1490 cells to kill cultured MCA-1490 cells, but it does not suppress the killing of cells from other MCA-induced sarcomas by immune T cells (Nelson *et al.*, 1980). It suppresses, in an antigen-specific way, the ability of Thy l⁺ lymph node cells from BALB/c mice immunized to MCA-1490 to inhibit the outgrowth of MCA-1490 cells in Winn assays as well as the ability of BALB/c mice to reject MCA-1490 cells after immunization with heavily irradiated tumor cells (Nelson *et al.*, 1980, 1985; Cory *et al.*, 1981). Furthermore, it suppresses the induction, and to a lesser extent the elicitation, of delayed-type hypersensitivity (DTH) to MCA-1490 cells in BALB/c mice; this suppression is also antigen-specific. The ability of K54SF to suppress can be removed by absorption with MCA-1490 cells, but not with cells from different BALB/c sarcomas, and it can be recovered by elution from the MCA-1490 cells used for absorption (Nelson *et al.*, 1980, 1985; Cory *et al.*, 1981).

In order to learn about the biology of K54SF and its molecular nature, it needed to be purified. "Unblocking" antibodies were believed to be useful for this purpose, in view of the postulate that they are directed to idiotypic determinants that are expressed on tumor-specific suppressor factors (K. E. Hellström *et al.*, 1977). To make such antibodies, mice were hyperimmunized with MCA-1490, their spleen cells fused with NS-1 myeloma cells, and the hybrids screened for antibodies capable of inducing DTH to MCA-1490 cells. This resulted in one hybridoma clone, which forms an IgG1 antibody, 4.72 (Forstrom *et al.*, 1983). Antibody 4.72 induces tumor-antigen-specific DTH to MCA-1490, which is mediated by Th 1⁺, Lyt 1⁺ lymphocytes. Its ability to induce DTH is genetically restricted to BALB/c mice, as compared to its congenic strains CB-20 and CAL-20, which have different allotypes (Nelson *et al.*, 1985; Forstrom *et al.*, 1983). Since the antibody does not bind to tumor cells, Forstrom *et al.* (1983) concluded that antibody 4.72 is most likely an antiidiotypic antibody specific for MCA-1490. Recently, another monoclonal antibody has been obtained, which shows similar characteristics, except for the fact that it was made using an antigenically different MCA sarcoma (MCA-1511) and is specific for that tumor.

In view of the evidence that antibody 4.72 is antiidiotypic (Nelson *et al.*, 1985; Forstrom *et al.*, 1983), Nelson *et al.* studied whether it would recognize an idiotype-specific determinant on K54SF (unpublished findings). Affinity columns have been prepared with Fab fragments of antibody 4.72, and they can remove the ability of preparations of K54SF to suppress DTH to MCA-1490; K54SF was recovered in eluates of the affinity columns. This approach is now being used to purify K54SF and investigate its molecular characteristics.

Interestingly, antibody 4.72 can be used to isolate, from sera of mice bearing MCA-1490, a factor that can specifically suppress DTH to MCA-1490 (K. Nelson, unpublished observations). This relates the present work on suppressor factors and antiidiotypic antibodies with past, more phenomenological studies on "blocking factors" and "unblocking antibodies" (I. Hellström *et al.*, 1969; I. Hellström and Hellström, 1970).

VI. IMMUNE MODULATION BY PLASMA TREATMENT: RATIONALE AND MAJOR FINDINGS

There are several possible ways to manipulate the immune response in favor of the tumor-bearing host based on the knowledge gained about circulating tumor antigens (IC), suppressor cells, and their interaction in modulating the immune response to tumors. For example, one may try to interfere with the activity of suppressor cells and their factors; as discussed previously, monoclonal antibodies reacting with tumor-antigen-specific suppressor factors may be used for this, as may whole-body irradiation, treatment with drugs such as cyclophosphamide, and injection of antisera to markers of suppressor cells.

Alternatively, one may try to physically remove circulating SBF in the form of antigens, IC, and/or suppressor factors. Different approaches for removal of SBF from plasma have been attempted. Most of these approaches have been directed toward removing IC and are based on the use of protein A from *Staphylococcus aureus* Cowan I (SAC), since protein A binds the Fc portion of most mammalian IgG (Forsgren and Sjöquist, 1966) and to IC (Kessler, 1975). It needs to be established, however, how efficiently these procedures remove IC, as compared to antibodies, and whether they also remove T-cell-derived suppressor factors; there is suggestive evidence that some suppressor factors have an affinity for protein A (R. K. Gershon, personal communication).

One of the first attempts to remove circulating SBF was made by Isbister *et al.* (1975), who drained the thoracic duct in a patient with advanced melanoma, removed the cell-free lymph, and returned the washed lymphocytes to the patient. There was a decrease of circulating SBF and some temporary slowing of tumor progression, but the results were not dramatic.

Hersey *et al.* (1976) plasmapheresed four patients with melanoma, replacing 4 liters of plasma at weekly intervals with plasma from normal donors. Three patients demonstrated an increase in antibody-dependent cellular cytotoxicity, but there were no clinical benefits. Israel *et al.* (1977) performed a similar study on 23 patients with a variety of disseminated tumors, including carcinomas of the breast, colon, melanoma, and thyroid. There were two to six exchanges of 4 liters of plasma in each patient. Eight patients had partial antitumor responses.

Based on evidence that protein A from SAC binds to both IgG (Forsgren and Sjöquist, 1966) and to IC associated with IgG (Kessler, 1975), Steele *et al.* (1974) used rats with transplanted, polyoma-virus-induced tumors to study whether incubation of sera from such rats with protein A could remove SBF. They found that circulating SBF were, indeed, removed and that antibodies could be subsequently detected that were cytotoxic *in vitro* to polyoma tumor cells when tested in the presence of complement (Steele *et al.*, 1974).

The finding of Steele *et al.* (1974) provided a rationale for developing immunoperfusion technology using protein A to remove SBF (IC) from plasma by an extracorporeal procedure. The first clinical study with this technique was performed by Bansal *et al.* (1978), who perfused plasma from a patient with colon carcinoma over heat-killed and formalin-stabilized SAC. They reported a decrease in serum SBF activity and the appearance of complement-dependent cytotoxic antibodies following treatment. Some decrease in tumor size was also reported, as was histological evidence of tumor destruction. There was relatively mild clinical toxicity resulting in chills and modest hypotension.

Terman *et al.* (1980*a*) used whole SAC as an immunoadsorbent to treat dogs with spontaneous mammary carcinoma. They reported partial tumor regressions in several dogs. A dramatic, tumor-necrotizing response was seen in some dogs that had been given a single, nontoxic dose of cytosine arabinoside after their plasma had been perfused over purified protein A, indicating that there was a synergistic effect of the two treatments (Terman *et al.*, 1980*b*). There were no beneficial effects when the protein A-deficient strain *Staphylococcus aureus* Wood 46 was employed.

Holohan *et al.* (1982) also reported that immunoadsorption of plasma from tumor-bearing dogs, using SAC, induced partial regression of mammary adenocarcinoma. The response was dependent on the site of tumor, and no complete regressions were observed.

Jones *et al.* extensively investigated extracorporeal immunoadsorption in leukemic cats. These studies are discussed in the next chapter.

Terman *et al.* (1981) subsequently developed an immunoadsorbent matrix consisting of protein A adsorbed onto collodion charcoal; they reported less toxic effects with such a matrix than when using whole SAC, and repeatedly treated five patients with breast adenocarcinoma. Objective partial responses were observed in four of the five patients. However, it was unclear to what extent these responses were due to the immunoadsorption, as compared to other therapies that the patients had received. It was also unclear whether they were due to removal of a factor (such as IC) or to introduction of some agent(s), such as protein A leaking off the column (K. E. Hellström and Hellström, 1981*b*; Balint and Jones, 1983).

Bensinger *et al.* (1982) employed large quantities (200 mg) of purified protein A that had been covalently coupled to an inert silica matrix as an immunoadsorbent. Five patients with breast adenocarcinoma were treated by extracorporeal immunoadsorption, and partial remission was reported in three patients. MacKintosh *et al.* (1983) gave 14 cancer patients a series of infusions of autologous plasma that had been perfused over purified protein A bound to Sepharose 4B. Objective tumor regressions were observed in two patients and stabilization of disease lasting from 4 to 12 weeks was noted in five other patients. At present

MacKintosh *et al.* have treated over 50 patients and have had no unmanageable toxicity (personal communication). Ray *et al.* (1980*a*,*b*) have performed extracorporeal immunoadsorption with whole-protein-A-bearing SAC. They reported some clinical improvement in one multiple myeloma patient who had hyperviscosity syndrome owing to abnormal IgG (Ray *et al.*, 1980*a*,*b*), and in one patient with chronic lymphocytic leukemia associated with autoimmune hemolytic anemia (Ray *et al.*, 1980*a*).

Messerschmidt *et al.* (1982*a*) first used extracorporeal immunoadsorption employing heat-killed and formalin-stabilized SAC in studies of dogs with mammary carcinomas. They reported an antitumor response rate of approximately 50% with tumor shrinkage. Subsequently Messerschmidt *et al.* (1982*b*) treated five patients by extracorporeal immunoadsorption using heat-killed and formalin-stabilized SAC. No beneficial effects were observed, and there were toxic effects in all patients, which varied in severity and included hypotension, leukopenia, fever, and diarrhea. These appeared to be related to the volume of plasma perfused. The findings of Messerschmidt *et al.* (1982*b*) were in contrast to earlier studies by Bansal *et al.* (1978) and Ray *et al.* (1980*a*,*b*) in which immunoperfusion over heat-killed and formalin-stabilized SAC was repeatedly performed without complications. It is possible that different SAC preparation procedures may result in adverse effects during treatments, caused by release of large amounts of bacterial products. Therefore, the therapeutic use of extracorporeal immunoadsorption with SAC must be approached with caution.

Miller *et al.* (1982) showed that incubation of sera from patients with acute myelogenous leukemia with protein A specifically increased their cytotoxic activity against leukemic blast cells *in vitro*. They employed both protein A-bearing SAC and purified protein A coupled to Sepharose.

A recent report by Gordon *et al.* (1983) suggests that bacterial products are released into plasma during immunoperfusion and that perfusion of plasma over non-protein-A-containing *Staphylococcus aureus* Wood 46 strain also causes tumor regression in dogs. The latter observation differs from that of Terman *et al.* in dogs (1980*a*) and F. R. Jones *et al.* in cats (unpublished).

VII. LYMPHOSARCOMA AND PERSISTENT FeLV INFECTION OF PET CATS: A MODEL TO STUDY IMMUNOLOGICAL RESPONSES DURING EXTRACORPOREAL IMMUNOADSORPTION TREATMENTS

Pet cats with feline leukemia virus (FeLV)-associated lymphosarcoma (LSA) have an expected lifespan of less than 3 months (Hardy *et al.*, 1975). Despite the occasional induction of temporary remission, multimodel chemotherapy (Cotter *et al.*, 1980) or several forms of immunotherapy (Carpenter and Holzworth, 1971; Squire and Bush, 1973; Hardy *et al.*, 1977) have not proven successful in significantly prolonging the lives of cats with LSA or in abrogating the persistent viremia. Furthermore, the prognosis for persistently FeLV-infected cats, even if free of LSA at the time of testing, is poor. One study showed that only 3 of 144 cats analyzed were able to clear their viremia spontaneously (Hardy *et al.*, 1976), and a follow-up study of 96 cats over a 3.5-year period indicated that 80 animals (83%) had died of an FeLV-associated disease (McClelland *et al.*, 1980). Of the cats that died, 26 (32%) succumbed to LSA, 7 (9%) succumbed to other FeLV-induced nonneoplastic diseases such as regenerative and nonregenerative anemia, and 47 (59%) died of other diseases, including feline infectious peritonitis, which is believed to be a secondary consequence of the immunosuppressive effects of the viral infection (Dorn *et al.*, 1967; Essex, 1980; McClelland *et al.*, 1980).

The fate of a healthy cat after exposure to FeLV depends upon its immunological response both to virus-envelope glycoprotein and to a virus-induced tumor-specific cell-surface antigen, the feline-oncornavirus-associated cell membrane antigen (FOCMA), which is expressed on the membranes of LSA cells (Essex *et al.*, 1976; Hardy *et al.*, 1976). Only about 40% of cats exposed to FeLV mount a measurable antibody response to the virus and become resistant to further challenge with the virus (Hardy *et al.*, 1973, 1976). Approximately half of the remaining cats become persistently infected and remain so for life. In terms of the antibody response to FOCMA, a prospective seroepidemiologic study of 51 cats in a single household over a 2.5-year period showed that the 43 cats that remained free of LSA all had high titers of antibody to FOCMA by the time of initial testing, while the 8 cats that subsequently developed LSA never developed significant levels of FOCMA antibodies (Essex *et al.*, 1975). It appears, therefore, that cats with a persistent FeLV infection with or without concomitant LSA are excellent candidates for a treatment that could make possible antibody responses to FeLV virion antigens and to LSA cell-surface antigens.

It was for such reasons that F. R. Jones *et al.* (1980) initiated studies to remove CIC from the plasma of FeLV-infected LSA cats. They assumed that such complexes acted as SBF and prevented the development of an effective immunity. Cats were treated by extracorporeal immunoadsorption using SAC in an attempt to remove IgG and IC.

F. R. Jones *et al.* (1984) have treated 16 FeLV-infected cats with LSA by extracorporeal immunoadsorption. Each cat was treated a minimum of 10 times on a biweekly schedule and was monitored for persistence of the FeLV virion antigens and for regression of LSA. Cats were considered to have cleared the FeLV infection when their peripheral blood leukocytes were negative for FeLV antigens in repeated immunofluorescent antibody (IFA) tests over a two-week period using a fixed-cell IFA test. Regression of LSA was determined by clearance of lymphoblasts from the blood, when present, or by reduction of the proportion of bone marrow lymphocytes to 20% and the absence of lymphoblasts. On the basis of these criteria, nine cats were determined to have cleared their viremia and to have regressed their LSA. Two other cats regressed their LSA but remained persistently viremic, and the remaining five cats failed to respond to either FeLV clearance or tumor regression. Most responses observed were long-term, with several responder cats remaining free of FeLV infection and in complete tumor remission for several years (one cat for more than four years). Five of the 16 cats received 250 or 300 rads of whole-body irradiation prior to extracorporeal immunoadsorption. Two of these cats were long-term survivors that remained LSA- and FeLV-free (F. R. Jones et al., 1980). It appears that whole-body irradiation neither positively nor negatively affected the outcome of the disease.

Current studies are concerned with determining what parameters distinguish responder and nonresponder cats, since this would help in determining, prior to therapy, how many treatments may be necessary to achieve FeLV clearance and/or LSA regression. In a retrospective analysis of three responder cats, one cat cleared the viremia after 14 treatments, while a second cat required 22 treatments, and a third cat needed 45 treatments (Snyder et al., 1984). Three other cats, given 14, 19, and 22 treatments, failed to clear their infections. These results led to a search for useful prognostic indicators for the treatment.

The FeLV-LSA system is particularly amenable to immunological analysis since the biology of the virus and that of the tumor cells are rather well understood. Like other retroviuses, FeLV comprises a 60–70 S RNA genome encapsulated in a protein core, which is in turn surrounded by an envelope. The envelope consists of a basement membrane containing the virally encoded protein p15E, embedded within the membrane, and a gp70 disulfide linked to p15E (Pinter and Honnen, 1983). Viral interference and neutralization tests have shown that there are at least three groups of FeLV envelope antigens (A, B, and C), which are distinct from each other and which comprise three different subgroups of FeLV (Sarma and Log, 1971, 1973; Jarrett et al., 1973). LSA cells from all viremic cats produce FeLV of subgroup A, while LSA cells from 50% of viremic cats produce FeLV-A and -B. Mixtures of FeLV-A and -C are found only in 1% of viremic cats. FeLV-B and -C are never found in the absence of FeLV-A under natural conditions (Sarma and Log, 1971, 1973; Jarrett et al., 1973; Hardy et al., 1976). Recently, antigens related to the envelope glycoprotein of FeLV-C were detected on all feline LSA cells, including those which were not producing infectious FeLV-C particles (Kedbrat et al., 1983; Snyder et al., 1983). These proteins were subsequently determined to be variants of FeLV-C gp70 that carry the antigenic determinants of the FeLV-specific cell membrane antigen (FOCMA) (Snyder et al., 1983). Despite the antigenic complexity of the FeLV-LSA system, the antibody responses to each of the above antigens can be monitored independently of the others (Snyder et al., 1983). Thus, the FeLV and FOCMA antibody responses can be determined in viremic cats subjected to extracorporeal immunoadsorption treatments (F. R. Jones et al., 1984; Snyder et al., 1984).

A quantitative analysis was performed to determine the levels of peripheral-blood-leukocyte-associated viral antigens, soluble viral antigens, FeLV-specific and FOCMA-specific antibodies, and FeLV-antigen-containing CIC in cats with different responses to the extracorporeal immunoadsorption treatments (F. R. Jones *et al.*, 1984; Snyder *et al.*, 1984). It was found that cats that responded by both clearance of FeLV infection and complete LSA regression developed antibodies to both the viral envelope protein gp70 and FOCMA during the course of treatments. No antibody responses to gp70 or FOCMA were found in cats that did not respond to LSA regression or FeLV clearance.

Serum antibodies in regressor cats were cytotoxic for several established LSA cell lines grown in culture and tested in the presence of complement (F. R. Jones *et al.*, 1984). This is significant because at least part of the antitumor effect of these antibodies may be due to complement-dependent cell lysis (Grant *et al.*, 1977). The cytolytic antibody response was observed in all cats that regressed their LSA following treatment, whether or not they also cleared their FeLV infection.

The antiviral response was studied in detail. Between 15 and 45 days after initiation of extracorporeal immunoadsorption with SAC, all cats had transient decreases in the proportion of FeLV-antigen-positive peripheral blood leukocytes. These fluctuations were observed over varying periods of time prior to the time points when some of the cats became consistently FeLV-negative. In some cats, FeLV antigen remained associated with bone marrow leukocytes or platelets for a certain time period after the blood leukocytes became negative. A good correlation was observed between quantitative levels of circulating gp70-related antigen in serum and the presence of cell-associated virus. In responder cats, all the blood and bone marrow leukocytes and platelets became consistently FeLV-negative and the gp70 antigen levels in serum became undetectable.

Low titers (1:10–1:20) of antibodies to gp70 in serum of responder cats were first detected at times when FeLV antigens were beginning to be cleared from blood leukocytes, and higher titers (1:40–1:80) were found in samples taken after the blood leukocytes became persistently FeLV-negative. There was a direct negative relationship between the levels of soluble antigen and antibody in serum (Snyder *et al.*, 1984).

In order to determine whether the induced antibodies were involved in clarifying at least a portion of the viral antigens, a quantitative method for measuring FeLV-specific CIC was developed (Snyder *et al.*, 1982), since it had become evident that the levels of total complement-fixing IC, as measured in the Raji cell radioimmunoassay (Day *et al.*, 1980) did not correlate with the levels of viral antigen and antibody in the sera of responder cats. The new assay demonstrated elevated levels of FeLV-IC until all detectable circulating viral antigen had disappeared from the serum. It was interesting to note that in one cat, in which treatment did not lead to clearance of virus, there was significant increase in the levels of FeLV-IC over time after initiation of treatment. This suggests that there was some stimulation of the antibody response and, possibly, that further treatment might also have led to viral clearance in that cat. Whether anti-FOCMA antibodies are involved in the clearance of tumor antigen after cell lysis is less clear, although IC-containing FOCMA proteins have been detected in the plasma of a treated LSA cat (F. R. Jones, H. W. Snyder, Jr., *et al.*, unpublished data).

There are many possible explanations of the antitumor and antiviral responses seen after extracorporeal immunoadsorption, and the actual mechanism may be a combination of several reactions (Table I). For example, a reduction in the concentration of IC in the plasma combined with a nonspecific stimulation of the immune response by protein A (or a contaminant of it) may result in an enhanced immune response against a particular antigen; the immune response may be stimulated by the induction of interferon formation and by complement activation, two events that have been detected after injection of protein A (Sjöquist and Stalenheim, 1969; Stalenheim *et al.,* 1972; Catalona *et al.,* 1981; Smith *et al.,* 1983). There is, indeed, some evidence for the release of protein A and/or other biologically active molecules from the columns used for treatment, and such molecules may enter the host and stimulate an immune response (Balint and Jones, 1983). Recent studies by Harper *et al.* (1985) suggest, however, that administration of purified protein A alone by intravenous infusion is not as effective as extracorporeal immunoadsorption. Of 15 FeLV-infected cats with LSA that were infused with protein A, five cats achieved complete or partial tumor remission, but in only one of these was the remission long-lasting (21 months), and none of the cats had any measurable antiviral response. This suggests that the removal of some molecules from plasma (e.g., IC), or some other event that takes place in the immunoadsorbent column, is necessary for the treatment to lead to long-lasting results. One may speculate that the *ex vivo* adsorption favorably triggers some tightly regulated feedback mechanism.

Table I. Extracorporeal Immunoadsorption with SAC: Possible Explanations of Therapeutic Benefits

Partial removal of "blocking factors"
  Reduction of circulating tumor antigens complexed with antibody
  Reduction of suppressor factors (which are immunologically specific or nonspecific)
Release of protein A
  Activation of the complement system
  Blast transformation of B and T lymphocytes
  Polyclonal activation of antibody synthesis
  Potentiation of natural killer cell activity
  Induction of interferon synthesis
  Rapid clearing of IC following introduction of protein A
Release of endotoxin
  Stimulation of immune response
  Hemorrhagic necrosis of tumor

VIII. EXTRACORPOREAL IMMUNOADSORPTION TREATMENTS OF AIDS-LIKE SYNDROMES

Acquired immune deficiency syndrome (AIDS) has been recently described. It is most frequent among homosexual males (Jaffae *et al.*, 1983). AIDS patients have profound cellular immunodeficiency, which is characterized by a marked decrease of helper T cells and a low helper to suppressor T-cell ratio, a decreased lymphocyte response to mitogens, subcutaneous anergy, high levels of CIC, antilymphocyte antibodies, and hypergammaglobulinemia (Schroff *et al.*, 1983; Groopman *et al.*, 1983; J. F. Jones *et al.*, 1983; Kiprov and Morand, 1982; Kiprov *et al.*, 1983, 1984). These abnormalities are believed to be responsible for the multiple opportunistic infections (particularly *Pneumocystis*) and malignancies (particularly Kaposi's sarcoma) that are common in this patient group (Groopman *et al.*, 1983). There is no effective treatment and the mortality rate is high.

It is of interest, therefore, that Kiprov *et al.* (1984) have observed some clinical responses against Kaposi's sarcoma in a patient treated with extracorporeal immunoadsorption using a protein A column on three occasions over a 7-day period. Three liters of plasma were perfused during each procedure. Twenty-five percent of the skin lesions showed a measurable decrease in size, central necrosis, and an erythematous halo after the second treatment, and there was healing of a large confluent ulcerated lesion on the right tibia. Microscopic examination of the lesions revealed a decrease of tumor cell density and collagen accumulation. Deposition of C3 in the tumors was observed using immunohistological techniques. The treatment was also found to be associated with decreased levels of IgG, IC, and antilymphocyte antibodies. Three days after the last perfusion, the level of IC increased and the patient died from his disease.

Our understanding of AIDS would improve if a good animal model were available. Thus far, it has not been possible to transmit AIDS to nonhuman primates or laboratory animals. We believe, however, that there are two possible naturally occurring syndromes that could serve as animal models for human AIDS, namely a FeLV-induced immunosuppression syndrome in pet cats, which could be called "FAIDS," and an AIDS-like disease in Simian monkeys ("SAIDS"), which is associated with a transmissible lymphoma.

There are numerous similarities between FeLV-induced immunosuppression in cats and human AIDS. Both syndromes are characterized by lymphopenia, reduced lymphocyte responses to mitogens and allogenic cells, cutaneous anergy, impaired antibody response, and secondary opportunistic infections (Anderson *et al.*, 1971; Perryman *et al.*, 1972; Mathes *et al.*, 1978; Hardy, 1980; Trainen *et al.*, 1983). The feline syndrome is caused by FeLV, which is a retrovirus with T-cell tropism. There is recent evidence suggesting that some human AIDS patients may be infected with HTLV, a human T-cell tropic retrovirus (Essex *et al.*, 1983; Gelmann *et al.*, 1983; Gallo *et al.*, 1983; Barré-Sinoussi *et al.*, 1983), thus furthering the analogy.

SAIDS is a disease in monkeys that has been detected at two different primate centers. It presents a remarkable facsimile to AIDS in its epidemiological, clinical, immunological, and pathological features (Letvin *et al.*, 1983; Hunt *et al.*, 1983; Hendrikson *et al.*, 1983; Gravell *et al.*, 1984). It is readily transmitted to monkeys by either cage contact or injection of tissue homogenates, whole blood, or filtered plasma (Hunt *et al.*, 1983; Gravell *et al.*, 1984). The experimentally induced disease is essentially identical to human AIDS, including the occurrence of Kaposi's-sarcoma-like skin lesions (Hunt *et al.*, 1983; Gravell *et al.*, 1984). The causative agent is, as yet, undetermined. Gravell *et al.* (1984) observed that the transmissible agent was small, according to filtration experiments with blood and plasma, and concluded that it was probably a virus; however, no virus has been isolated in preliminary attempts by standard cell culture techniques.

IX. CONCLUSIONS

Most tumors grow progressively even when they express tumor-specific antigens that are recognized by the host and that can, under favorable circumstances, induce tumor rejection. Circulating antigen released from the tumor, alone and in the form of IC, can inhibit ("block") the development of an otherwise effective tumor immunity. This inhibition appears to be primarily the result of a suppressor cell response, and circulating suppressor factors with tumor antigen specificity seem to be important mediators of that response.

A seemingly straightforward approach to cancer therapy is to physically remove (some of) those circulating factors that inhibit the development of an effective antitumor immunity. Extracorporeal immunoadsorption of plasma on protein A from SAC has been introduced for this purpose and has been performed with the primary intention of removing IC. The data are most clear-cut in cats with FeLV-associated lymphosarcoma, in which there is a correlation between decreased levels of IC, increased levels of antitumor antibodies, and clinical benefit. Although some provocative results have been obtained in man, the value of extracorporeal immunoadsorption for the treatment of human cancer remains to be established.

The mechanisms responsible for the beneficial effects sometimes observed following *ex vivo* plasma adsorption need to be further investigated. Possible explanations include removal of IC and/or suppressor factors, and the introduction into the tumor-bearing individual of some immunomodulating agent, such as protein A or endotoxin, leaking from the immunoadsorbent columns during use. These mechanisms may be best approached in animal models like FeLV-LSA, in which immunological reagents are available, and by selecting those types of human malignancies in which some information can be gained about circulating antigens and antibodies (AIDS patients with Koposi's sarcoma and leukemic patients with HTLV infection may fit into this category).

ACKNOWLEDGMENTS

This work has been supported in part by grants from the National Institutes of Health to K.E.H. (CA 19148), F.R.J. (CA 36678), and H.W.S. (CA 16599, CA 24357). The work of H.W.S., J.P.B., and F.R.J. was also supported by grants from Imré Corporation and the Cancer Research Institute, Inc. H.W.S. is a Scholar of the Leukemia Society of America. We thank Lois H. Yoshida for excellent assistance with this project and Phyllis Harps for expert typing of the manuscript.

X. REFERENCES

Amlot, P., Pussel, B., Slaney, J. M., and Williams, B. D., 1978, Correlation between immune complexes and prognostic factors in Hodgkin's disease, *Clin. Exp. Immunol.* **31**:166.

Anderson, L. J., Jarrett, W. F. H., Jarrett, O., and Laird, H. M., 1971, Feline leukemia virus infection of kittens: Mortality associated with atrophy of the thymus and lymphoid depletion, *J. Natl. Cancer Inst.* **44**:339.

Asherson, G. L., and Zembala, M., 1976, Suppressor T-cells in cell mediated immunity, *Br. Med. Bull.* **32**:158.

Baldwin, R. W., and Robins, R. A., 1977, Induction of tumor-immune responses and their interaction with the developing tumor, in: *Contemporary Topics in Molecular Immunology*, Vol. 6 (R. R. Porter and G. L. Ada., eds.), pp. 177–207, Plenum Press, New York.

Baldwin, R. W., Price, M. R., and Robins, R. A., 1972, Blocking of lymphocyte-mediated cytotoxicity for rat hepatoma cells by tumor-specific antigen–antibody complexes, *Nature New Biol.* **238**:185.

Baldwin, R. W. Price, M. R., and Robins, R. A., 1973, Inhibition of hepatoma-immune lymph node cell cytotoxicity by tumor-bearer serum, and solubilized hepatoma antigen, *Int. J. Cancer* **11**:527.

Balint, J., Jr., 1982, Immune complexes with antiglobulin activity in sera of Moloney sarcoma bearing rats, *Clin. Exp. Immunol.* **48**:70.

Balint, J., Jr., and Jones, F. R., 1983, Perfusion of canine serum over *Staphylococcus aureus* Cowan I: Evidence for release of protein A and changes in specific antibody activity, *Immunol. Commun.* **12**:573.

Bansal, S. C., Bansal, B. R., Thomas, H. L., Siegel, P. D., Shoads, J. E., Cooper, D. R., Terman, D. S., and Mark, R., 1978, *Ex vivo* removal of serum IgG in a patient with colon carcinoma, *Cancer* **42**:1.

Barré-Sinoussi, F., Chermann, J. C., Rey, F., Nugeyre, M. T., Chamaret, S., Gruest, J., Daugnet, C., Axler-Blin, C., Vezinet-Brun, F., Rouzioux, C., Rozenbau, W., and Montagnier,

1983, Isolation of a T-lymphotropic retrovirus from a patient at risk for acquired immune deficiency syndrome (AIDS), *Science* 220:868.

Bensinger, W. I., Kinet, J. B., Hennen, G., Franckenne, F., Schaus, C., Saint-Remy, M., Hoyoux, P., and Mahieu, P., 1982, Plasma perfused over immobilized protein A for breast cancer, *N. Engl. J. Med.* 306:935.

Berke, G., 1980, Interaction of cytotoxic T lymphocytes and target cells, *Prog. Allergy* 27:69.

Brandeis, W. E., Nelson, L., Wang, Y., Good, R. A., and Day, N. K., 1978, Circulating immune complexes in sera of children with neuroblastoma: Correlation with stage of disease, *J. Clin. Invest.* 62:1201.

Catalona, W. T., Ratliff, T. L., and McCool, R. E., 1981, Gamma interferon induced by *S. aureus* protein A augments NK and ADCC, *Nature* 291:77.

Carpenter, J. L., and Holzworth, J., 1971, Treatment of leukemia in the cat, *J. Am. Vet. Med. Assoc.* 158:1130.

Carpentier, N. A., Fiere, D. M., Schuh, D., Ghislaine, T., Lange, T. A., and Lambert, P.-H., 1982, Circulating immune complexes and the prognosis of acute myeloid leukemia, *N. Engl. J. Med.* 307:1174.

Cerrotini, J.-C., and Brunner, K. T., 1974. Cell-mediated cytotoxicity, allograft rejection and tumor immunity, *Adv. Immunol.* 18:67.

Cory, J., Nelson, K., Forstrom, J. W., Hellström, I., and Hellström, K. E., 1981, A T cell hybridoma suppressor factor which binds tumor antigen, in: *Monoclonal Antibodies and T-Cell Hybridomas* (G. J. Hammerling, U. Hammerling, and J. F. Kearney, eds.), pp. 503–508, Elsevier/North-Holland, Amsterdam.

Cotter, S. M., Essex, M., McLane, M. F., Grant, C. K., and Hardy, W. D., Jr., 1980, Chemotherapy and passive immunotherapy in naturally occurring feline mediastinal lymphoma, in: *Feline Leukemia Virus* (W. D. Hardy, Jr., M. Essex, and A. J. McClelland, eds.), pp. 219–225, Elsevier/North-Holland, New York.

Day, N. K., O'Reilly-Felice, C., Hardy, W. D., Jr., Good, R. A., and Withkin, S. S., 1980, Circulating immune complexes associated with naturally occurring lymphosarcoma in pet cats, *J. Immunol.* 125:2363.

Daynes, R. A., and Spellman, C. W., 1977, Evidence for the generation of suppressor cells by ultraviolet radiation, *Cell. Immunol.* 31:182.

Dorn, C. R., Taylor, D. O. N., and Hubbard, H. H., 1967, Epizootiologic characteristics of canine and feline leukemia and lymphosarcoma, *Am. J. Vet. Res.* 28:993.

Enker, W. E., and Jacobitz, J. L., 1980, *In vivo* splenic irradiation eradicates suppressor T cells causing the regression and inhibition of established tumor, *Int. J. Cancer* 25:819.

Essex, M., 1980, Feline leukemia and sarcoma viruses, in: *Viral Oncology* (G. Klein, ed.), pp. 205–229, Raven Press, New York.

Essex, M., Sliski, A., Cotter, S. M., Jakowski, R. M., and Hardy, W. D., Jr., 1975, Immunosurveillance of naturally occurring feline leukemia, *Science* 190:790.

Essex, M., Sliski, A., Cotter, S. M., and Hardy, W. D., Jr., 1976, The immune response to leukemia virus and tumor-associated antigen in cats, *Cancer Res.* 36:640.

Essex, M., McLane, M. F., Lee, T. H., Folk, L., Howe, C. W. S., Mullins, J. I., Cabradillo, C., and Frances, D. P., 1983, Antibodies to cell membrane antigens associated with T-cell leukemia virus in patients with AIDS, *Science* 220:859.

Fisher, M. S., and Kripke, M. L., 1982, Suppressor T lymphocytes control the development of primary skin cancers in ultraviolet irradiated mice, *Science* 216:1133.

Forsgren, A., and Sjöquist, J., 1966, Protein A from *S. aureus:* I. Pseudo-immune reactions with human gamma globulin, *J. Immunol.* 97:822.

Forstrom, J. W., Nelson, K. A., Nepom, G. T., Hellström, I., and Hellström, K. E., 1983, Immunization to a syngeneic sarcoma by a monoclonal antiidiotypic antibody, *Nature* 303:627.

Fujimoto, S., and Tada, T., 1978, I Region expression on cytotoxic and suppressor T cells against syngeneic tumors in the mouse, in: *Cancer Immunotherapy and Its Immunological Basis* (Y. Yamamura, M. Kitagawa, and I. Azuma, eds.), pp. 11–20, University Park Press, Baltimore, Maryland.

Gallo, R. C., Sarin, P. S., Gelmann, E. P., Robert-Guroff, M., Richardson, E., Kalyanaraman, V. S., Mann, D., Sidhu, G. D., Stahl, R. E., Zolla-Pazner, S., Liebowitch, I., and Popovic, M., 1983, Isolation of a human T cell leukemia virus in acquired immune deficiency syndrome (AIDS), *Science* **220:**865.

Gelmann, E. P., Popovic, M., Blayney, D., Masur, H., Sidhu, G., Stahl, R. E., and Gallo, R. C., 1983, Proviral DNA of a retrovirus, human T-cell leukemia virus, in two patients with AIDS, *Science* **220:**862.

Gershon, R. K., 1974, T cell control of antibody production, in: *Contemporary Topics in Immunobiology*, Vol. 3 (M. D. Cooper and N. L. Warner, eds.), pp. 1–40. Plenum Press, New York.

Gershon, R. K., Carter, R. L., and Kondo, K., 1967, On concomitant immunity in tumor-bearing hamsters, *Nature* **213:**674.

Gershon, R. K., Mokyr, M. B., and Mitchell, M. S., 1974, Activation of suppressor T cells by tumor cells and specific antibody, *Nature* **250:**594.

Gordon, B. R., Matus, R. E., Saal, S. D., MacEwen, E. G., Hurwitz, A., Stengel, K. H., and Rugin, A. L., 1983, Protein A independent tumoricidal responses in dogs after extracorporeal perfusion of plasma over *Staphylococcus aureus*, *J. Natl. Cancer Inst.* **70:** 1127.

Grant, C. K., DeBoer, D. J., Essex, M., Worley, M. B., and Higgins, J., 1977, Antibodies from healthy cats exposed to feline leukemia virus lyse feline lymphoma cells slowly with cat complement, *J. Immunol.* **119:**401.

Gravell, M., London, W. T., Houff, S. A., Madden, D. L., Dalakas, M. C., Sever, J. L., Osborn, K. G., Maul, D. H., Hendrickson, R. V., Manx, P. A., Lerche, N. W., Prahalada, S., and Gardner, M. B., 1984, Transmission of simian acquired immunodeficiency syndrome (SAIDS) with blood or filtered plasma, *Science* **233:**74.

Greene, M. L., 1980, The genetic and cellular basis for regulation of the immune response to tumor antigens, in: *Contemporary Topics in Immunobiology*, Vol. 11 (N. L. Warner, ed.), pp. 81–116, Plenum Press, New York.

Greene, M. L., Dorf, M. E., Pierres, M., and Benacerraf, B., 1977, Reduction of syngeneic tumor growth by an anti-IJ-antiserum, *Proc. Natl. Acad. Sci. USA* **74:**5118.

Groopman, J. D., Weinstein, W. M., Fahey, J. L., and Detels, R., 1983, The acquired immunodeficiency syndrome, *Ann. Intern. Med.* **99:**208.

Gupta, R. K., Leitch, A. M., and Morton, D. L., 1983, Nature of antigens and antibodies in immune complexes isolated by Staphylococcal protein A from plasma of melanoma patients, *Cell Immunol. Immunother.* **16:**40.

Gutterman, J. U., 1977, The C1q binding test for soluble immune complexes: Clinical correlations obtained in patients with cancer, *J. Natl. Cancer Inst.* **58:**1205.

Hardy, W. D., Jr., 1980, Feline leukemia virus disease, in: *Feline Leukemia Virus* (W. D. Hardy, Jr., M. Essex, and A. J. McClelland, eds.), pp. 3–31, Elsevier/North-Holland, New York.

Hardy, W. D., Jr., Hirshaut, Y., and Hess, P., 1973, Detection of the feline leukemia virus and other mammalian oncornaviruses by immunofluorescence, in: *Unifying Concepts of Leukemia* (R. M. Dutcher, and L. Chieco-Bianchi, eds.), pp. 778–799, Karger, Basel.

Hardy, W. D., Jr., Hess, P. W., MacEwen, E. G., Hayes, A., Kassel, R. L., Day, N., and Old, L. J., 1975, Treatment of feline lymphosarcoma with feline blood constituents, in *Comparative Leukemia Research* (J. Clemmesen and D. S. Yohn, eds.), pp. 518–521, Karger, Basel.

Hardy, W. D., Jr., Hess, P. W., MacEwen, E. G., McClelland, A. J., Zuckerman, E. E., Essex,

M., Cotter, S. M., and Jarrett, O., 1976, Biology of the feline leukemia virus in the natural environment, *Cancer Res.* 36:582.

Hardy, W. D., Jr., McClelland, A. J., MacEwen, E. G., Hess, P. W., Hayes, A. A., and Zuckerman, E. E., 1977, The epidemiology of feline leukemia virus (FeLV), *Cancer* 39:1850.

Harper, H. D., Sjöquist, J., Hardy, W. D., Jr., and Jones, F. R., 1985, Antitumor activity of protein A administered intravenously to pet cats with leukemia or lymphosarcoma, *Cancer* (in press).

Hayami, M., Hellström, I., Hellström, K. E., and Yamanouchi, K., 1972, Cell-mediated destruction of Rous' sacomas in Japanese quails, *Int. J. Cancer* 10:507.

Heimer, R., and Klein, G., 1976, Circulating immune complexes in sera of patients with Burkitt's lymphoma and nasopharyngeal carcinoma, *Int. J. Cancer* 18:310.

Hellström, I., 1967, A colony inhibition (CI) technique for demonstration of tumor cell destruction by lymphoid cells *in vitro, Int. J. Cancer* 2:65.

Hellström, I., and Hellström, K. E., 1969, Studies in cellular immunity and its serum mediated inhibition in Moloney virus induced mouse sarcomas, *Int. J. Cancer* 4:587.

Hellström, I., and Hellström, K. E., 1970, Colony inhibition studies on blocking and nonblocking serum effects on cellular immunity to Moloney sarcomas, *Int. J. Cancer* 5:195.

Hellström, I., and Hellström, K. E., 1971, Colony inhibition and cytotoxicity assays, in: *In Vitro Methods in Cell-Mediated Immunity* (B. R. Bloom and P. R. Glade, eds.), pp. 409–414, Academic Press, New York.

Hellström, I., Hellström, K. E., and Pierce, G., 1968, *In vitro* studies of immune reactions against autochthonous and syngeneic mouse tumors induced by methylcholanthrene and plastic discs, *Int. J. Cancer* 3:467.

Hellström, I., Hellström, K. E., Evans, C. A., Heppner, G., Pierce, G. E., and Yang, J. P. S., 1969, Serum mediated protection of neoplastic cells from inhibition by lymphocytes immune to their tumor specific antigens, *Proc. Natl. Acad. Sci. USA* 62:362.

Hellström, I., Hellström, K. E., and Sjögren, H. O., 1970, Serum mediated inhibition of cellular immunity to methylcholanthrene induced murine sarcomas, *Cell. Immunol.* 1:18.

Hellström, I., Hellström, K. E., and Bernstein, I. D., 1979, Tumor enhancing suppressor activator T cells in spleens and thymuses of tumor immune mice, *Proc. Natl. Acad. Sci. USA* 76:52.

Hellström, I., Hellström, K. E., and Nelson, K., 1983, Antigen-specific suppressor ("blocking") factors in tumor immunity, in: *Biomembranes*, Vol. 11: *Pathological Membranes* (A. Nowotny, ed.), pp. 365–388, Plenum Press, New York.

Hellström, K. E., and Brown, J. P., 1979, Tumor antigens, in: *The Antigens* (M. Sela, ed.), pp. 1–82, Academic Press, New York.

Hellström, K. E., and Hellström, I., 1970, Immunological enhancement as studied by cell culture techniques, *Annu. Rev. Microbiol.* 24:373.

Hellström, K. E., and Hellström, I., 1974, Lymphocyte-mediated cytotoxicity and blocking serum activity to tumor antigens, in: *Advances in Immunology*, Vol. 18 (F. J. Dixon, ed.), pp. 209–277, Academic Press, New York.

Hellström, K. E., and Hellström, I., 1978, Evidence that tumor antigens enhance tumor growth *in vivo* by interacting with a radiosensitive (suppressor?) cell population, *Proc. Natl. Acad. Sci. USA* 75:436.

Hellström, K. E., and Hellström, I., 1979, Enhancement of tumor outgrowth by tumor-associated blocking factors, *Int. J. Cancer* 23:336.

Hellström, K. E., and Hellström, I., 1981a, Cell-mediated suppression of tumor immunity has a nonspecific component. I. Evidence from transplantation tests, *Int. J. Cancer* 27:481.

Hellström, K. E., and Hellström, I., 1981b, Does perfusion with treated plasma cure cancer? *N. Engl. J. Med.* 305:1215.

Hellström, K. E., and Möller, G., 1965, Immunological and immunogenetic aspects of tumor transplantation, *Prog. Allergy* 9:158.

Hellström, K. E., Hellström, I., and Nepom, J. T., 1977, Specific blocking factors—are they important? *Biochim. Biophys. Acta* 473:121.

Hellström, K. E., Hellström, I., Kant, J. A., and Tamerius, J. D., 1978, Regression and inhibition of sarcoma growth by interference with a radiosensitive T cell population, *J. Exp. Med.* 148:799.

Hendrickson, R. V., Maul, D. H., Osborn, K. G., Sever, J. L., Madden, D. L., Ellingsworth, L. R., Anderson, J. H., Lowenstine, L., and Gardner, M. D., 1983, Evidence of acquired immunodeficiency in Rhesus monkeys, *Lancet* 1:388.

Heppner, G. H., 1969, Studies on serum-mediated inhibition of cellular immunity to spontaneous mouse mammary tumor, *Int. J. Cancer* 4:608.

Hersey, P., Edwards, A., Adams, E., Hoister, J., Murray, E., Biggs, J., and Milton, G. W., 1976, Antibody-dependent, cell-mediated cytotoxicity against melanoma cells induced by plasmapheresis, *Lancet* 1:825.

Hewitt, H. B., Blake, E. R., and Walder, A. S., 1976, A critique of the evidence for active host defense against cancer based on personal studies of 27 tumors of spontaneous origin, *Br. J. Cancer* 33:241.

Hofken, H., Meredith, I. D., Robins, R. A., Baldwin, R. W., Davies, C. J., and Blamey, R. W., 1978, Immune complexes and prognosis of human breast cancer, *Lancet* 1:672.

Holohan, T. V., Phillips, T. M., and Bowles, C., 1982, Regression of canine mammary carcinoma after immunoadsorption therapy, *Cancer Res.* 42:3663.

Hunt, R. D., Blake, B. J., Chalifoux, L. V., Sehgal, P. K., King, N. W., and Letvin, N. L., 1983, Transmission of naturally occurring lymphoma in macaque monkeys, *Proc. Natl. Acad. Sci. USA* 80:5085.

Isbister, W. H., Noonan, F. P., Halliday, W. J., and Clunie, G., 1975, Human thoracic duct cannulation: Manipulation of tumor-specific blocking factors in a patient with malignant melanoma, *Cancer* 35:1465.

Israel, L., Edelstein, R., Mannoni, P., and Radot, E., 1977, Plasmapheresis in patients with disseminated cancer. Clinical results and correlation with changes in serum proteins, *Cancer* 40:3145.

Jaffe, H. W., Choi, K., Thomas, P. A., Haverkos, H. W., Auerbach, D. M., Guinan, M. E., Rogers, M. F., Spira, T. J., Darrow, W. W., Kramer, M. A., Friedman, S. M., Monroe, J. M., Friedman-Kien, A. E., Laubenstein, L. J., Marmor, M., Safai, B., Dritz, S. K., Crispi, S. J., Fannin, S. L., Orkwis, J. P., Kelter, A., Rushing, W. R., Thacker, S. B., and Curran, J. W., 1983, National case–control study of Kaposi's sarcoma and *Pneumocystis carinii* pneumonia in homosexual men: Part I, Epidemiological results, *Ann. Intern. Med.* 99:145.

Jarrett, O., Laird, H. M., and Hay, D., 1973, Determinants of the host range of feline leukemia viruses, *J. Gen. Virol.* 20:169.

Jennette, J. C., and Feldman, J. D., 1977, Sequential quantitation of circulating immune complexes in syngeneic and allogeneic rats bearing Moloney sarcomas, *J. Immunol.* 118:2269.

Jones, F. R., 1978, *In vivo* studies of the mechanisms underlying enhancement and the reversal of tumor growth in mice employing X-irradiation and adoptive transfer of lymphoid cells, Ph.D. thesis, University of Washington, Seattle.

Jones, F. R., Yoshida, L. H., Ladiges, W. C., and Kenney, M. A., 1980, Treatment of feline leukemia and reversal of FeLV by *ex vivo* removal of IgG: A preliminary report, *Cancer* 46:675.

Jones, F. R., Grant, C. K., and Snyder. H. W., Jr., 1984, Lymphosarcoma and persistent FeLV infection of pet cats: A system to study responses during extracorporeal treatments, *J. Biol. Resp. Modif.* 3:286.

Jones, J. F., Minnich, L. M., Lucas, D. O., Fulginiti, V. A., Ingham, Z., Langford, M. P., and Stanton, G. J., 1983, Serum interferon in Navajo children with severe combined immunodeficiency disease inhibits lymphoblastogenesis, *J. Clin. Immunol.* 3:14.

Kaliss, N., 1958, Immunological enhancement of tumor homografts in mice: A recent review, *Cancer Res.* 18:992.

Kall, M. A., Hellström, I., and Hellström, K. E., 1975, Different responses of lymphoid cells from tumor-bearing as compared to tumor-immunized mice when sensitized to tumor specific antigens *in vitro, Proc. Natl. Acad. Sci. USA* 72:5086.

Katz, D. H., 1977, *Lymphocyte Differentation, Recognition, and Regulation,* Academic Press, New York.

Kedbrat, S. S., Rasheed, S., Lutz, H., Gonda, M. A., Ruscetti, S., Gardner, M. B., and Prensky, W., 1983, Feline oncornavirus-associated cell membrane antigen: A viral and not a cellularly coded transformation-specific antigen of cat lymphomas, *Virology* 124:445.

Kessler, S. W., 1975, Rapid isolation of antigens from cells with a staphylococcal protein A antibody adsorbent: Parameters of the interaction of antibody–antigen complexes, *J. Immunol.* 115:1617.

Kiprov, D. D., and Morand, P., 1982, Lymphocyte subpopulations and mitogenic response studies in homosexuals with acquired immunodeficiency syndrome, *Immunobiology* 163:337.

Kiprov, D. D., Dan, P. C., and Morand, P., 1983, The effect of phasmapheresis and drug immunosuppression on T-cell subset as defined by monoclonal antibodies, *J. Clin. Apheresis* 1:57.

Kiprov, D. D., Lippert, R., Jones, F. R., Lagios, M. D., Balint, J. P., and Cohen, R. J., 1984, Extracorporeal perfusion of plasma over immobilized protein A in patient with Kaposi's sarcoma and acquired immunodeficiency, *J. Biol. Resp. Modif.* 3:341.

Klein, G., and Klein, E., 1977, Rejectability of virus-induced tumors and nonrejectability of spontaneous tumors: A lesson in contrasts, *Transplant. Proc.* 9:1095.

Klein, G., Sjögren, H. O., Klein, E., and Hellström, K. E., 1960, Demonstration of resistance against methylcholanthrene-induced sarcomas in the primary autochthonous host, *Cancer Res.* 20:2561.

Kripke, M. L., Lofgreen, J. S., Beard, J., Jessup, J. M., and Fisher, M. S., 1977, *In vivo* immune responses of mice during carcinogenesis by ultraviolet irradiation, *J. Natl. Cancer Inst.* 59:1227.

Letvin, N. L., Eaton, D. A., Aldrich, W. R., Sehgal, P. K., Blake, B. J., Schlossman, S. F., King, N. W., and Hunt, R. D., 1983, Acquired immunodeficiency syndrome in a colony of macaque monkeys, *Proc. Natl. Acad. Sci. USA* 80:2718.

McClelland, A. J., Hardy, W. D., Jr., and Zuckerman, E. E., 1980, Prognosis of healthy feline leukemia virus infected cats, in: *Feline Leukemia Virus* (W. D. Hardy, Jr., M. Essex, and A. J. McClelland, eds.), pp. 121–126, Elsevier/North-Holland, New York.

MacKintosh, F. R., Bennett, K., Schiff, S., Shields, J., and Hall, S. W., 1983, Treatment of advanced malignancy with plasma perfused over Staphylococcol protein A, *West. J. Med.* 139:36.

Mathes, L. E., Olsen, R. G., Hebebrand, L. C., Hoover, E. A., and Schaller, J. P., 1978, Abrogation of lymphocyte blastogenesis by a feline leukemia virus protein, *Nature* 274:687.

Messerschmidt, G. L., Bowles, C., and Alsaker, R., 1982a, Long-term followup of dogs with spontaneous mammary tumors treated with *ex vivo* plasma perfusion over *Staphylococcus aureus* Cowan I, *Proc. Am. Assoc. Cancer Res.* 23:279.

Messerschmidt, G., Bowles, C., Dean, D., Parker, M., Lester, R., Dowling, R., Holohan, T., Osborn, L., Schaff, B. F., McCormack, K., Corbitt, R., Phillips, T., Glasstein, E., and Deisseroth, A., 1982b, Phase II trial of *S. aureus* Cowan I immunoperfusion, *Cancer Treatment Rep.* 66:2027.

Mikulska, Z. B., Smith, C., and Alexander, P., 1966, Evidence for an immunological reaction of the host directed against its own actively growing primary tumor, *J. Natl. Cancer Inst.*, 36:29.

Miller, W. J., Branda, R. F., Hurd, D. D., Wachsman, W., Nelson, N. L., and Jacob, H. D., 1982, Protein A adsorption of acute myelogenous leukemia serum induces *in vitro* blast lysis, *Blood* 59:1344.

Möller, E., 1965, Antagonistic effects of humoral isoantibodies on the *in vitro* cytotoxicity of immune lymphoid cells, *J. Exp. Med.* 122:11.

Mulé, J. J., Hellström, I., and Hellström, K. E., 1982, Cell surface phenotypes of radio-labeled immune long-lived lymphocytes that selectively localize in syngeneic tumors, *Am. J. Pathol.* 107:142.

Naor, D., 1979, Suppressor cells: Permitters and promotors of malignancy? in: *Advances in Cancer Research*, Vol. 29 (G. Klein and S. Weinhouse, eds.), pp. 45–125, Academic Press, New York.

Nelson, K., 1975, Products of murine spleen cells that specifically modulate cell-mediated immunity to syngeneic tumor cells, Ph.D. thesis, University of Washington, Seattle.

Nelson, K., Pollack, S. B., and Hellström, K. E., 1975a, Specific anti-tumor responses by cultured immune spleen cells. I *In vitro* culture method and initial characterization of factors which block immune cell-mediated cytotoxicity *in vitro*, *Int. J. Cancer* 15:806.

Nelson, K., Pollack, S. B., and Hellström, K. E., 1975b, Specific anti-tumor responses by cultured immune spleen cells. III. Further characterization of cells which synthesize factors with blocking and antiserum dependent cellular cytotoxic (ADC) activities, *Int. J. Cancer* 16:539.

Nelson, K., Pollack, S. B., and Hellström, K. E., 1975c, *In vitro* synthesis of tumor-specific factors with blocking and antibody-dependent cellular cytotoxicity, *Int. J. Cancer* 16:932.

Nelson, K., Cory, J., Hellström, I., and Hellström, K. E., 1980, A T-T hybridoma product specifically suppresses tumor immunity, *Proc. Natl. Acad. Sci. USA* 77:2866.

Nelson, K., Hellström, I., and Hellström, K. E., 1985, Tumor antigen-specific suppressor factors made by T cell hybridomas, in: *T-Cell Hybridomas* (M. J. Taussig, ed.), pp. 129–138, CRC Press, Boca Raton, Florida.

Nepom, J. T., 1977, Serum blocking factors: Purification and properties, Ph.D. thesis, University of Washington, Seattle.

Nepom, J. T., Hellström, I., and Hellström, K. E., 1976, Purification of partial characterization of a tumor-specific blocking factor from sera of mice with growing chemically induced sarcomas, *J. Immunol.* 117:1846.

Nepom, J. T., Hellström, I., and Hellström, K. E., 1977, Antigen-specific purification of blocking factors from sera of mice with chemically induced tumors, *Proc. Natl. Acad. Sci. USA* 74:4605.

Nepom, J. T., Hellström, I., and Hellström, K. E., 1983, Suppressor mechanisms in tumor immunity, *Experientia* 39:235.

North, R. J., 1982, Cyclophosphamide facilitated adoptive immunotherapy of an established tumor depends on elimination of suppressor cells, *J. Exp. Med.* 155:1063.

Old, L. J., and Boyse, E., 1964, Immunology of experimental tumors, *Annu. Rev. Med.* 25:167.

Oldstone, M. B. A., Theofilopoulos, A. N., Gunven, P., and Klein, G., 1975, Immune complexes associated with neoplasia: Presence of Epstein–Barr virus antigen–antibody complexes in Burkitt's lymphoma, *J. Natl. Cancer Inst.* 54:223.

Paranjpe, M. S., Boone, C. W., and Takeichi, N., 1976, Specific paralysis of the anti-tumor cellular immune response produced by growing tumors studied with a radioisotope footpad assay, *Ann. N. Y. Acad. Sci.* 276:254.

Perryman, L. E., Hoover, E. A., and Yohn, D. S., 1972, Immunologic reactivity of the cat: Immunosuppression in experimental feline leukemia, *J. Natl. Cancer Inst.* **49**:1357.

Pinter, A., and Honnen, W. J., 1983, Topography of murine leukemia virus envelope protein: Characterization of transmembrane components, *J. Virol.* **46**:1056.

Prehn, R., and Main, D., 1957, Immunity to methylcholanthrene-induced sarcomas, *J. Natl. Cancer Inst.* **18**:768.

Rao, V. S., Bennett, J. A., Shen, F. W., Gershon, R. K., and Mitchell, M. S., 1980, Antigen-antibody complexes generate Lyt-1 inducers of suppressor cells, *J. Immunol.* **125**:63.

Ray, P. K., Idiculla, A., Rhoads, J. R., Jr., Bessa, E., Bassett, J. G., and Cooper, D. R., 1980a, Immunoadsorption of IgG molecules from the plasma of multiple myeloma and autoimmune hemolytic anemia patients, *Plasma Ther.* **1**:11.

Ray, P. K., Idiculla, A., Bessa, E., Idiculla, A., and Rhoads, J. E., Jr., 1980b, Efficient removal of abnormal immunoglobulin G from the plasma of a multiple myeloma patient, *Cancer* **45**:2633.

Rotter, V., and Trainin, N., 1975, Inhibition of tumor growth in syngeneic chimeric mice mediated by a depletion of suppressor T cells, *Transplantation* **20**:68.

Sarma, P. S., and Log, T., 1971, Viral interference in feline leukemia–sarcoma complex, *Virology* **44**:352.

Sarma, P. S., and Log, T., 1973, Subgroup classification of feline leukemia and sarcoma viruses by viral interferences and neutralization tests, *Virology* **54**:160.

Schroff, R. W., Gottlieb, M. S., Prince, H. E., Chai, L. L., and Fahey, J. L., 1983, Immunological studies of homosexual men with immunodeficiency and Kaposi's sarcoma, *Clin. Immunol. Immunopathol.* **27**:300.

Sjögren, H. O., 1965, Transplantation methods as a tool for detection of tumor-specific antigens, *Prog. Exp. Tumor Res.* **6**:289.

Sjögren, H. O., Hellström, I., Bansal, S. C., and Hellström, K. E., 1971, Suggestive evidence that the "blocking antibodies" of tumor-bearing individuals may be antigen-antibody complexes, *Proc. Natl. Acad. Sci. USA* **68**:1372.

Sjöquist, J., and Stalenheim, G., 1969, Protein A from *Staphylococcus aureus*. IX. Complement-fixing activity of protein A–IgG complexes, *J. Immunol.* **103**:467.

Smith, E. M., Johnson, H. M., and Blalock, J. E., 1983, *Staphylococcus aureus* protein A induces the production of alpha-interferon in human lymphocytes and alpha/beta-interferon in mouse spleen cells, *J. Immunol.* **130**:773.

Snyder, H. W., Jr., Jones, F. R., Day, N. K., and Hardy, W. D., Jr., 1982, Isolation and characterization of circulating feline leukemia virus immune complexes removed from plasma of persistently infected pet cats by *ex vivo* immunoadsorption, *J. Immunol.* **128**:2726.

Snyder, H. W., Jr., Singhal, M. C., Zuckerman, E. E., Jones, F. R., and Hardy, W. D., Jr., 1983, The feline oncornavirus-associated cell membrane antigen (FOCMA) is related to, but distinguishable from, FeLV-C gp70, *Virology* **131**:315.

Snyder, H. W., Jr., Singhal, M. C., Hardy, W. D., Jr., and Jones, F. R., 1984, Clearance of feline leukemia virus from persistently infected pet cats treated by extracorporeal immunoadsorption is correlated with an enhanced antibody response to FeLV, *J. Immunol.* **132**:1538.

Squire, R. A., and Bush, M., 1973, The therapy of canine and feline lymphosarcoma, in: *Unifying Concepts of Leukemia* (R. M. Dutcher and L. Chieco-Bianchi, eds.), pp. 189–197, Karger, Basel.

Stalenheim, G., Gotze, O., Cooper, N. R., Sjöquist, J., and Muller-Eberhard, H. J., 1972, Consumption of human complement by complexes of IgG with protein A of *Staphylococcus aureus, Immunochemistry* **10**:501.

Steele, G., Jr., Ankerst, J., and Sjögren, H. O., 1974, Alteration of *in vitro* anti-tumor activity of tumor bearer sera by adsorption with *Staphylococcus aureus* Cowan I, *Int. J. Cancer* 14:83.

Tamerius, J., Nepom, J., Hellström, I., and Hellström, K. E., 1976, Tumor-associated blocking factors: Isolation of sera of tumor-bearing mice, *J. Immunol.* 116:724.

Terman, D. S., Yamamota, Y., Mattioli, M., Cook, G., Tillquist, R., Henry, J., Poser, M. R.. and Daskal, Y., 1980a, Extensive necrosis of spontaneous canine mammary adenocarcinoma after extracorporeal perfusion over *Staphylococcus aureus* Cowan I, *J. Immunol.* 124:795.

Terman, D. S., Yamamoto, T., and Tillquist, R. L., 1980b, Tumoricidal response induced by cytosine arabinoside after plasma perfusion over protein A, *Science* 209:1257.

Terman, D. S., Young, J. B., and Shearer, W. T., 1981, Preliminary observations of the effects on breast adenocarcinoma of plasma perfusion over immobilized protein A, *N. Engl. J. Med.* 305:1195.

Theofilopoulos, A. N., and Dixon, F. J , 1980, Immune complexes in human disease, *Am. J. Pathol.* 100:531.

Theofilopoulos, A. N., Andrews, B. S., Urist, M. M., Morton, D. L., and Dixon, F. J. J., 1977, The nature of immune complexes in human cancer sera, *J. Immunol.* 199:657.

Tilkin, A. F., Schaaf, L. A., Fontaine, N., Van Acker, A., Boccadoro, M., and Urbain, J., 1981, Reduced tumor growth after low-dose irradiation or immunization against blastic suppressor cells, *Proc. Natl. Acad. Sci. USA* 78:1809.

Trainen, Z., Wenicke, D., Unger-Waron, H., and Essex, M., 1983, Suppression of the humoral antibody response in natural retrovirus infections, *Science* 220:858.

Tucker, D. F., Begent, R. H., and Hogg, N. M., 1978, Characterization of immune complexes in serum by adsorption on Staphylococcal protein A: Model studies and application to sera of rats bearing Gross virus induced lymphoma, *J. Immunol.* 121:1644.

Umiel, T., and Trainin, N., 1974, Immunological enhancement of tumor growth by syngeneic thymus-derived lymphocytes, *Transplantation* 18:244.

Vaagc, J., 1972, Specific desensitization of resistance against a syngeneic methylcholanthrene-induced sarcoma in CH3HF mice, *Cancer Res.* 32:193.

Chapter 7

Trials of Staphylococcal Protein A-Treated Plasma Infusions in Cancer Therapy: Clinical Effects and Implications for Mode of Action

F. Roy MacKintosh, Kim Bennett, and Stephen W. Hall

Department of Internal Medicine
University of Nevada School of Medicine
Reno, Nevada 89520

I. INTRODUCTION AND BACKGROUND

Protein A, a cell wall protein of some strains of *Staphylococcus aureus*, was found to bind Fc receptors of some classes of IgG from many species (Forsgren and Sjoquist, 1966; Sjoquist, 1973). Its potential role in cancer therapy arose with demonstrations of the role of immunoglobulins as blocking factors (of cell-mediated cytotoxicity) in the serum of tumor-bearing animals (Hellström *et al.*, 1969; Ankerst, 1971; Bansal *et al.*, 1972, 1976). Some feel that the blocking factor is an antigen–antibody complex (Sjögren *et al.*, 1971). Blocking activity could be demonstrated by *in vitro* cytotoxicity testing and could be removed by exposure of sera from tumor-bearing animals to *S. aureus* bearing protein A (Steele *et al.*, 1974).

These findings stimulated clinical trials of cancer therapy in animals (e.g., Terman *et al.*, 1980; Ray *et al.*, 1981; Jones *et al.*, 1980; Holohan *et al.*, 1982) and in humans (Bansal *et al.*, 1978; Ray *et al.*, 1982a; Terman *et al.*, 1981; Bensinger *et al.*, 1982; MacKintosh *et al.*, 1983b; Messerschmidt *et al.*, 1982). In some of these studies, clinically significant responses have been observed in patients with advanced carcinomas of the breast, colon, and lung, and other tumor types. Response rates in humans reported by the individual investigators have ranged from 0% (Messerschmidt *et al.*, 1982) to 60% (Terman *et al.*, 1981) in series with five or more patients. These studies have been phase I studies, and

239

it is not realistic to assess response rates in such a setting. Toxic effects have included fever, chills, hypotension, and bronchospasm. Toxicity has ranged from lethal (Messerschmidt *et al.*, 1982) to severe but manageable (Terman *et al.*, 1981; Bansal *et al.*, 1978; Ray *et al.*, 1982*a*) to moderate (MacKintosh *et al.*, 1983*b*).

There has been variation in the materials used for the *ex vivo* perfusions of plasma over protein A as well as in the volume of plasma infused and in the probable stability of the protein A preparations used for the *ex vivo* perfusions. Volumes of plasma used have ranged from an attempted total exchange (Messerschmidt *et al.*, 1982) to treatment volumes as low as 20 cc (Terman *et al.*, 1981). Materials used have been *S. aureus* itself (Bansal *et al.*, 1978; Ray *et al.*, 1982*a*), protein A complexed with collodion charcoal (Terman *et al.*, 1981), and protein A covalently linked to silica gel (Bensinger *et al.*, 1982) or to agarose (MacKintosh *et al.*, 1983*b*).

There has been only limited information regarding the immunological effects of these treatments in humans (Bansal *et al.*, 1978; Ray *et al.*, 1982*a*). However, the quantities of protein A used have never been sufficient to remove the IgG from more than about 20% of the patients' plasma even with the most aggressive protocols used, and responses have been observed with adsorptions involving a much smaller percentage of the patients' IgG.

Holohan *et al.* (1982) performed a detailed investigation of the quantitative effects of the *ex vivo* perfusions on putative blocking factors and also included important controls related to specificity of the observed effects. They treated dogs with spontaneous breast cancer with *ex vivo* perfusion of autologous plasma over protein A-bearing *S. aureus* and included additional control groups treated with perfusions without *S. aureus* and perfusions of normal plasma over *S. aureus*. The latter two treatments produced no antitumor effects. While there was a nonsignificant trend favoring response in dogs who had improved removal of purported blocking factors, it was ultimately stated by the authors that "removal of all blockers was neither a necessary nor sufficient condition for initiation of tumor regression" (Holohan *et al.*, 1982, p. 3666). Plasmapheresis should be a way to remove blocking factors regardless of their biochemical nature. It has been tested as the therapy for advanced malignancy (e.g., Israel *et al.*, 1977; Retsas *et al.*, 1981; Salinas *et al.*, 1981), but the limited results have not warranted extensive pursuit of this modality.

The possibility of a direct activation of humoral antitumor effects through protein A interactions with sera from tumor-bearing animals was suggested by Steele *et al.* (1974) and further supported by others (Miller *et al.*, 1982; MacKintosh *et al.*, 1983*a*, 1984). Steele's study was an evaluation *in vitro* of the ability of protein A to remove factors in serum that block lymphocyte-mediated cytotoxicity, and this effect was indeed demonstrated. However, when sera from tumor-bearing rodents were passed over protein A-bearing *S. aureus* capable of adsorbing about 20% of the total IgG, it was found that these treated sera had direct cytotoxicity against appropriate target cells. The effect appeared to be complement-mediated in that it was abrogated by 56°C heating for 30 min. Miller reported a series of experiments examining cytocidal effects of protein A-treated plasma against blast cells of acute myeloid leukemia (AML) (Miller et al., 1982). These studies indicated that protein A was effective whether bound to agarose or used with intact S. aureus Cowan I (SAC). The effect was specific in that it was necessary to utilize AML patient plasma to obtain cytotoxicity, the treated sera were nontoxic to normal cells, and S. aureus Wood 46 (SAW) not bearing protein A was not able to induce cytotoxicity. These investigators used amounts of protein A sufficient to adsorb 50% of the IgG present, and when larger amounts of protein A were used the effect was lost. Heating at 56°C did not eliminate toxicity in this system, but trypsin digestion did. These investigators concluded that cytotoxic antibodies were likely to be involved in tumor cell killing. A humoral mechanism for tumor regressions observed after protein A-treated plasma was infused was also raised by Terman et al. (1981). They observed substantial effects of small volumes of plasma treated with amounts of protein A inadequate to adsorb a significant percentage of the immunoglobulins present. They found no cellular inflammatory infiltrate in biopsy specimens after treatment and did find immunoglobulin and complement bound to tumor cell surfaces (Terman et al., 1980, 1981).

The concept that humoral cytotoxic activity arises from interactions of protein A with sera of specific tumor-bearing hosts is supported by in vitro and animal studies in which a variety of control sera failed to reproduce the tumoricidal effects of protein A-treated patient sera (e.g., Miller et al., 1982; Steele et al., 1974; Holohan et al., 1982). The origin of this specificity remains uncertain, although the occurrence of tumor-associated antigens and the presence of antitumor antibodies in tumor-bearing hosts may provide a basis for this specificity. The presence of immunoglobulins and complement (Terman et al., 1981) on tumor cells after but not before treatment would support the concept of a protein A-mediated interaction with serum yielding an increase in the effective titer of antitumor antibodies.

It has become clear that perfusions of plasma over protein A–collodion charcoal or SAC may leach protein A and/or other bacterial materials, which may be toxic and/or therapeutic in the patient (Ray and Bandyopadhyay, 1983). The negative results reported by investigators using SAW as a control (e.g., Steele et al., 1974; Ray et al., 1982b; Miller et al., 1982) support the concept that protein A itself is the active meterial. Holohan et al. (1982) observed no antitumor effects in control dogs who received infusions of normal plasma passed over S. aureus bearing protein A. Direct intravenous infusions of relatively pure protein A have also produced tumoricidal effects in some cases (Ray and Bandyopadhyay, 1983; Charles Bowles, personal communication, 10/17/83). However, the mechanism of these effects remains unclear. Direct toxicity of protein A for tumor cells could not be demonstrated (Ray and Bandyopadhyay, 1983). Interactions of protein A with immunoglobulins in patient plasma remian a possible explanation of these effects.

Thus a considerable amount of data from several groups of investigators supports the concept of a humoral effect dependent on interaction of protein A with sera of tumor-bearing hosts as one possible component of clinically observed tumoricidal effects. Here we review in more detail the methodology of prior studies and review our own experience in the clinical treatment of advanced malignancy with infusions of protein A-treated autologous plasma and in the generation of *in vitro* cytotoxicity in a model system.

II. METHODOLOGY

A. Clinical Trials

Patients selected for these clinical trials had advanced malignancy refractory to standard therapy and have had at least one course of chemotherapy. Informed consent is obtained according to institutional guidelines. During the trials, they receive no other systemic therapy. Patients are considered evaluable for toxicity after one infusion of treated plasma and for response after five infusions. Treatments are usually administered in an outpatient setting twice weekly until progression. For each patient, the quantity of protein A used and volume of plasma infused is gradually increased to toxicity or to maximal tolerance of repeated phlebotomy. The usual dose limit is $\frac{1}{2}$ to 1 unit of plasma passed over 30–50 mg protein A infused twice weekly. Treated plasma infusions are prepared from whole blood obtained by phlebotomy using standard blood donor sets (CPDA anticoagulant) attached to plasma transfer packs. Red blood cells are separated and reinfused. Plasma is centrifuged (30 min, 3000g, 8°C, passed over a suitable quantity of protein A-agarose (Pharmacia) at ambient temperature (20°C), and then filtered through a 0.22-μm sterile cartridge filter. The filtered plasma is collected at ice temperature and packaged in blood product administration sets. Generally, these are stored frozen (–70°C) and are thawed immediately before use by immersion in warm (37°C) water. The processing of plasma is carried out in a laminar flow tissue culture hood. The treated plasma is sterile and is nonpyrogenic in a normal volunteer. Protein A is regenerated after use by washing alternately with 0.1 M glycine-acetate (pH 3) and normal saline until absorbance (280 nm) is zero. Each patient's protein A-agarose column is stored in saline at 4°C when not in use.

As our initial intent was to perform a phase I study, it was necessary to choose an arbitrary measure of dose, as the mechanism of action of this therapy remains uncertain. We considered the "dose" at each infusion to be the product of volume (in ml of plasma) and ratio of protein A to plasma used (in mg per 100 ml plasma) in preparation of the infusion. Individual infusions varied from 35 to 7500 arbitrary units.

B. *In Vitro* Cytotoxicity Testing

We have evaluated protein A-produced cytotoxicity *in vitro* using an ovarian cancer cell line, designated MES/OV-13. This line was established in 1980 from an omental metastasis removed from a patient with ovarian adenocarcinoma (MacKintosh *et al.*, 1981). The line grows well adherent to plastic in a variety of standard culture media. We routinely use a 50/50 mix of McCoy's-Waymouth's 751 to which is added 10% newborn calf serum (NBCS). The doubling time is 16 hr. The line is mycoplasma-free, tumorigenic in nude mice, and is histologically typical of adenocarcinoma both when grown as agar colonies and in nude mice. It binds an antiovarian carcinoma antibody (Bast *et al.*, 1981).

For cytotoxicity testing, cells growing in late log phase are harvested [Hank's balanced salt solution (HBSS), pronase 0.03 mg/ml and DNase 0.003 mg/ml, 5 min, ambient temperature], washed, and suspended in HBSS with 10% NBCS. Toxic exposures are generally 1 hr at $37°C$ at 5×10^3 cells/ml, and cells are then washed twice, resuspended in culture medium at 2.5×10^3/ml with 0.3% noble agar, and plated at 0.5 ml per well in 24-well plastic plates (Costar) in triplicate. Colonies are counted manually after 7–10 days incubation ($37°C$, 5% CO_2) using an inverted microscope.

Material for portein A-activated cytotoxicity testing has been derived from ascitic fluid from two patients with ovarian carcinoma. Samples of matierials to be treated with protein A are passed over protein A bound to agarose (Pharmacia) or silica gel (Imré) at ambient temperature, collected over ice, and frozen immediately at $-70°C$. All samples to be used for a particular experiment are thawed simultaneously. The toxic exposures use materials anticoagulated by chelation, as otherwise a single-cell suspension is not maintained. Final culture media then have 20% fresh single donor human AB+ serum added.

III. RESULTS

A. Phase I Clinical Trial

Forty-four patients enrolled in phase I trials have received approximately 600 infusions of protein A-treated autologous plasma. The most relevant clinical and treatment parameters are summarized in Table I. Twenty of 44 patients experienced one or more episodes of acute toxicity associated with therapy (Table I).

Table I. Clinical Parameters of Patients in Phase I Trial[a]

History/age/sex	KPS	Sites	N	T	Resp.	T prog	Surv.	mg SPA	Arb. units	Acute toxicity	Max. vol.
1. Melanoma/38/F	70	DG	72	36	PR	34	70+	25–100	480–2600	None	135
2. Breast/65/M	60	ON	38	16	PR	14	20	12–50	385–1680	N	105
3. Paragangioma/53/F	50	LOPS	27	12	MR	12	30	5–40	100–1100	NP	120
4. Melanoma/38/F	60	HDNLC	25	11	MR	14	24	50–100	700–7500	None	250
5. Ovary/63/F	60	V	25	10	Prog	10	18+	20	300–4000	F	540
6. Salivary/34/M	90	L	22	11	S	24	30+	20–39	560–3000	None	165
7. Melanoma/35/M	70	HC	20	10	Prog	10	18	20	280–1450	None	180
8. Sarcoma/54/F	90	L	20	12	Prog	12	34+	20–40	500–2640	F	470
9. Myeloma/68/M	70	M	18	7	S	10	28	50–100	750–4000	None	155
10. Ad. lung/54/F	50	LOCH	17	8	PR	8	24	10–30	200–1000	None	80
11. Renal/64/M	40	LOS	16	7	Prog	7	9	25–100	480–3900	B	100
12. Colon/58/M	90	H	16	8	Prog	8	21	20–50	300–1250	None	70
13. Colon/43/M	90	H	16	8	Prog	8	22	15–50	260–1750	F	70
14. Breast/70/F	50	P	16	10	Prog	15	18	12–35	250–1500	FCNVDB	125
15. Sq. lung/54/M	80	L	15	8	Prog	10	29	5–50	100–2400	None	240
16. Melanoma/57/M	80	DN	15	6	Prog	6	13	50	560–4500	None	100
17. Melanoma/59/M	50	GHD	14	7	Prog	7	15+	10–36	300–2000	None	150
18. Colon/35/F	70	H	13	6	Prog	7	40	11–60	200–2000	F	125
19. Colon/43/F	50	HG	13	8	Prog	8	10	10–40	300–1050	None	100
20. Kaposi/28/M	90	D	13	8	Prog	8	8+	25	250–1942	None	230
21. Ad. lung/53/M	70	ODL	13	6	Prog	6	6+	10–30	180–1200	None	120
22. Breast/70/F	90	D	12	6	Prog	6	10+	10–24	200–600	None	400
23. Sq. lung/77/M	50	PL	12	9	PR	9+	9	5–16	200–720	FCNB	100
24. Colon/70/M	60	HL	12	6	Prog	6	8	30–50	500–3000	None	125

No. Diagnosis/Age/Sex	KPS	Sites	N	T	Resp	T prog	Surv	Arb. units	Max. vol.	Acute toxicity	mg SPA
25. Pancreas/55/M	70	HV	10	3	Prog	3	3+	20	300–550	C	100
26. Gastric/33/M	60	HN	10	5	Prog	5	12	30–100	450–3000	F	150
27. Colon/68/M	60	HL	10	3	Prog	3	5	50	850–1900	None	100
28. Sq. H&N/65/M	80	N	10	4	PR	16	27	6–16	120–750	F	110
29. Sq. lung/66/M	60	OL	10	6	S	6+	6+	12–90	200–3000	F	100
30. Breast/43/F	40	OL	9	9	Prog	12	20	2–8	85–800	F	100
31. Cervix/37/F	60	N	8	4	Prog	4	14	20–30	300–2250	None	225
32. Sq. lung/53/M	70	DO	8	4	Prog	4	16	6	100–200	FCNPV	100
33. Renal/44/M	40	DLO	6	2	Prog	2	2	12	200–1050	None	150
34. Melanoma/55/M	50	N	5	2	Prog	2	6	20–29	660–1250	None	200
35. Colon/54/F	40	HL	5	1	Prog	1	1	12–34	250–1000	F	100
36. Melanoma/63/M	40	DLO	4	2	NE	—	2	50	1150–3800	None	115
37. Breast/37/F	60	DLOH	4	2	NE	—	2	10–20	150–800	None	110
38. Colon/71/M	40	PLH	4	2	NE	—	3	20	280–740	None	140
39. Sarcoma/12/F	50	LP	3	2	NE	—	7	20	355–595	FC	85
40. Breast/42/F	40	HO	3	4	NE	—	6	4	35–95	Ca^{2+}	85
41. Ad. lung/54/M	40	LO	3	2	NE	—	2	20	400–800	Ca^{2+}	110
42. Ad. lung/30/M	20	L	2	1	NE	—	1	4	60–120	None	120
43. Sq. H&N/57/M	30	ND	2	1	NE	—	1	10	100	None	110
44. Ovary/54/F	40	V	1	1	NE	—	4	40	260	FCNV	200

[a]Abbreviations: KPS, Karnofsky performance score of beginning therapy; N, number of infusions; T, duration of therapy (weeks); Resp, best response using standard criteria; T prog, time to progression (weeks); Surv, time to death (weeks); mg SPA, range of quantities of protein A utilized in preparation of one unit of plasma; Arb. units, range of dose administered (see Section II); Max. vol., largest volume (ml) administered as a single infusion.

Acute toxicity: B, bronchospasm; C, chills; Ca^{2+}, hypercalcemia; D, diarrhea; F, fever; N, nausea; P, pain at tumor sites; V, vomiting.

Sites of disease: C, central nervous system; D, skin; G, GI tract; H, liver; L, lung; M, marrow; N, nodes; O, osseus; P, pleura; S, soft tissue mass; V, visceral mass.

Best response: PR, partial remission; MR, minor or mixed regression; S, stable; Prog, progression; NE, not evaluable by response.

Table II. Summary of Responses of Evaluable
Patients by Tumor Primary Site[a]

	N	PR	MR
Breast	4	1	0
Colon	7	0	0
Melanoma	6	1	1
Lung	6	2	0
Miscellaneous	12	1	1
	35	5	2

[a]Abbreviations: N, number of available patients; PR, partial
regression; MR, mixed or minor regression.

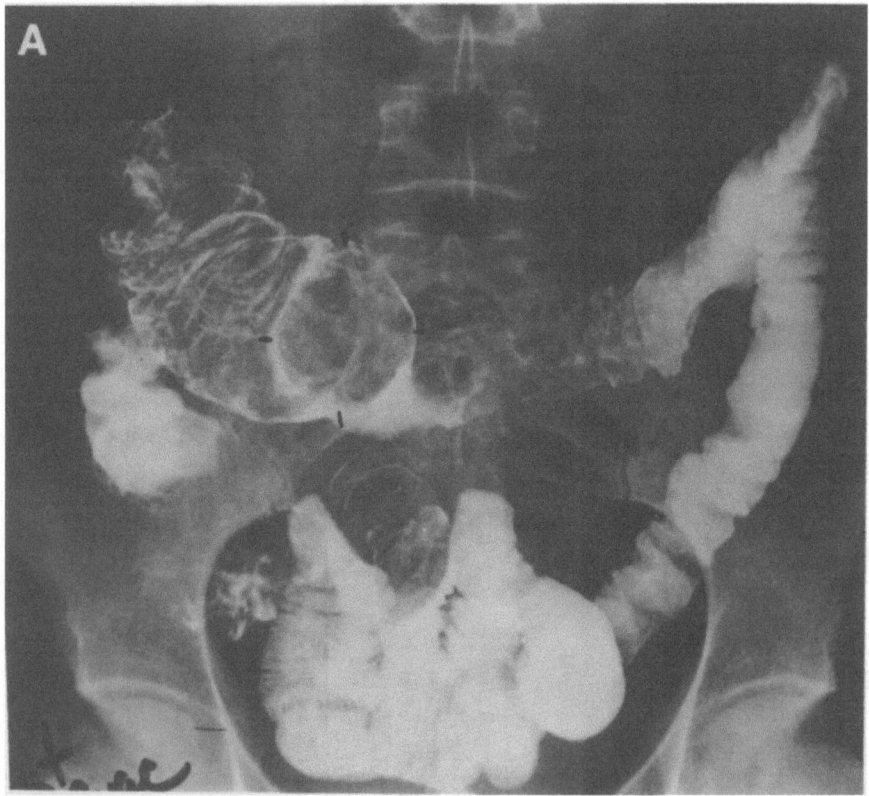

Figure 1. Barium enema examinations before (A) and 2 months after (B) patient No. 1 began
therapy with treated plasma. Initially a large mass at the hepatic flexure is causing intussus-

There were no deaths attributed to therapy and no significant hypotension. Toxicities generally were apparent within 1 hr and resolved by 2-3 hr. Two patients (Nos. 5 and 8) had fever up to 6 hr after infusions of treated plasma, and two patients (Nos. 40 and 41) had elevations of serum calcium noted 3-7 days after infusions. For individual patients, increased dose measured in arbitrary units (see Section II) was generally associated with increased toxicity, if any toxicity was observed. However, there was a considerable idiosyncratic element to the toxicity experienced by individual patients. For example, patient No. 32 experienced severe toxicity regularly with infusions of 50 ml plasma treated at 4 mg/100 ml (200 arbitrary units). Patient No. 4 experienced no observable toxicity at any dosage achieved. Patient No. 23 experienced no toxicity at doses of 200 units, but regularly had fevers and chills at doses of 400 units or more. This occurred with infusions of 50 ml treated at 12 mg/100 ml and with infusions of 100 ml

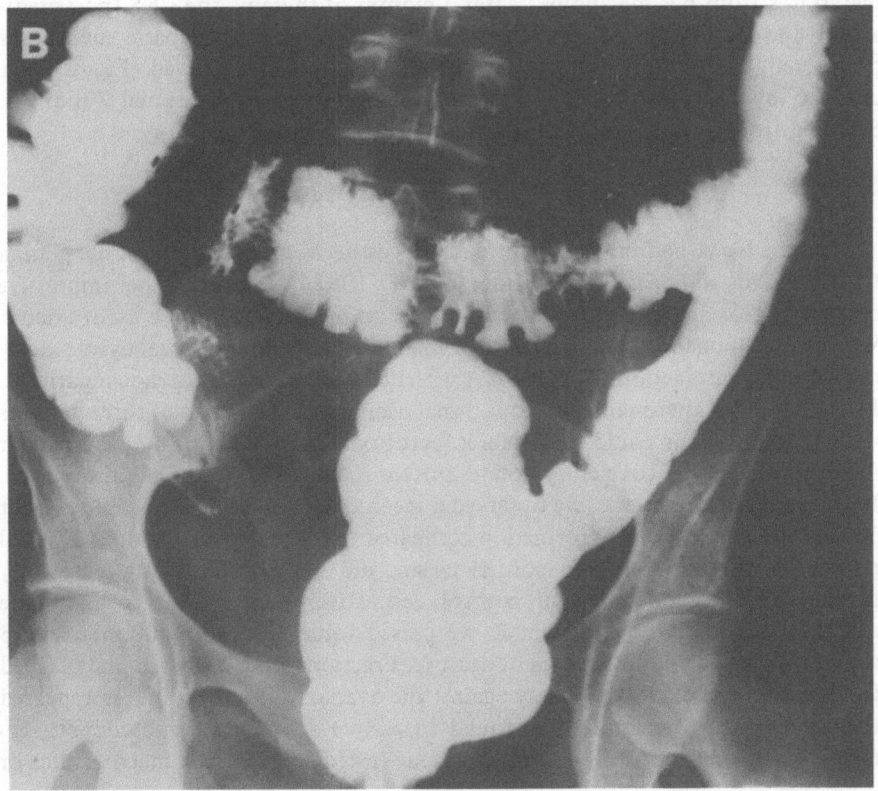

ception. After therapy, the projected area of the mass has decreased by 50% and there is no longer radiological or clinical evidence of intussusception.

treated with 4–6 mg/100 ml. Seven patients experienced objective improvement (5 PR, one mixed, and one minor response) lasting 8–34 weeks. Distribution of responders by tumor site of origin is indicated in Table II. Clinical histories of two of these patients (Nos. 3 and 23) have been reported (MacKintosh *et al.*, 1982*a*).

Patient No. 1 had recurrent melanoma with multiple subcutaneous nodules up to 5 × 7 cm and a colon lesion at the hepatic flexure, causing severe abdominal pain from intussusception at the start of treated plasma infusions (Fig. 1A). After 2 months, repeat barium enema (Fig. 1B) showed a decrease in the size of the colon lesion by 50% and resolution of the intussusception. This correlated with clinical relief of pain as well. Over the first 6 months of therapy, all her subcutaneous nodules resolved except the largest, which shrank to 1 × 2 cm. At that time, she had excisional biopsy of this skin lesion and right hemicolectomy. Progression was noted in subcutaneous nodules and the central nervous system (CNS) after 8 months.

Patient No. 4 had hepatic, lymphatic, pulmonary, CNS, and subcutaneous metastases from her melanoma. After 2 months of therapy, the CNS (postirradiation) and dermal/lymphatic metastases were unchanged. Hepatic metastases progressed, and multiple pulmonary nodules completely resolved (Fig. 2). Her chest X ray continued to be interpreted as normal for an additional 3 months. She died from hepatic progression 6 months after beginning therapy.

B. *In Vitro* Cytotoxicity Testing

Patient No. 1 had pretreatment data suggesting *in vitro* toxicity of her plasma to autologous tumor cells (MacKintosh *et al.*, 1983*a*). Because of her impressive clinical improvement, we sought to develop an *in vitro* model for cytotoxicity. We used an human ovarian cancer cell line as a target for humoral cytotoxicity produced by interactions of protein A with body fluids of ovarian cancer patients. In preliminary experiments, we found that ascitic fluid from two of three patients with ovarian cancer could be rendered cytotoxic to the cell line by passage over modest amounts of covalently bound protein A (10 ml fluid to 1 mg protein A). In three such experiments, we observed a mean 68% reduction (i.e., colony count 32% of control) of colony formation compared to untreated ascitic fluid. Normal plasma or protein A-treated normal plasma did not significantly alter colony formation (97% and 115% of control, respectively). In seeking to assess the optimal ratio of fluid to protein A, we passed volumes of 200–400 ml over 0.5 mg of protein A bound to silica or agarose. Fractions were collected and assayed for toxicity in a clonogenic assay against the ovarian cancer cell line. It appeared that the toxicity produced was found in early fractions, and subsequently increased and persisted at the maximal volume tested (Fig. 3). The matrix (silica or

Figure 2. Chest X rays before (A) and 2 months after (B) patient No. 4 began therapy with treated plasma. Multiple small nodules are present in the lung bases bilaterally before therapy.

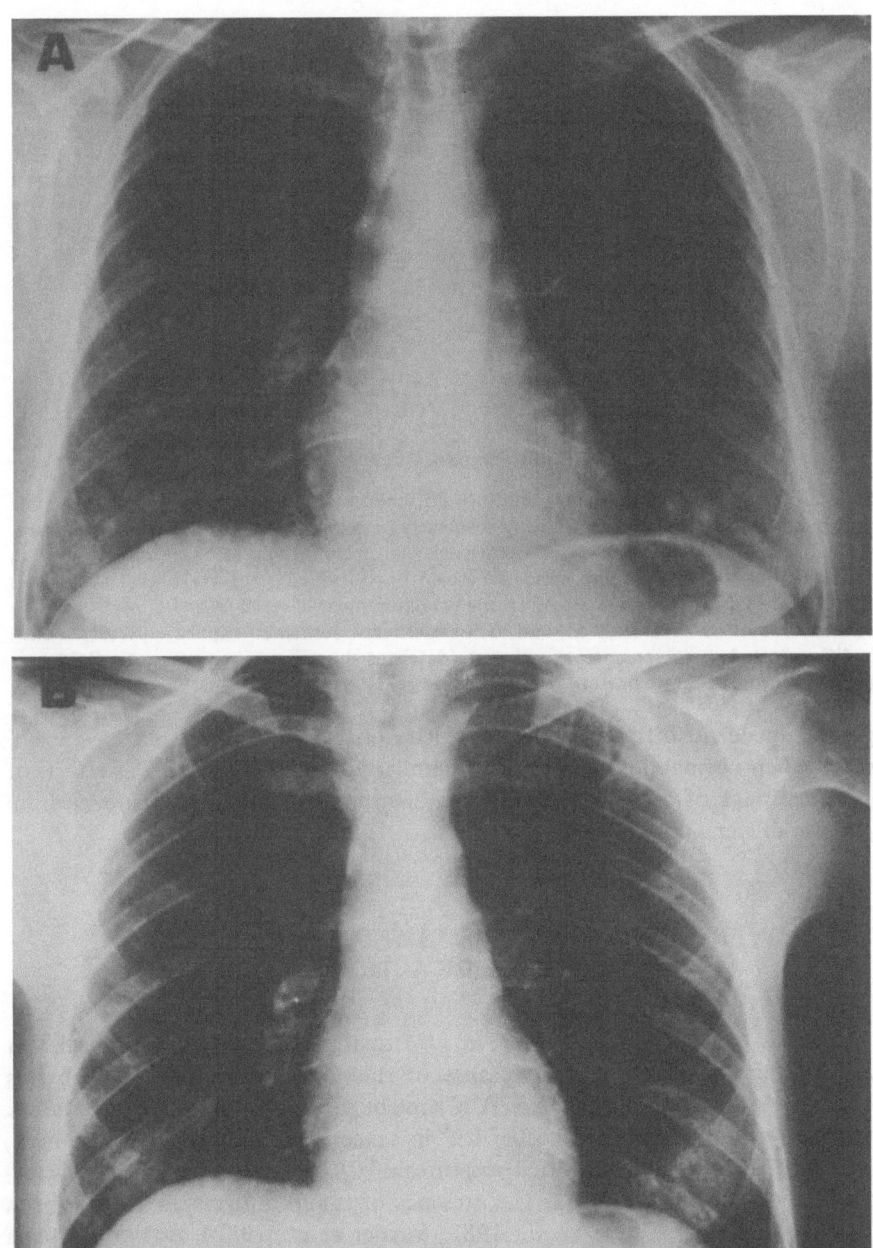

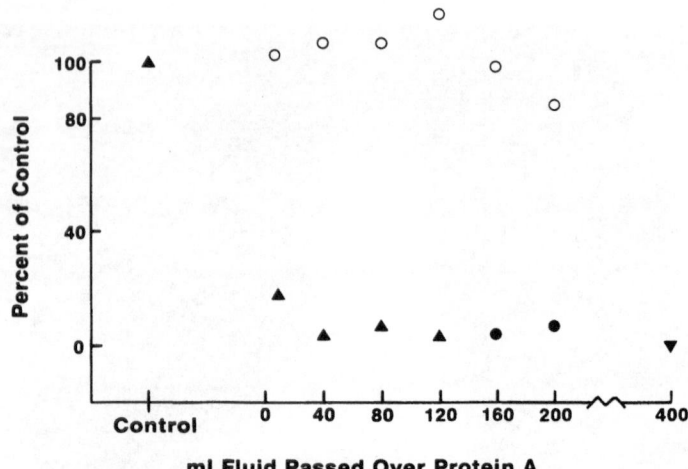

Figure 3. Ovarian cancer patients' ascitic fluid (solid symbols) or random donor plasma (open symbols) was passed over 0.5 mg covalently linked protein A and fractions collected. Selected fractions were assayed for cytotoxicity in a clonogenic assay against an ovarian cancer cell line. Results are expressed as percent of control colony formation. The symbols denote means of 5 (▲), 4 (●), 2 (○), or one (▼) experiment. Overall mean colony formation for controls was 85 colonies/well, and each experiment contained triplicate plates for each condition tested. In a separate experiment (data not shown), passage of ascitic fluid over agarose beads not bearing protein A produced no toxicity to the cell line.

agarose) made no difference in the toxicity observed, and no toxicity was observed when normal donor plasma was similarly treated (Fig. 3). The effects of heat treatment of ascites or of the sera incorporated into the culture medium were variable and continue to be studied.

IV. DISCUSSION OF RESULTS AND IMPLICATIONS FOR MODE OF ACTION

Clinical trials of therapy using *ex vivo* treatment of cancer patient plasma with protein A were initiated because of the concept that immunoglobulins or circulating immune complexes (CIC) might serve as inhibitors of antitumor immune response. The presence of CIC in cancer patients is well documented, and there is some indication that measures of CIC are related to prognosis (reviewed by Gauci *et al.*, 1981). The presence of tumor antigens in CIC has been demonstrated (e.g., Gupta *et al.*, 1983; Snyder *et al.*, 1982). However, others suggest that antiidiotype antibody against antitumor antibody is a significant component of CIC (Lewis *et al.*, 1971; Morgan *et al.*, 1979; Retsas *et al.*, 1981). As yet, there has not been direct evidence that CIC play a pathogenetic role in tumor progression in patients.

Clinical trials of *ex vivo* perfusion of plasma over protein A-bearing materials have used amounts of protein A too small to adsorb a significant fraction of the patients' immunoglobulin (Table III), and only if we postulate a remarkable increase in specific binding of CIC as compared to IgG monomers and rapid exchange during the exposure of plasma to protein A can a substantial removal of CIC be expected. However, this combination of increased binding and rapid exchange seems unlikely based on the limited data available (Kessler, 1975). In addition, it would not explain the therapeutic and toxic effects observed with infusions of very small volumes (20–200 ml) of plasma treated with covalently bound protein A (MacKintosh *et al.*, 1983*a*).

In comparing results among clinical trials, it is apparent that the use of whole, fixed SAC or purified protein A complexed to collodion charcoal (PACC) results in more toxicity than covalently linked preparations. This has led to the demonstration of leaching of protein A from these noncovalently bound materials in potentially significant quantities (2–5 μg from 5 μg SAC) (Balint and Jones, 1983). Direct infusion of 12 g protein A has produced tumor regressions in a rat system (Ray and Bandyopadhyay, 1983), but these investigators could not demonstrate any direct effect of protein A on tumor cells. It thus appears that interaction of protein A with patient plasma and/or the host immune system is necessary to produce tumor cell killing. A variety of mechanisms can be proposed to explain the tumoricidal effects observed. In view of the variability of host–tumor interactions (Rossen, 1981), it may be that differing mechanisms are operative in different patients, and that none of them are operative in some patients.

In vitro studies of humoral cytotoxicity have implicated an interaction of protein A with tumor bearers' sera which may (Steele *et al.*, 1974) or may not (Miller *et al.*, 1982) involve complement. Protein A from various sources is active in these systems, but the source of plasma must be specific to the tumor. Possible mechanisms of cytotoxicity that could be entertained include release of cytotoxic antibody from CIC (either tumor antigen or antiidiotype CIC) on exposure to protein A, or formation of cytotoxic complexes of antitumor antibody with complement components or protein A itself. Direct infusion of portein A could mediate these possible interactions as well as could *ex vivo* perfusions.

The possibility that other staphylococcal toxins may be involved in the reported studies of protein A has not been excluded. However, the Wood 46 strain has usually produced no antitumor effects when used as a control (Steele *et al.*, 1974; Miller *et al.*, 1982; Ray *et al.*, 1982*b*), nor did perfusion of normal plasma over SAC (Holohan *et al.*, 1982). Purified protein A from two sources (Pharmacia, Imré) has been equally effective in our *in vitro* system. A definitive test of the role of protein A should be possible using protein A produced by cloning staphylococcal DNA sequences in yeast (Repligen, Cambridge, Massachusetts).

Evaluation of the immunological effects of *ex vivo* perfusions of plasma over protein A-bearing materials (with or without infusion of protein A) remains problematic. Quantitation of IgG indicates an increase (Ray *et al.*, 1982*b*) or a decrease (Ray *et al.*, 1982*a*). CIC-like material in plasma of treated animals or

Table III. Tumoricidal Activity of Protein A-Treated Plasma in Relation to Source and Amount of Protein A

Reference	Subjects	Protein A source[a]	Quantity of IgG adsorbed	Percent IgG bound[b]	Tumoricidal effects[c]
Sjoquist (1973)	Rat tumor cells	SAC	Not specified	20–30%	+ (25–45%)
Miller et al. (1982)	Human AML blasts[d]	SAC	5 mg	49%	+ (57%)
	Human AML blasts	Agarose	4 mg	40%	+ (36%)
Present report	Human ovarian cell line	Agarose or silica gel	10 mg	0.5%	+ (68–100%)
Ray et al. (1981)	Rat (DMBA breast ca.)	SAC	30 mg	3–5%	+ (1/7 CR)
Holohan et al. (1982)	Dog (breast ca.)[d]	SAC	4 mg/kg	0.65%	+ (5/10 PR)
Snyder et al. (1982)	Dog (breast ca.)	SAC	5 mg/kg	0.8%	+ (7/12 PR)
Jones et al. (1980)	Cat (FeLV)[d]	SAC	150 mg	3–5%	+ (2/5 CR)
Bansal et al. (1978)	Colon ca. (1)[e]	SAC	22500 mg	10–30%	+ (PR)
Ray et al. (1982a)	Colon ca. (1)	SAC	2500 mg	2–6%	+ (PR)
Steele et al. (1974)	Breast ca. (5)	PACC	100 mg	0.2%	+ (3/5 PR)
Messerschmidt et al. (1982)	Misc. (5)	SAC	500 mg	4%	– (0/5)
Present report	Misc. (35 eval.)	Agarose	200–1000 mg	0.5–1.5%	+ (5 PR, 2 MR)

[a]*Abbreviations:* SAC, *S. aureus* Cowan I; PACC, protein A–collodion charcoal; agarose, protein A covalently bound to agarose (Sepharose); silica, protein A covalently bound to silica gel.

[b]Percent bound relates to whole sample of plasma (*in vitro*) or whole plasma volume (*in vivo*). If insufficient data are given to calculate, an estimate is made based on typical normal values.

[c]*Abbreviations:* CR, complete regression; PR, partial regression; MR, minor or mixed regression.

[d]Negative controls with normal plasma/SAC and/or tumor-bearer sera/Wood 46 were included.

[e]Number of patients.

patients may be decreased (Holohan *et al.*, 1982; Jones *et al.*, 1980; Ray *et al.*, 1982*a*), but measurements of CIC-like material in treated plasma may show an increase (Balint *et al.*, 1982). Tumor biopsy specimens may show evidence of humoral effector mechanisms (Terman *et al.*, 1981) or of cellular inflammatory infiltration (Holohan *et al.*, 1982). Any of these observations may be important to the genesis of the observed effects or may be unrelated incidental findings. The difficulty of performing *in vitro* tests of tumor immunity is substantial, and there is a paucity of data indicating a quantitative correlation of such effects with clinical benefit. Holohan *et al.* (1982) did report a trend favoring antitumor response in dogs who had greater reduction of "blocking" CIC.

In summary, numerous groups of investigators have demonstrated *in vitro* or *in vivo* antitumor effects of protein A-bearing materials in a variety of animal and human tumors. The mechanism of these effects remains unknown. It appears that the immediate priorities for further investigations are as follows:

1. Certain identification of protein A as the active material responsible for therapeutic effects.
2. Establishing appropriate *in vitro* and/or animal models for evaluation of the mechanism of tumoricidal effects.
3. Establishing relevant paramenters for optimizing the interaction of plasma with protein A for producing tumoricidal effects, using an *in vitro* model.
4. Using this information to devise predictive tests for entering patients on future clinical trials.

Based on the information presented and discussed, it appears that these are reasonable goals that should be attained within the next one or two years. It will then be possible to assess realistically the possible role of protein A in cancer treatment programs.

V. SUMMARY

The data presented here indicate that patients with advanced cancer exhibit a modest but definite objective response rate to biweekly infusions of autologous plasma treated with purified, covalently bound staphylococcal protein A in a relatively nontoxic treatment program. The possibility that responses could be enhanced by alteration of treatment parameters, improved patient selection, and/or combined therapy remains to be explored.

In vitro studies indicate that tumor cell killing can be produced in an ovarian cancer cell line using ascitic fluid of some ovarian cancer patients that has been treated with small amounts of protein A covalently linked to silica gel or agarose. This may be a suitable model system for exploration of possible humoral mechanisms of protein A-associated tumoricidal effects.

The available literature indicates an antitumor effect of protein A-treated patient plasma in a variety of *in vitro* systems, as well as in animal and human tumors *in vivo*. Preliminary investigations of the mechanism of these effects are inconsistent and support the view that several different mechanisms of tumor cell killing may be operative in different settings.

VI. REFERENCES

Ankerst, J., 1971, Demonstration and identification of cytotoxic antibodies and antibodies blocking the cell mediated antitumor immunity against adenovirus 12-induced tumors, *Cancer Res.* 31:997–1003.

Balint, J., Jr., and Jones, F. R., 1983, Perfusion of canine serum over *Staphylococcus aureus* Cowan I: Evidence for release of portein A and changes in specific antibody activity, *Immunol. Commun.* 12:573–591.

Balint, J. P., Shearer, W. T., Ikeda, Y., Nagai, T., Meek, K. D., and Terman, D. S., 1982, Generation of bioreactive immunoglobulin oligomers in serum of dogs with breast adenocarcinoma after perfusion over staphylococcal protein A (SPA), *Clin. Res.* 30:532A.

Bansal, S. C., Hargreaves, R., and Sjogren, H. O., 1972, Facilitation of polyoma tumor growth in rats by blocking sera and tumor eluates, *Int. J. Cancer* 9:97–108.

Bansal, S. C., Bansal, B. R., and Boland, J. P., 1976, Blocking and unblocking serum factors in neoplasia, *Curr. Top. Microbiol. Immunol.* 75:45–76.

Bansal, S. C., Bansal, B. R., Thomas, H. L., Siegel, P. D., Rhoads, J. E., Copper, D. R., Terman, D. S., and Mark, R., 1978, *Ex-vivo* removal of serum IgG in a patient with colon carcinoma, *Cancer* 42:1–18.

Bast, R. C., Jr., Feeney, M., Lazarus, H., Nadler, L. M., Colvin, R. B., and Knapp, R. C., 1981, Reactivity of a monoclonal antibody with human ovarian carcinoma, *J. Clin. Invest.* 68:1331–1337.

Bensinger, W. I., Hutchinson, F., Kinet, J. P., Hennen, G., Franckenne, F., Schaus, C., Saint-Remy, M., Hoyoux, P., and Nahieu, P., 1982, Plasma perfused over immobilized protein A for breast cancer, *N. Engl. J. Med.* 306:935–936.

Forsgren, A., and Sjoquist, J., 1966, Protein A from *Staphylococcus aureus* I: Pseudoimmune reaction with human globulin, *J. Immunol.* 97:822–827.

Gauci, L., Caraux, J., and Serrou, B., 1981, Immune complexes in the context of the immune response in cancer patients, in: *Immune Complexes and Plasma Exchanges in Cancer Patients* (B. Serrou and G. C. Rosenfeld, eds.), pp. 37–98, Elsevier/North-Holland, Amsterdam.

Gupta, R. K., Lectch, A. M., and Norton, D. L., 1983, Tumor associated antigen in eluates of protein A columns used for *ex vivo* immunoadsorption of melanoma patients, *Proc. Am. Assoc. Cancer Res.* 24:791.

Hellström, I., Hellström, K. E., Evans, C. A., Heppner, G. H., Pierce, G. E., and Yang, J. P. S., 1969, Serum mediated protection of neoplastic cells from inhibition by lymphocytes immune to their tumor-specific antigens, *Proc. Natl. Acad. Sci. USA* 62:362–368.

Holohan, T. V., Phillips, T. M., Bowles, C., and Deisseroth, A., 1982, Regression of canine mammary carcinoma after immunoadsorption therapy, *Cancer Res.* 42:3663–3668.

Israel, L., Edelstein, R., Mannoni, P., Radot, E., and Greenspan, E. M., 1977, Plasmapheresis in patients with disseminated cancer: Clinical results and correlation with changes in serum protein, *Cancer* 40:3146–3154.

Jones, F. R., Yoshida, L. H., Ladiges, W. C., and Kenny, M. A., 1980, Treatment of feline leukemia and reversal of FeLV by *ex vivo* removal of IgG: A preliminary report, *Cancer* 46:675-684.

Kessler, S. W., 1975, Rapid isolation of antigens from cells with a staphylococcal protein A-antibody adsorbent: Parameters of the interaction of antibody-antigen complexes with protein A, *J. Immunol.* 115:1617-1624.

Lewis, M. G., Phillips, T. M., Cook, K. B., and Blake, J., 1971, Possible explanation for loss of detectable antibody in patients with disseminated malignant melanoma (Letter to the Editor), *Nature* 232:52-53.

MacKintosh, F. R., Louie, A. C., Evans, T. L., Amylon, M. D., and Sikic, B. I., 1981, Clonal heterogeneity in a human ovarian adenocarcinoma, *Proc. Am. Soc. Clin. Oncol.* 22:379.

MacKintosh, F. R., Bennett, K., and Hall, S. W., 1983a, Tumoricidal effects of staphylococcal protein A (SPA) treated plasma *in vitro*: Clinical correlation and possible mechanism of action, *Proc. Am. Assoc. Cancer Res.* 13:780.

MacKintosh, F. R., Bennett, K., Schiff, S., Shields, J., and Hall, S. W., 1983b, Treatment of advanced malignancy with plasma perfused over staphylococcal protein A, *West. J. Med.* 139:36-40.

MacKintosh, F. R., Bennett, K., and Hall, S. W., 1984, Clinical response to protein A treated plasma infusions and *in vitro* correlation, *J. Biol. Resp. Modif.* 3:336-340.

Messerschmidt, G., Bowles, C., Dean, D., Parker, M., Lester, R., Dowling, R., Holohan, T., Osborne, L., Schaff, B. F., McCormack, K., Corbitt, R., Phillips, T., Glatstein, E., and Deisseroth, A., 1982, Phase I trial of *Staphylococcus aureus* Cowan I Immunoperfusion, *Cancer Treatment Rep.* 66:2027-2031.

Miller, W. J., Branda, R. F., Hurd, D. D., Wachsman, W., Nelson, N. L., and Jacob, H. S., 1982, Protein A adsorption of acute myelogenous leukemia serum induces in vitro blast lysis, *Blood* 59:1344-1347.

Morgan, A. C., Jr., Rossen, R. D., and Twomey, J. J., 1979, Naturally occurring circulating immune complexes: Normal human serum contains idiotype-anti-idiotype complexes dissociable by certain IgG antiglobulins, *J. Immunol.* 122:1672-1680.

Ray, P. K., and Bandyopadhyay, S., 1983, Inhibition of rat mammary tumor growth by purified protein A—A potential anti-tumor agent, *Immunol. Commun.* 12:453-464.

Ray, P. K., McLaughlin, D., Mohammed, J., Idiculla, A., Rhoads, J. E., Jr., Mark, R., Bassett, J. G., and Cooper, D. R., 1981, *Ex vivo* immunoadsorption of IgG or its complexes— A new modality of cancer treatment, in: *Immune Complexes and Plasma Exchanges in Cancer Patients* (B. Serrou and G. C. Rosenfeld, eds.), pp. 197-208, Elsevier/North-Holland, Amsterdam.

Ray, P. K., Idiculla, A., Mark, R., Rhoads, J. E., Jr., Thomas, H., Bassett, J. G., and Cooper, D. R., 1982a, Extracorporeal immunoadsorption of plasma from a metastatic colon carcinoma patient by protein A-containing nonviable *Staphylococcus aureus*, *Cancer* 49:1800-1809.

Ray, P. K., Raychaudhuri, S., and Allen P., 1982b, Mechanism of regression of mammary adenocarcinomas in rats following plasma adsorption over protein A-containing *Staphylococcus aureus*, *Cancer Res.* 42:4970-4974.

Retsas, S., Thomas, C. R., Chambers, J. D., Newston, K. A., and Hobbs, J. R., 1981, The effect of plasmapheresis on the clinical and immune status of patients with renal adenocarcinoma, in: *Immune Complexes and Plasma Exchanges in Cancer Patients* (B. Serrou and G. C. Rosenfeld, eds.), pp. 271-276, Elsevier/North-Holland, Amsterdam.

Rossen, R. D., 1981, Immune complexes and cancer—Unmasking the hidden humoral immune response to neoplastic tissue, *Cancer Bull.* 33(5):221-226.

Salinas, F. A., Silver, H. K. B., Grossman, L., and Thomas, J. W., 1981, Plasmapheresis: A new approach in the management of advanced malignant melanoma, in: *Immune Com-

plexes and Plasma Exchanges in Cancer Patients (B. Serrou and G. C. Rosenfeld, eds.), pp. 253–270, Elsevier/North-Holland, Amsterdam.

Sjögren, H. O., Hellström, I., Bansal, S. C., and Hellström, K., 1971, Suggestive evidence that blocking antibodies of tumor individuals may be antigen–antibody complexes, *Proc. Natl. Acad. Sci. USA* **68**:1372–1375.

Sjoquist, J., 1973, Structure and immunology of protein A, in: *Streptococci and Staphylococcal Infection* (J. Jiljaszewica and W. Hryneiwicz, eds.), pp. 83–92, S. Karger, Basel.

Snyder, H. W., Jr., Jones, F. R., Day, N. K., and Hardy, W. D., Jr., 1982, Isolation and characterization of circulating feline leukemia virus-immune complexes from plasma of persistently infected pet cats removed by *ex vivo* immunosorption, *J. Immunol.* **128**:2726–2730.

Steele, G., Jr., Ankerst, J., and Sjögren, H. O., 1974, Alteration of *in vitro* antitumor activity of tumor-bearer sera by absorption with *Staphylococcus aureus* Cowan I, *Int. J. Cancer* **14**:83–92.

Terman, D., Yamamoto, T., Mattioti, M., Cook, G., Gillquist, R., Henry, J., Poser, R., and Daskal, Y., 1980, Extensive necrosis of spontaneous canine mammary adenocarcinoma after extracorporeal perfusion over *S. aureus* Cowan, *J. Immunol.* **124**:795–805.

Terman, D. S., Shearer, W. T., Ayus, C., Mattioli, C., Lehane, D., Espada, R., Howell, J. F., Yamamoto, T., Zaleski, H. I., Frommer, P., Henry, J. F., Feldman, L., Miller, L., Tillquist, R., Cook, G., and Daskal, Y., 1981, Preliminary observations of the effects on breast adenocarcinoma of plasma perfused over immobilized protein A, *N. Engl. J. Med.* **305**:1195–1199.

Chapter 8

Protein A Immunoadsorption/Immunoactivation: A Critical Review

Mehmet F. Fer

Section of Hematology/Oncology
University of Kentucky Medical Center
Lexington, Kentucky 40536

and

Robert K. Oldham

Biological Therapy Institute
Franklin, Tennessee 37064

I. INTRODUCTION

Over the past several years, reports have been published describing antitumor effects of autologous plasma after contact with protein A or bacterial products containing protein A (Bansal *et al.*, 1978; Bensinger *et al.*, 1981; Holohan *et al.*, 1982; Jones *et al.*, 1980; Terman *et al.*, 1980, 1981). Although the efficacy of these manipulations, the best reagents to use, and the mechanism of action are all unclear, considerable enthusiasm regarding the effects of protein A has been generated. This chapter will review the available information on protein A-related plasma immunoadsorption/immunoactivation studies for cancer therapy and to summarize current thoughts and controversies.

The discovery in serum from cancer patients of "blocking factors" capable of inhibiting cell-mediated cytotoxicity against tumor cells led to interest in removing these factors as a means of restoring immunocompetence (Baldwin *et al.*, 1972, 1973; Hellström and Hellström, 1970; Sjögren *et al.*, 1971). These factors were generally thought to be antigen–antibody complexes (Baldwin *et al.*, 1972;

Sjögren *et al.*, 1971). Since protein A, a component of the bacterial cell wall of *Staphylococcus aureus* Cowan type I (SAC), can bind nonspecifically to the Fc portion of human IgG (subclassess 1, 2, and 4) (Forsgren and Sjoquist, 1966; Kronvall and Frommel 1970), it has offered a logical reagent for removing immune complexes from tumor-bearing host sera by affinity binding *ex vivo*. Steele *et al.* (1974) demonstrated that exposure of host serum to protein A-bearing SAC *in vitro* can reduce the inhibitory effects of host serum on cellular cytotoxicity. Subsequently, a number of studies were directed at pursuing this concept with *in vivo* experiments and clinical trials. The first patient was treated by Bansal *et al.* (1978) for metastatic carcinoma of the colon with autologous plasma perfused over heat- and formalin-killed, protein A-bearing SAC. The effects described were dramatic, with the development of acute inflammation over subcutaneous metastases and eventual tumor shrinkage (Bansal *et al.*, 1978). Toxicity was significant, with fever, chills, tachycardia, and hypotension. Follow-up trials were then initiated in both animal models and man using killed SAC or the presumed active ingredient, protein A, on columns, enabling the *ex vivo* exposure of autologous plasma to these agents. Antitumor effects were observed in dogs with spontaneous mammary carcinomas (Holohan *et al.*, 1982; Jones *et al.*, 1984; Terman *et al.*, 1980), in feline leukemia virus (FeLV)-associated neoplasms of cats (Day *et al.*, 1984; Jones *et al.*, 1980, 1984), and more recently in chemically induced mammary tumors of rats (Sukumar *et al.*, 1984). In clinical trials, the most impressive antitumor effects were reported in a small group of patients with breast cancer treated by Terman *et al.* at the Baylor College of Medicine (Terman *et al.*, 1981). Less dramatic effects have been reported in other trials against various tumors, including malignant melanoma and lung and colon cancers (Bensinger *et al.*, 1984; Korec *et al.*, 1984; MacKintosh *et al.*, 1983, 1984; Ray *et al.*, 1982) The response rates in these studies have been variable, but this is not surprising since the materials and technical procedures have varied considerably. Along with the *in vivo* experiments, *in vitro* studies to elucidate the mechanisms of action and to predict responses have been performed (MacKintosh *et al.*, 1984; Miller *et al.*, 1982). We will first review the descriptive studies in animal models, followed by discussions of the clinical results, *in vitro* studies, and proposed mechanisms of action.

II. *IN VIVO* STUDIES IN LABORATORY ANIMALS

Following the observation of marked antitumor effects in the first patient treated by Bansal *et al.*, studies were pursued by Terman *et al.* (1980) in dogs bearing spontaneous mammary carcinoma. In 12 dogs with mammary adenocarcinoma, perfusion of autologous plasma was performed over SAC (1 g/kg) at a rate of 15–30 ml/min. In all 12 dogs there was apparent tumor necrosis as early as 4 hr following plasma therapy (Terman *et al.*, 1980). In all six dogs with measurable tumors, necrosis was apparent by 24 hr. Healing of ulcerated lesions reportedly occurred within 18 days after commencing therapy. Sequential biopsies at 4 and 48 hr showed that at 4 hr following therapy there was a minimal leukocytic infiltration with deposits of IgG and C3. At 48 hr there was extensive infiltration by leukocytes, mostly of the polymorphonuclear type. Toxicity included mild fever and leukocytosis in 6 of the 12 dogs. Immunological changes included decreases in circulating IgG and C3 levels following the perfusions. Although the IgG levels rebounded back to previous levels shortly after therapy, C3 levels remained low for up to 48 hr. Circulating immune complex (CIC) levels were increased following the perfusions and stayed high for up to 72 hr. Circulating immunoglobulins reactive with the tumor in each animal (but not with other canine tumors or normal mammary tissue) were demonstrated in sera from dogs shortly after plasma therapy. No information on long-term results was presented in this paper.

Antitumor responses with SAC perfusion of plasma in this animal model were later confirmed by Holohan *et al.* at the National Cancer Institute (Holohan *et al.*, 1982). These investigators studied ten dogs with spontaneous mammary carcinoma by perfusing the total calculated plasma volume weekly over SAC paste (0.2 g/kg) at a rate of 40–60 ml/min. Five of ten dogs had a partial response. Toxicity included fever in 15% of the procedures. There were no responses in five controls treated with plasma perfused over chambers containing no SAC or in five controls treated with normal dog plasma perfused over SAC. Biopsies performed at 18, 55, and 65 days after therapy revealed histological evidence of inflammation and tumor necrosis. Nevertheless, all dogs had residual tumor at the end of the trial. In two responders who died during the study, autopsy showed extensive tumor involvement in the visceral sites in spite of regressions in soft tissues. Circulating IgG levels were unaffected by immunoadsorption over SAC. Tumor-associated antibodies were demonstrated prior to therapy in all ten animals and clearly were not predictors of antitumor response.

Another interesting tumor model has been FeLV-associated neoplasms. Jones *et al.* (1980) first reported their experience in treating five cats with low-dose radiotherapy plus extracorporeal immunoadsorption over heat- and formalin-killed SAC paste. Perfusions were performed over 20–30 mg of SAC. Blood (35–45 ml) was drawn from the cats, and the plasma was separated by centrifugation, exposed to SAC, mixed with the remainder of the blood components, and returned to the animals. The procedure was performed once or twice weekly. Following this therapy, three of five cats improved. Two of the five cats were in complete remission at 7 and 8 months following therapy. A third cat was tumor-free for 6 months and one cat had died because of bleeding during the immunoadsorption procedure. Interestingly, all five cats became seronegative for FeLV-2 associated antigens following therapy (Jones *et al.*, 1980). These results are impressive, considering the natural history of feline leukemia, which is generally fatal within 2-4 months. An expanded experience by the same group has been reported, with viral clearance and durable tumor regressions in 9 out of 16 treated cats (Jones *et al.*, 1984).

Day *et al.* (1984) have independently studied over 50 cats with FeLV-associated disease, utilizing silica filters on which purified protein A was covalently linked. This system offers the advantage of specifically testing for protein A-related changes, as opposed to the trials by Jones *et al.* (1980), in which the whole bacteria SAC was used. Although the percentage of responses was not stated in this paper, some of the cats reportedly achieved impressive remissions, accompanied by decreases in CIC levels, increases in complement levels, and a decrease in the circulating Gp70 antigen associated with FeLV infection. Increases in circulating interferon levels were observed in this study. With prolonged therapy, two cats developed a complement-dependent cytotoxic antibody that showed some specificity for FeLV-infected lumphoblastoid cells. This complement-mediated cytotoxicity was inhibited by a monoclonal antibody directed against an epitope on the Gp70 envelope protein of the virus.

The question has been raised of whether leaching of protein A from the plasma perfusion systems may have facilitated some of the antitumor responses previously summarized. Another consideration has been that, if protein A is indeed the active reagent producing these effects, similar consequences might result from direct injections of protein A into the circulation, without requiring an *ex vivo* exposure chamber. These questions have been addressed in a series of animal studies conducted by our group at the National Cancer Institute (Cohen *et al.*, 1984). In these experiments, a number of tumor models were chosen, including the canine transmissible venereal tumor, a transplantable guinea pig breast carcinoma, and a transplantable murine melanoma. These tumors were chosen partly because of their immunogenicity, with the assumption that if the reported phenomena are immunologically mediated these models should provide an adequate opportunity for the development of similar effects. In studies with the canine transmissible venereal tumor, Cohen administered protein A at a dose of 100 g/kg body weight intravenously twice weekly, for a total of ten treatments. Control dogs were treated with injections of normal saline. There were no decreases in the tumor volumes attributable to protein A therapy. There were transient increases in the polymorphonuclear cells in the peripheral blood 24 hr after the first protein A injection, with a decrease in lymphocyte and monocyte counts. These parameters returned to pretreatment levels by 24 hr after the last protein A dose. In the guinea pig experiments, strain 2 guinea pigs were transplanted with a mammary tumor and observed. When tumors achieved a diameter of 10-15 mm, the animals were treated once weekly for a month with intravenous protein A (0.25 or 0.06 mg/guinea pig). Controls were treated with normal saline alone. There were no decreases in the tumor size in either group (Cohen *et al.*, 1984). In the murine model, C3H mice bearing transplantable K1735 malignant melanoma were treated three times weekly for three weeks with intravenous protein A along a broad dose range (0.06, 0.25, 1, 4, 16, and 64 g protein A per mouse). Again there were no alterations in tumor growth compared to saline-treated controls. Thus in the systems tested the interaction of protein A with plasma *in vivo* did not produce antitumor effects.

The role of protein A in producing antitumor effects has been extensively studied by Gordon *et al.* in canine spontaneous tumor systems by comparing perfusion over SAC with that over non-protein A-bearing *S. aureus* Wood 46 (SAW) (Gordon *et al.*, 1983, 1984). These investigators observed that regression of tumors occurred in six of nine dogs following the reinfusion of dog plasma incubated with either SAC or SAW. Of the seven dogs treated by plasma perfusion over SAC (protein A-bearing), three had mammary carcinoma, one had melanoma, and three had lymphoma. There were partial responses in three dogs (two with lymphoma, one with mammary carcinoma) and a complete response in one dog with lymphoma. Of seven dogs perfused with plasma exposed to SAW, there were six partial responses (three with lymphoma, one with melanoma, one with carcinoma of the lung, and one with mamary carcinoma). Antitumor response correlated with the presence of toxicity; responding dogs had fever, diarrhea, and lethargy, while the three nonresponders had little toxicity. There was marked complement consumption in all treated animals. Complement activation *in vitro* was demonstrated when saline extracts obtained from SAW were added to dog plasma. Histological findings in responding dogs showed disruption of cell membranes without a prominent inflammatory infiltrate. Based on these findings, these investigators suggested that the observed phenomena might be related to *Staphylococcus*-derived products other than protein A.

The role of protein A in generating antitumor activity has also been questioned by Sukumar *et al.* (1984), who conducted experiments in *N*-methyl nitrosourea-induced mammary carcinomas in rats. In this study, seven rats were treated with autologous plasma exposed to protein A convalently linked to Sepharose and developed marked reductions in tumor size compared to untreated controls within 2 weeks of therapy. However, six control rats treated by plasma exposed to inactivated CNBr–Sepharose also showed comparable reduction in tumor size. Incubation of plasma with inactivated Sepharose or normal plasma exposed to CNBr–Sepharose did not result in antitumor effects. When plasma from tumor-bearing rats was exposed to protein A–Sepharose or Sepharose alone and administered to other rats, there were some reductions in tumor size. These results have led to the suggestion that inactivated CNBr–Sepharose may have effects comparable to protein A–Sepharose and that the presence of protein A may not be critical (Sukumar *et al.*, 1984).

III. CLINICAL STUDIES

The technical features, antitumor responses, toxicity, and immunological consequences of plasma therapy observed in clinical trials are summarized in Tables I–IV.

Table I. Comparison of Immunoadsorption Techniques in Clinical Trials

Study	Type of immunoadsorbent[a]	Quantity of immunoadsorbent	Amount of plasma perfused per procedure	Perfusion method	Frequency of treatments	Total number of treatments given per patient
Bansal et al. (1978)	S. aureus paste	30–75 g	900–1800 ml	Continuous-flow	1–2×/wk	20
Terman et al. (1981)	PA-CC	0.6–6 mg	5–300 ml	Previously stored	1–2×/wk	5–12[b]
Bensinger et al. (1984)	PA-silica	100–200 mg	Total calculated plasma volume	Continuous-flow	1–3×/wk	20
Korec et al. (1984)	PA-PAGB	60 mg	600 ml	Continuous-flow	2×/wk × 3 wk 1×/wk × 2 wk	8
Messerschmidt et al. (1982a,b)	S. aureus paste	1 g/kg	686–3517 ml	Continuous-flow	1×/1–2 wk	1–2[c]
Messerschmidt et al. (1984)	PA-CC	5 mg	50–450 ml	Previously stored	—	—
MacKintosh et al. (1983)	PA-Sepharose	2–100 mg	35–500 ml	Previously stored	2×/wk	—
Fer et al. (1984)	PA-CC	0.6–7.5 mg	50–200 ml	Previously stored plasma	2–3×/wk	18
Bertram et al. (1984)	PA-CC	<40 mg	100 ml	Previously stored	1–3×/wk	—

[a] Abbreviations: PA-CC, protein A on collodion charcoal; PA-PAGB, protein A on polyacrylamide-coated glass beads.
[b] One patient was removed from study after a single procedure because of toxicity.
[c] Two patients died owing to pulmonary toxicity after the first procedure.

Table II. Results of Plasma Immunoadsorption Clinical Trials[a]

Study	Tumor types studied	Number of evaluable patients	Partial responses[b]	Other objective responses[c]
Bansal et al. (1984)	Colon	1	–	1
Terman et al. (1981)	Breast	4	1	3
Bensinger et al. (1984)	Malignant melanoma	7	–	3
	Breast	3	–	1
	Other (lung, colon, renal, sarcomas, CML, thymoma)	8	–	–
Kinet et al.[d]	Breast	6	1	2
MacKintosh et al. (1983)	Lung	6	2	–
	Colon	7	–	–
	Breast	4	1	–
	Malignant melanoma	5	1	1
	Miscellaneous	10	1	1
Korec et al. (1984)	Colon	5	–	2
	Malignant melanoma	2	–	–
	Ovary	1	–	1
	Prostate, breast	2	–	–
Messerschmidt et al. (1982a,b)[e]	Esophagus (2), colon, melanoma, synovial sarcoma	5	–	–
Messerschmidt et al. (1984)	Breast (6), colon (3), glioma, unknown primary	8	–	–
Fer et al. (1984)	Breast	5	–	–
Total reviewed		89	7	15

[a] Protein A used as immunoadsorbent except where indicated.
[b] As defined by 50% tumor shrinkage.
[c] 50% tumor shrinkage.
[d] Quoted by Bensinger et al. (1984).
[e] SAC used in perfusion apparatus. Two of five patients died of toxicity.

The first patient treated by Bansal et al. (1978) was a 57-year-old man with metastatic colon cancer and peritoneal carcinomatosis. Twenty perfusion procedures were conducted over a 5-month period with SAC, using an on-line continuous-flow perfusion system. There was considerable toxicity, including peripheral vasoconstriction, 50–70 min after the procedure, with an increase in blood pressure and shaking chills followed by burning pain over the tumor. This was followed by fever and peripheral vasodilation manifested by hypotension and tachy-

Table III. Clinical Toxicity in Plasma Immunoadsorption Studies[a]

Fever, chills
Initial rise in blood pressure followed by hypotension and tachycardia
Nausea, vomiting, diarrhea
Bronchospasm, tachypnea, dyspnea
Tumor pain

[a]Toxicity has been more severe with SAC compared to systems containing purified protein A.

cardia. An inflammatory reaction around an umbilical metastasis was apparent
several hours following the procedure. When a second-look laparotomy was performed at the end of therapy, the peritoneal seeding demonstrated previously
was not present, although there were residual pelvic and retroperitoneal masses.
A liver metastasis contained areas of necrosis and fibrosis mixed with residual
viable tumor. Immunological consequences included a decrease in IgG and CIC

Table IV. Immunological Changes during Clinical Protein A Immunoadsorption Trials[a]

Study	Changes observed
Bansal et al. (1978)[b]	IgG, IgM, immune complex levels Reduction in serum blocking activity and appearance of complement-dependent serum cytotoxicity Transient increase in surface-Ig-bearing lymphocytes and E-rosetting lymphocytes
Terman et al. (1981)	Deposits of IgG, IgM, IgA, and C3 in tumor biopsies
Bensinger et al. (1984)	10–20% decreases from baseline in IgA, IgM, IgC, C3, C4, and CH50; 70% increase in C1q binding; elevated interferon levels in six patients posttherapy
Korec et al. (1984)	Up to 70% drop in circulating lymphocyte count, rebound by 36 hr; increase in OKT4:OKT8-positive T cells
Bertram et al. (1984)	Mitogenicity in perfused plasma in four of six patients
Fer et al. (1984)	No significant change in natural killer cell activity, antibody-dependent cellular cytotoxicity, T-cell subpopulations, CH50, immunoglobulins, and serum interferon levels
Kiprow et al. (1984)[c]	Deposits of C3 and Ig in Kaposi's sarcoma lesions; reduction in CIC, antilymphocyte antibodies, and blocking factors to mitogen stimulation; no improvement in helper/suppressor-T-cell ratios

[a]Comparability of these studies is limited since different materials and methods were used.
[b]One patient reported, SAC used as immunoadsorbent.
[c]One patient with acquired immune deficiency syndrome

levels with an increase in IgM. Transient reductions in serum blocking activity were demonstrated by a microlymphocytotoxicity assay, using a cell line derived from the patient's tumor as target cells (Bansal *et al.*, 1978; Hellström and Hellström, 1976).

The next series of patients was reported by Terman *et al.* (1981), who treated five patients with recurrent breast cancer using a cartridge system containing protein A immobilized over a charcoal collodion matrix (PACC); 5-300 ml of previously stored autologous plasma was perfused over 0.6-5 mg of immobilized protein A. Although the dose of protein A used initially was 5 mg, this was steadily decreased in additional patients in order to reduce cardiovascular toxicity. Toxicities were similar to those observed by Bansal *et al.* and included fever, chills, hypotension, tachycardia, nausea, and vomiting. One patient with extensive lung metastases developed respiratory distress and had to discontinue therapy. All of the remaining four patients demonstrated reductions in tumor size, with three partial responses and one less than partial response. Inflammatory changes were described over chest wall recurrences, with necrosis seen on biopsies. Histological examination revealed cytoplasmic swelling, loss of cytoplasmic elements, and a decrease and fragmentation of nuclear chromatin. Biopsies performed 24–48 hr after therapy showed deposits of IgG, IgM, IgA, and C3 in the postperfusion samples compared to those obtained prior to therapy. Cells contained densely stained nuclei and vacuolated cytoplasm. Interstitial edema was present. With additional treatment, affected cells showed decreases in nucleoplasm density and condensation of peripheral chromatin, although overall the severity of nuclear changes varied. After the initial responses became apparent, these patients were treated by other forms of therapy, such as chemotherapy, radiation therapy, and surgery. Thus, the long-term effects of plasma therapy in these patients cannot be evaluated.

Two trials at the National Cancer Institute have been attempted to reproduce these impressive antitumor effects (Fer *et al.*, 1984; Messerschmidt *et al.*, 1982*a,b*). The first trial conducted by Messerschmidt *et al.* initially involved the use of heat- and formalin-killed SAC in the perfusion systems (Messerschmidt *et al.*, 1982*a*). Five patients were treated using this material, and approximately 24–60% of the calculated total plasma volume was perfused over the SAC. Patients included in this study had a variety of tumors, including one synovial carcinoma, one melanoma, and one patient each with esophageal, breast, and colon carcinoma. None of the patients exhibited an antitumor response, while toxicity was formidable in all, with two toxic deaths. Shortly after perfusion, the initial effects would include an increase in the mean arterial blood pressure, followed in 30-60 min by a marked decrease in the systemic vascular resistance and severe hypotension. Fluids and vasoconstrictor agents were usually needed to maintain the systolic blood pressure above 60 mm Hg. In spite of hyperventilation manifested by tachypnea and decreasing P_{CO_2}, the patients generally became hypoxic. Two patients, both of whom had pulmonary metastases, died of respiratory failure. Granulocytopenia occurred, at times below 500 granulocytes/mm^3, and would resolve by 12–24 hr after plasma therapy. Platelets dropped by 50% in all of the patients. One patient required platelet transfusions. The trial was stopped after five patients owing to the severe toxicity. Under a revised protocol eight additional patients were treated by previously stored autologous plasma passed over PACC, in a technique similar to that used by Terman *et al.* (1981) and Messerschmidt *et al.* (1982b); 50–450 ml of plasma was perfused over 5 mg of immobilized protein A. Unlike the trial utilizing the whole bacterial product, this procedure was free of toxicity, but again there were no antitumor responses.

The negative results obtained by Messerschmidt *et al.* (1982b) are in clear contrast to the dramatic effects reported by the Baylor group. It was suggested by Terman that the marked differences in the outcomes of those two studies could be explained by some technical differences in the materials used in the two studies. Since the mechanism of action for the observed effects was unclear, it was conceivable that relatively minor technical differences could have accounted for an important alteration in the outcome. Thus, a second trial was initiated at the National Cancer Institute by our group, this time using precisely the same materials and methods provided by the investigators at Baylor (Fer *et al.*, 1984). Since the major purpose of this study was to reproduce the results observed at Baylor, a similar patient population with measurable, recurrent breast cancer refractory to standard therapy was chosen. No simultaneous or subsequent chemotherapy, radiotherapy, or surgery was performed in this trial. Since the major toxicities observed in previous studies had all included cardiovascular and respiratory problems, patients were screened to ensure adequate cardiovascular and pulmonary functions. Two plasma collection procedures were performed, when approximately 800 ml of plasma was stored in 100-ml aliquots. Twelve treatments were then given over 6 weeks, starting with 0.6 mg of protein A and 50 ml of plasma, escalating stepwise to 1.25 mg of protein A and 100 ml of plasma. The first four patients on the study exhibited no antitumor responses, no inflamatory changes over the chest wall lesions, and no toxicity. Extensive immunological monitoring was performed during the study at several times before and after plasma therapy, including total serum complement, CIC levels, natural killer cell activity, antibody-dependent cellular cytotoxicity, and T-cell helper/ suppressor ratios as determined by lymphocyte surface markers and flow cytometry. There was no significant change attributable to plasma therapy in any of these values (Fer *et al.*, 1984). The low dose range chosen was due to the severe toxicity observed during the Baylor trial. In the absence of toxicity, it was felt that further dose escalations should be conducted to exceed the higher dose levels used at Baylor. Thus, the initial four patients were retreated with six additional plasma perfusions over 2 weeks, again in an escalating dose schedule starting from 2.5 mg of protein A and 100 ml of plasma up to 7.5 mg of protein A and 200 ml of plasma. Again, there was no toxicity, no antitumor effects, and no evidence of biological response modifier activity.

A possible explanation for the discrepancies between the observations made at Baylor and those in this NCI trial may lie in the preparation methods for protein A. The methods for the production of protein A used in these trials have been modified by the vendor (Pharmacia, Inc.) from those in use at the time of the Baylor study to increase the yield and purity. Thus, it is possible that other bioactive staphylococcal products that previously co-purified with protein A may have been eliminated from the current preparations.

Bensinger *et al.* (1984) have treated twenty patients with various types of cancer in a phase I study with autologous plasma passed in a continuous-flow system over protein A covalently bound to silica. Protein A (100–200 mg) was bound to 50–100 g of silica matrix and plasma therapy was administered 1–3 times/week. Each patient received a total ranging from 1 to 20 treatments. Toxicity was mild, including fever and chills in approximately one-half of the patients and nausea in one-third. In 25% of the procedures, patients experienced pain over tumor sites, and there was a blood pressure drop during 18% of the perfusions. Seventeen percent of the perfusions were associated with respiratory symptoms, and one patient had to discontinue therapy because of severe respiratory problems. Modest antitumor responses were seen in four of the twenty patients in the series. Three of seven patients with malignant melanoma and one of three patients with breast cancer had greater than 25% reduction in tumor size, only one patient with melanoma having a greater than 50% tumor shrinkage. Nonresponders included a patient with squamous cell carcinoma of the lung, two with carcinoma of the colon, two sarcomas, and one patient each with Ewing sarcoma, renal cell carcinoma, and chronic myelogenous leukemia. Detailed laboratory analyses during therapy showed posttreatment platelet count reductions of 23% in most patients, with reductions in the 10–20% range in hematocrit and in quantitative assays for IgA, IgM, IgG, C3, C4, and CH50 levels. C1q bindings assays showed a 70% increase in immune complexes postperfusion compared to pretreatment values. Six patients in this series had increases in interferon levels following plasma therapy.

In a collaborative study by the investigators at Seattle and the University of Liège in Belgium, eleven additional patients were treated in a similar fashion or by use of "inactivated" columns containing the same matrix with heat-denatured protein A, which does not bind to Fc portions of human IgG (Bensinger *et al.*, 1984). Five of the eight patients treated by use of the "active" columns manifested objective tumor shrinkage, while none of the three patients treated with "inactivated" columns had a response, suggesting that the antitumor activity of the system tested requires an intact Fc-binding capability by protein A. Of the six breast cancer patients in the study, three had tumor shrinkage exceeding 50% and qualifying for a partial response. In the Belgian study, circulating protein A levels in patient serum was measured by radioimmunoassay. Minute quantities of protein A were detected in these studies in less than 25% of the perfusions. Although the presence of protein A in serum correlated with toxicity, it did not predict response.

Messerschmidt *et al.* (1984) are conducting a trial using protein A covalently bound to silica, similar to the materials used by Bensinger *et al.* In three patients 300-1200 ml plasma was perfused over 200 mg of protein A without antitumor responses.

Yet a different column has been used at Georgetown University by Korec *et al.* in a phase I study (Korec *et al.*, 1984). Eleven patients were treated with approximately 600 ml of autologous plasma perfused over approximately 60 mg of protein A bound to polyacrylamide-coated glass beads. A continuous-flow system was used whereby plasma was passed over the columns at 5 ml/min, combined with the remaining blood components, and returned to the patient. Most patients underwent eight treatments over 5 weeks. Toxicity included fever and chills in 22% of the patients, nausea and vomiting in 13%, and a greater than 35 mm Hg drop in blood pressure in 5% of the perfusions. Similar to descriptions elsewhere, chills would start after 20-250 ml of plasma was perfused and would last for 15-20 min, followed by a rise in temperature and a drop in blood pressure. Hypotensive episodes were generally less than 10 min in duration but would at times be followed by orthostatic hypotension for up to 40 min. Antitumor effects were again modest, with one colon cancer patient exhibiting a 40% reduction in tumor size as assessed by ultrasound. There were four other patients with colon carcinoma in this series, one of whom had resolution of intestinal obstruction. Both of these patients had declines in their carcinoembryonic antigen levels. An additional patient with ovarian carinoma also had resolution of intestinal obstruction. Laboratory analyses during the study revealed that up to a 70% drop occurred in the number of circulating total lymphocytes immediately following plasma therapy, followed by a rebound to 150-200% of the baseline values by 36 hours. The T-cell surface markers assessed by immunofluorescence flow cytometry showed that the ratio of OKT4 to OKT8 positive cells was increased. In patients with more severe chills and fever there was neutropenia followed by leukocytosis 24 hr later. There were no changes in immunoglobulin, C3, and C4 levels associated with therapy.

MacKintosh *et al.* (1983, 1984) have treated 32 patients at the University of Nevada with autologous plasma exposed to protein A bound covalently to Sepharose. These investigators have infused 35-500 ml (median 90 ml) of previously stored autologous plasma passed over 2-100 mg (median 30 mg) of protein A-Sepharose, at a rate of 5-20 ml/min, twice weekly. There were seven objective tumor responses in 32 evaluable patients. Five of those qualified for partial response with over 50% reduction in tumor size. One patient had a minor response and another a mixed response. Responses were seen in carcinoma of the breast, squamous carcinoma of the lung, adenocarcinoma of the lung, and two patients with malignant melanoma. Tumors in soft tissue and in lung were more responsive (nine responses in 28 patients) compared to other sites. Side effects were mild, and 55% of the patients had no toxicity. Toxicity included fever, chills, nausea, vomiting, diarrhea, and bronchospasm, similar to the problems reported by others. Hypercalcemia and elevated liver function tests were also reported among the side effects. Clonogenic assays were performed in this study in four patients with autologous tumor cells exposed to patient plasma passed over protein A-Sepharose. Cells were incubated with untreated plasma as controls. Two patients had ovarian carcinoma and ascites fluid was used instead of plasma. Two others had malignant melanoma. In one patient with malignant melanoma a decrease in colony formation by 44% correlated with a partial response lasting 8 months. Two patients who failed to show suppression of colony formation by treated plasma had no response to therapy. A fourth patient was not evaluable. These results are obviously preliminary. If this assay proves to be useful as a predictor of response to plasma therapy, it will provide a novel guide for the selection of patients for clinical trials.

Bertram *et al.* (1984) are conducting a study with a PACC system similar to that used by Terman and in the NCI trials. In the first six patients treated in this phase I trial, patient plasma exposed to PACC has resulted in the appearance of mitogenicity in plasma from four of the six patients. The plasma gave strong mitogenicity after passage over PACC. No data were presented in this paper correlating the induced mitogenicity to the clinical outcome.

Korec *et al.* (1984) have treated three patients with mitomycin C-induced thrombotic thrombocytopenic purpura with *ex vivo* plasma immunoadsorption, using the system described previously. Reportedly, two of these patients showed marked recovery with improvement of platelet counts and hematocrit. Both were doing well at the time of the report, having survived this disease, which previously has been uniformly fatal (Zimmerman *et al.*, 1982).

Kiprow *et al.* (1984) have treated a 44-year-old patient with the acquired immune deficiency syndrome and Kaposi's sarcoma with plasma perfused over protein A-silica. After three treatments were given over a week, there was central necrosis and hemorrhage in metastatic lesions, with erythema around cutaneous lesions. Some early healing occurred over a confluent lesion, although the patient died 3 days after the last procedure owing to advanced disease. Toxicity was minor, and similar to that reported in other trials. Biopsies taken after the last procedure showed deposits of C3 and immunoglobulins. There was a 46% decrease in the platelet count over the treatment period without other hematological changes. There was no improvement in the helper/suppressor-T-cell ratios. There were reductions in CIC levels, antilymphocyte antibodies, and blocking factors to mitogen stimulation. These anectodal findings need further corroboration.

IV. *IN VITRO* INVESTIGATIONS

In vitro systems offer the clear advantage of allowing specific questions to be asked in a controlled manner. Thus, the value of *in vitro* studies in elucidating the consequences of plasma immunoadsorption/immunoactivation cannot be overemphasized. Miller *et al.* (1982) have demonstrated that protein A adsorption of serum from patients with acute myelogenous leukemia (AML) induces lysis of blast cells in short-term cultures. In this study, AML serum was immunoadsorbed with one of the following: (1) protein A-bearing SAC, (2) non-protein A-bearing SAW, or (3) purified protein A bound to Sepharose 4B beads. Plasma was then added to target cells in tissue culture and cell viability assessed after 24 hr by trypan blue exclusion. Cell viability was expressed as percent viability in test cultures compared to controls incubated with nonadsorbed plasma. Cell viability was reduced to 42% by protein A–Sepharose. There was no reduction in viability when SAW was used, or when normal donor plasma was substituted for patient plasma. These experiments suggest that the cytotoxicity elicited in leukemic serum by the immunoadsorption procedure resulted from exposure to protein A, although reduction in cell viability was more marked when the whole bacterial paste was used. When untreated sera were added to immunoadsorbed patient sera, there was an increase in the leukemic blast viability, suggesting that untreated serum either contained substances that support viability or block cytotoxicity, and that these factors might be removed or inactivated by the procedure. When normal peripheral blood mononuclear cells were incubated with SAC-treated AML sera or autologous normal sera, there was no decrease in viability, suggesting that the cytotoxic effect is selective for AML cells. These authors then investigated the possible mechanisms of action by a series of experiments. To test the hypothesis that the cytotoxic effect may require serum complement, AML sera were heat-inactivated at 56°C for 30 min prior to immunoadsorption. A similar reduction in viability (40%) was seen with or without heat inactivation, suggesting that complement is not essential for the cytotoxic effect. To test whether mononuclear cells contaminating the blast cells may take part in an antibody-dependent cell-mediated cytotoxicity (ADCC), additional procedures were used to remove the adherent cell population (mainly monocytes) from the target cells. Cytotoxicity remained unhampered, suggesting that ADCC is not involved. Similarly, removal of T lymphocytes by sheep red cell rosetting from target cells also did not improve viability. To test the role of immunoglobulins in cytotoxicity, the immunoglobulin fraction of AML sera was purified chromatographically. This immunoglobulin fraction reduced cell viability (to 26% of the control) only if adsorbed with SAC, suggesting either that a cytotoxic component was activated or that a component essential for cell viability was removed. When treated sera were exposed to trypsin, cytotoxicity was eliminated, suggesting that the mediator may be a protein. When multiple immunoadsorption procedures were performed to remove increasing amounts of IgG, maximal cytotoxicity was noted after one or two adsorptions, while further adsorption caused improved viability. The authors suggested that the initial adsorptions may allow the expression of cytotoxicity while additional procedures may in fact remove the active substance, which could, for example, be a cytotoxic immunoglobulin. Although the mechanism of the cytotoxicity demonstrated in these experiments remains unclear, it appeared to be protein-mediated (probably immunoglobulin-mediated), did not require complement, and did not rely on the presence of effector cells. The authors hypothesized that the immunoadsorption procedures might selectively block an antibody or an immune complex leaving a cytotoxic antibody (possibly of the IgG3 subclass, binding poorly to protein A), which by repeated procedures could itself be eliminated (Miller, et al., 1982). An alternate possibility raised is the removal or alteration of a necessary growth factor from AML sera.

The investigators at Baylor have proposed that these antitumor effects may result from the formation of protein A–IgG oligomers during the perfusion procedure (Langone et al., 1978a). It has been shown previously that IgG and protein A will combine to form complexes in a configuration dependent on the molar ratios of the two substances (Langone et al., 1978b; Langone, 1984). In the case of protein A excess, these complexes are in a one-to-one molecular ratio while in the presence of immunoglobulin excess the configuration of these complexes will be $(IgG)_2 (protein A)_2$, resembling IgM. The Baylor group has illustrated that protein A is eluted in nanogram to microgram amounts from the collodion charcoal matrix during perfusion of plasma over these columns in complexes with IgG, in the IgM-like configuration (Langone et al., 1978b; and Balint et al., 1984). It has been well illustrated that such protein A–IgG oligomers activate human complement (Langone et al., 1978b; Langone, 1984). Thus, it has been hypothesized that such complexes, formed during the *ex vivo* exposure of plasma to protein A, can result in some of the same biological effects when infused into the patient (Langone et al., 1978a). At this point these thoughts remain hypothetical.

V. DISCUSSION AND CONCLUSIONS

It is clear from the studies summarized that the role of protein A immunoadsorption/immunoactivation as a form of cancer therapy requires much further clarification before such procedures can be considered effective. In many of the studies conducted to date, different techniques and materials have been used with different animal models or human diseases. Perfusions have been performed over protein A or SAC paste or non-protein A-bearing staphylococci or matrices alone, with variable results. Furthermore, the quantities of plasma perfused have ranged from only a few milliliters to the total calculated plasma volume. Some studies have applied previously stored frozen plasma while others have utilized continuous-flow plasmapheresis procedures in which the plasma was removed, exposed to the agent, and immediately returned to the host. The question of a removal process exists in continuous-flow perfusions, in which large quantities of plasma are passaged, while removal cannot be the mechanism of action when previously stored aliquots of frozen plasma are used. In these studies, it has been generally accepted that the effects must be secondary to activation of an un-known factor. Whether this is a humoral component or involves cellular mecha-nisms is unclear. Leaching of various components of the columns used is another distinct possibility.

The role of protein A in these perfusion systems in controversial. Addi-tionally, studies by Sukumar *et al.* (1984) have demonstrated that plasma per-fused over a non-protein A-bearing Sepharose matrix can induce changes in tumor-bearing rats comparable to those due to plasma passaged over protein A–Sepharose. On the other hand, even if one assumes that protein A is a critical component or co-factor in certain systems, the mechanism of action is still unclear, because of its diverse biological effects, such as binding to Fc portions of immunoglobulins; generation of C3A, C4A, and C5A in human serum; and inducing B- and T-cell mitogenesis, interferon production, and interleukin synthesis. Why all of these biological effects would result in tumor damage as opposed to general systemic consequences is unknown.

Based on the studies summarized previously, it is clear that plasma immuno-adsorption/immunoactivation can result in certain tumor reductions in a variety of systems, including humans and animal models. In humans the responses have been modest. Studies conducted with SAC have been more toxic compared to those utilizing protein A, but more effective in the animal models studied.

Much of the previous trials have emphasized observations, without great success in identifying mechanisms of action. The major questions that now need to be addressed include the following:

1. Is protein A a crucial component of the systems tested? Experiments by Gordon *et al.* (1983) would suggest that it is not, while most other inves-tigators have relied on certain effects of protein A in their study designs.
2. If the crucial component is not protein A, or if protein A requires other co-factors for certain effects, what are these substances? One would think, based on studies using SAC, that other *Staphylococcus*-derived products could be important. However, if Sukumar's data prove to apply to other systems, inactivated Sepharose alone might produce similar antitumor effects. The common denominator in all of these studies is tumor-bearer plasma, and it is possible that a broad range of materials can trigger a certain mechanism (or mechanisms) mediated by a plasma factor. Anti-tumor effects of bacterial products have been observed since the experi-ments of Cooley (1906) at the turn of the century. Pursuit of specific bacterial products with antitumor activity has been an attractive quest, but one thus far without success.
3. Independent of the hypothesized immunoactivation processes, can the removal of "blocking factors" be a mechanism of antitumor activity? This

is a question that cannot be easily answered, since any procedure performed to "remove" these substances can also activate other mechanisms.

With the large number of questions that remain to be answered, serious doubts have been expressed as to whether clinical trials are appropriate at this point. Purists would state that the answers will come from detailed laboratory studies. On the other hand, proponents of clinical studies emphasize that, given the complexity of and vast interspecies differences in immune networks, the effects of an as yet undetermined "agent" cannot be tested adequately in the laboratory alone, since the choice of animal models or *in vitro* systems might result in misleading outcomes not relevant to the human condition. Nevertheless, all would agree that the number of variables that await testing can only be studied in laboratory experiments. It would be reasonable to conduct clinical trials only when detailed studies of the biological effects can be accomplished. The choice of animal systems and human tumors to be studied would be important. A chemically induced or transplantable tumor in a small animal model would clearly offer advantages since large numbers of animals could be studied. In this regard, the *N*-methyl-nitrosourea-induced mammary carcinoma of rats is of interest. FeLV-associated lymphosarcomas also appear to represent a suitable model, although accrual of those animals bearing spontaneous tumors is often slow. In humans, relatively "immunogenic" tumors such as malignant melanoma and renal cell carcinoma would appear to be suitable tumors for these trials. These tumors (1) often present with measurable lesions, (2) have well defined antigens defined by a variety of monoclonal antibodies (particularly in the case of malignant melanoma), (3) have no "standard" therapy, so that patients can be placed on investigational immunotherapy prior to the administration of immunosuppressive chemotherapy or radiation, (4) often occur in younger individuals who are likely to tolerate potential toxicity, and (5) have responded to other forms of immunotherapy in previous trials. Obviously, since the mechanisms of action involved in plasma therapy are not well understood, the choice of tumors to be studied cannot be made dogmatically. All patients studied should have measurable lesions for assessments of objective responses, which should be made separately from observations of biological effects, such as inflammation, edema, or healing of ulcers. We have previously commented on certain similarities between the histological changes induced by delayed-type hypersensitivity reactions after active specific immunotherapy and those seen with plasma treated with protein A (Oldham, 1984). These observations and those relative to the problem of drug delivery (Hanna *et al.*, 1983) may point to new approaches for cancer therapy. The immunological consequences of plasma therapy with respect to the complement system, immune complexes, lymphokine and cytokine production, leukocyte chemotactic factors, cellular immune functions, and a variety of other variables should be carefully monitored. It is now known that a series of cytotoxic factors can be elaborated under certain conditions in animal models and probably in humans, ranging from tumor necrosis factor to cytotoxins released by macrophages and lymphocytes (Carswell *et al.*, 1975; Kull *et al.*, 1981). Only through a series of detailed and systematic studies will a better understanding emerge of what plasma immunoadsorption procedures may promise for the treatment of cancer.

VI. REFERENCES

Baldwin, R. W., Price, M. R., and Robins, R. A., 1972, Blocking of lymphocyte-mediated cytotoxicity for rate hepatoma cells by tumor-specific antigen–antibody complexes, *Nature* 238:185–187.

Baldwin, R. W., Price, M. R., and Robins, R. A., 1973, Significance of serum factors modifying cellular immune responses to growing tumors, *Br. J. Cancer* (Suppl.) 28:37–47.

Balint, J., Ikeda, Y., Langone, J. J., Shearer, W. T., Daskal, I., Meek, K., Cook, G., Henry, J., and Terman, D. S., 1984, Tumoricidal response following perfusion of plasma over immobilized protein A: Identification of immunoglobulin oligomers in serum after perfusion and their partial characterization, *Cancer Res.* 44:734–743.

Bansal, S. C., Bansal, B. R., Thomas, H. L., Siegel, P. D., Rhoads, J. E., Cooper, D. R., Terman, D. S., and Mark, R., 1978, Ex-vivo removal of serum IgG in a patient with colon carcinoma: Biochemical, immunological and histological observations, *Cancer* 42:1–18.

Bensinger, W. I., Kinet, J. P., Hennen, G., Franckenne, F., Schaus, C., Saint-Remy, M., Hoyoux, P., and Mahieu, P., 1981, Plasma perfused over immobilized protein A for breast cancer, *N. Engl. J. Med.* 306:935–937.

Bensinger, W. I., Buckner, C. D., Clift, R. A., and Thomas, E. D., 1984, Clinical trials with staphylococcal protein A, *J. Biol. Resp. Modif.* 3:347–351.

Bertram, J., Hengst, J. C. D., and Mitchell, M. S., 1984, Staph protein A immunoadsorptive column induces mitogenicity in perfused plasma, *J. Biol. Resp. Modif.* 3:235–240.

Carswell, E. A., Old, L. J., Kassel, R. L., Green, S., Fiore, N., and Williamson, B., 1975, Induced serum factor that causes necrosis of tumors, *Proc. Natl. Acad. Sci. USA* 72:3666–3670.

Cohen, D., Fer, M. F., Pearson, J. W., and Herberman, R. B., 1984, Treatment of canine transmissible venereal tumor by intraveneous administration of protein A, *J. Biol. Resp. Modif.* 3:271–277.

Cooley, W. B., 1906, Late results of the treatment of inoperable sarcoma by the mixed toxins of erysipelas and bacillus prodigiosus, *Am. J. Med. Sci.* 131:375–430.

Day, N. K., Engelman, R. W., Liu, W. T., Trang, T., and Good, R. A., 1984, Remission of lymphoma leukemia in cats following ex-vivo immunosorption therapy using Staphylococcus protein A, *J. Biol. Resp. Modif.* 3:278–285.

Fer, M. F., Beman, J. A., Stevenson, H. C., Maluish, A., Moratz, C., Delawter, T., Foon, K., Herberman, R. B., Oldham, R. K., Terman, D. S., Young, J. B., and Daskal, Y., 1984, A trial of autologous plasma perfused over Protein A in patients with breast cancer, *J. Biol. Resp. Modif.* 3:352–358.

Forsgren, A., and Sjoquist, J., 1966, "Protein A" from *S. aureus.* I. Pseudoimmune reaction with human gamma-globulin, *J. Immunol.* 97:822–827.

Gordon, B. R., Matus, R. E., Saal, S. D., MacEwen, E. G., Hurwitz, A. I., Stenzel, K. H., and Rubin, A. L., 1983, Protein A-independent tumoricidal responses in dogs after extracorporeal perfusion of plasma over *Staphylococcus aureus, J. Natl. Cancer Inst.* 70:1127–1133.

Gordon, B. R., Matus, R. E., Hurvitz, A. I., MacEwen, E. G., Saal, S. D., Stenzel, K. H., Rubin, A. L., and Hyden, H., 1984, Perfusion of plasma over *S. aureus*: Release of bacterial products is related to regression of tumor, *J. Biol. Resp. Modif.* 3:266–270.

Hanna, M. G., Jr., Key, M. E., and Oldham, R. K., 1983, Biology of cancer therapy: Some new insights into adjuvant treatment of metastatic solid tumors, *J. Biol. Resp. Modif.* 2:295–309.

Hellström, I., and Hellström, K. E., 1970, Colony inhibition studies on blocking and non-blocking serum effects on cellular immunity to Moloney sarcomas, *Int. J. Cancer* 5:195–201.

Hellström, I., and Hellström, K. E., 1976, Microcytotoxicity assay of cell mediated tumor immunity and blocking serum factors, in: *In Vitro Methods of Cell Mediated and Tumor Immunity* (R. B. Bloom and J. R. David, eds.), pp. 553–591, Academic Press, New York.

Holohan, T., Phillips, T. M., Bowles, C., and Deisseroth, A., 1982, Regression of canine mammary carcinoma after immunoadsorption therapy, *Cancer Res.* 42:3663–3668.

Jones, F., Yoshida, L., Ladiges, W., and Kenny, M., 1980, Treatment of feline leukemia and reversal of FeLV by *ex vivo* removal of IgG: A preliminary report, *Cancer* 46:675–684.

Jones, F. R., Grant, C. K., and Snyder, H. W., 1984, Lymphosarcoma and persistent feline leukemia virus infection of pet cats: A system to study responses during extracorporeal treatments, *J. Biol. Resp. Modif.* 3:286–292.

Kiprow, D. D., Lippert, R., Jones, F. R., Lagios, M. D., Balint, J. P. and Cohen, R. J., 1984, Extracorporeal perfusion of plasma over immobilized protein A in a patient with Kaposi's sarcoma and acquired immunodeficiency, *J. Biol. Resp. Modif.* 3:341–346.

Korec, S., Smith, F. P., Schein, P. S., and Phillips, T. M., 1984, Clinical experiences with extra-corporeal immunoperfusion of plasma from cancer patients, *J. Biol. Resp. Modif.* 3:330–335.

Kronvall, G., and Frommel, D., 1970, Definition of staphylococcal protein A reactivity for human immunoglobulin G fragments, *Immunochemistry* 7:124–127.

Kull, F. C., Jr., and Cuatrecasas, P., 1981, Possible requirement of internalization in the mechanism of in vitro cytoxicity in tumor necrosis serum, *Cancer Res.* 41:4885–4890.

Langone, J. J., 1984, Complexes containing *Staphylococcus aureus* protein A: Composition and biological activity, *J. Biol. Resp. Modif.* 3:241–246.

Langone, J. J., Boyle, M. D. P., and Borsos, T., 1978*a*, Studies on the interaction between protein A and immunoglobulin G. I. Effect of protein A on the functional activity of IgG, *J. Immunol.* 121:327–332.

Langone, J. J., Boyle, M. D. P., and Borsos, T., 1978*b*, Studies on the interaction between protein A and immunoglobulin G. II. Composition and activity of complexes formed between Protein A and IgG, *J. Immunol.* 121:333–338.

MacKintosh, F. R., Bennett, K., Schiff, S., Shields, J., and Hall, S. W., 1983, Treatment of advanced malignancy with plasma perfused over staphylococcal protein A, *West. J. Med.* 139:36–42.

MacKintosh, F. R., Bennett, K., and Hall, S. W., 1984, Clinical response to protein-A tested plasma infusions and in vitro correlation, *J. Biol. Resp. Modif.* 3:336–340.

Messerschmidt, G., Bowles, C., Dean, D., Parker, M., Lester, R., Dowling, R., Holohan, T., Osborne, L., Schaff, B. F., McCormack, K., Corbitt, R., Phillips, T., Glatstein, E., and Deisseroth, A., 1982*a*, Phase I trial of *Staphylococcus aureus* Cowan I immunoperfusion, *Cancer Treat. Rep.* 66:2027–2031.

Messerschmidt, G. L., Steis, R., Dowling, R., Parrillo, J., Parker, M., Shelhammer, J., Brown, R., Herberman, R., Maluish, A., Phillips, T., Voith, M., Diehl, L., Bowles, C., Young,

R. C., Glatstein, E., and Deisseroth, A., 1982b, Phase I trials of ex-vivo plasma perfusion with *Staphylococcus aureus* Cowan strain I and protein A charcoal in malignancies, *Proc. Soc. Clin. Oncol.* 1:80.

Messerschmidt, G. L., Bowles, C. A., Henry, D., and Deisseroth, A. B., 1984, Clinical trials with *Staphylococcus aureus* and protein A in the treatment of malignant disease, *J. Biol. Resp. Modif.* 3:325–329.

Miller, W. J., Branda, R. F., Hurf, D. D., Wachsman, W., Nelson, N. L., and Jacob, H. S., 1982, Protein A adsorption of acute myelogenous leukemia serum induces in vitro blast lysis, *Blood* 59:1344–1347.

Oldham, R. K., 1984, Introduction, *J. Biol. Resp. Modif.* 3:229–230.

Ray, P. K., Idiculla, A., Mark, R., Rhoads, J. E., Thomas, H., Bassett, J. G., and Cooper, D. R., 1982, Extracorporeal immunoadsorption of plasma from a metastatic colon carcinoma patient by protein A containing non-viable *Staphylococcus aureus*, *Cancer* 49:1800–1809.

Sjögren, H. O., Hellström, I., Bansal, S. C., and Hellström, K. E., 1971, Suggestive evidence that the "blocking antibodies" of tumor-bearing individuals may be antigen–antibody complexes, *Proc. Natl. Acad. Sci. USA* 68:1372–1375.

Steele, G., Jr., Ankerst, J., and Sjögren, H. O., 1974, Alteration of in vivo antitumor activity of tumor-bearer sera by absorption with *Staphylococcus aureus* Cowan I, *Int. J. Cancer* 14:83–92.

Sukumar, S., Zbar, B., Terata, N., and Langone, J., 1984, Plasma therapy of primary rat mammary carcinoma, *J. Biol. Resp. Modif.* 3:303–315.

Terman, D. S., Yamamoto, T., Mattioli, M., Cook, G., Tillquist, R., Henry J., Poser R., and Daskal, Y., 1980, Extensive necrosis of spontaneous canine mammary adenocarcinoma after extracorporeal perfusion over *Staphylococcus aureus* Cowan I: Description of acute tumoricidal response–Morphologic, histologic, immunohistochemical, immunologic, and serologic findings, *J. Immunol.* 124:795–805.

Terman, D. S., Young, J. B., Shearer, W. T., Ayus, C., Lehane, D., Mattioli, C., Espada, R., Howell, J. F., Yamamoto, T., Zaleski, H. I., Miller, L., Frommer, P., Feldman, L., Henry, J. F., Tillquist, R., Cook, G., and Daskal, Y., 1981, Preliminary observations of tumoricidal response following plasma perfusion over immobilized protein A in adenocarcinoma of the breast, *N. Engl. J. Med.* 305:1195–1200.

Zimmerman, S. E., Smith, F. P., Phillips, T. M., Coffey, R. J., and Schein, P. S., 1982, Gastric carcinoma and thrombotic thrombocytopenic purpura: Association with plasma immune complex concentrations, *Br. Med. J.* 284:1432–1434.

Index

277